Mayo Clinic Cardiology: Concise Textbook

Fourth Edition

Mayo Clinic Cardiology: Concise Textbook

FOURTH EDITION

Editors-in-Chief

Joseph G. Murphy, MD

Margaret A. Lloyd, MD

Associate Editors

Peter A. Brady, MB, ChB, MD

Lyle J. Olson, MD

Raymond C. Shields, MD

MAYO CLINIC SCIENTIFIC PRESS   OXFORD UNIVERSITY PRESS

MAYO
CLINIC

The triple-shield Mayo logo and the words MAYO, MAYO CLINIC, and MAYO CLINIC
SCIENTIFIC PRESS are marks of Mayo Foundation for Medical Education and Research.

OXFORD
UNIVERSITY PRESS

Oxford University Press is a department of the University of Oxford.
It furthers the University's objective of excellence in research, scholarship,
and education by publishing worldwide.

Oxford   New York

Auckland   Cape Town   Dar es Salaam   Hong Kong   Karachi
Kuala Lumpur   Madrid   Melbourne   Mexico City   Nairobi
New Delhi   Shanghai   Taipei   Toronto

With offices in

Argentina   Austria   Brazil   Chile   Czech Republic   France   Greece
Guatemala   Hungary   Italy   Japan   Poland   Portugal   Singapore
South Korea   Switzerland   Thailand   Turkey   Ukraine   Vietnam

Oxford is a registered trademark of Oxford University Press in the UK and
certain other countries.

Published by Oxford University Press, Inc.
198 Madison Avenue, New York, New York 10016
www.oup.com

Library of Congress Cataloging-in-Publication Data

Mayo Clinic cardiology : concise textbook / editors-in-chief, Joseph G. Murphy, Margaret A. Lloyd ; associate editors, Peter A.
Brady, Lyle J. Olson, Raymond C. Shields. — 4th ed.
    p. ; cm.
Cardiology
Includes bibliographical references and index.
Summary: "Organized to present a comprehensive overview of the field of cardiology in an accessible, reader-friendly format
that can be covered in about 12 months, this new edition contains roughly 50% new material, the cardiac pharmacology
section has been completely reworked, cardiovascular trials have been included, and the entire book has been updated to reflect
current practice guidelines and recent developments. The book is peppered throughout with numerous tables and clinical
pearls that aid the student, as well as the teacher, to remain focused"—Provided by publisher.
ISBN 978-0-19-991571-2 (alk. paper)
I. Murphy, Joseph G.   II. Lloyd, Margaret A.   III. Mayo Clinic.   IV. Title: Cardiology.
[DNLM: 1. Heart Diseases—Examination Questions. 2. Heart Diseases—Outlines. WG 18.2]

616.1'20076—dc23
2012025452

9 8 7 6 5 4 3 2
Printed in China
on acid-free paper

Dedication

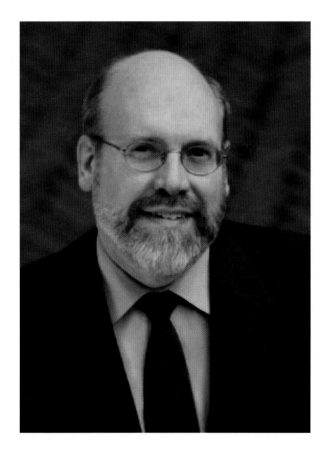

This book is dedicated to our friend and colleague, Mark Callahan, MD, who tragically died shortly before completion of this edition. Mark was a dedicated Mayo Clinic clinician and educator who inspired all of his colleagues and a generation of Mayo Medical School students, cardiology residents, and fellows. His passions were the clinical care of patients, medical teaching, and health care in underserved countries, as evidenced by his multiple trips to Haiti. He contributed to multiple editions of this textbook. We will always miss Mark for his integrity, dedication to serving others, and endless good humor.

Joseph G. Murphy, MD
Margaret A. Lloyd, MD

Preface

It has been a great honor to serve as editors-in-chief of this, the fourth, edition of *Mayo Clinic Cardiology: Concise Textbook*. Large textbooks are never the work of 1 or 2 individuals but rather the product of a group of dedicated authors and a team of publications professionals, as has been the case for this book. This textbook is unique in several regards in that it comes almost entirely from a single institution but was written by a diverse faculty of more than 100 physicians, many with an international background. Mayo Clinic contributors practice at multiple Mayo Clinic locations—Minnesota (Rochester, Austin, and Mankato); Scottsdale, Arizona; and Jacksonville, Florida.

This textbook is primarily a teaching and learning textbook of cardiology rather than a comprehensive reference textbook of cardiology. Our concise textbook specifically addresses the learning needs of cardiology fellows-in-training seeking initial cardiovascular board certification and those of busy clinicians in cardiology practice seeking cardiovascular board recertification. It will also be useful for international physicians studying for examinations of the Royal Colleges of Physicians, anesthesiologists, critical care physicians, internists and general physicians with a special interest in cardiology, and coronary care and critical care nurses.

In response to welcome feedback from readers of the 3 previous textbook editions, we have reduced the size of the textbook by several hundred pages while striving to produce a readable textbook with features that facilitate its use as a review tool,

including highlighted entries of key points. Newer electronic search methods have made textbook references less timely; thus, we deleted most chapter references but have included selected readings when appropriate.

This textbook is designed to present the field of cardiology in a reader-friendly format that can be studied over about 12 months. Many small cardiology textbooks are bare-bones compilations of facts that do not explain the fundamental concepts of cardiovascular disease, and many large cardiology textbooks describe the field of cardiology in great detail. *Mayo Clinic Cardiology: Concise Textbook* is designed to be a bridge between these approaches. We sought to present a solid framework of ideas with sufficient depth to make the subjects interesting yet concise, aimed specifically toward fellows-in-training or practicing clinicians wanting to update their knowledge. The book contains more than 1,000 figures, many of which are in color, to supplement the text. Summary points in each chapter facilitate review of key facts.

We appreciate comments and suggestions from our readers about how we might improve this textbook.

Joseph G. Murphy, MD
murphy.joseph@mayo.edu

Margaret A. Lloyd, MD
lloyd.margaret@mayo.edu
Mayo Clinic

Echocardiography

A Case-Based Review

Echocardiography

A Case-Based Review

Garvan C. Kane, MD, PhD

Co-Director, Echocardiography Laboratory
Consultant, Division of Cardiovascular Diseases
Assistant Professor of Medicine
Mayo Clinic
Rochester, Minnesota

Jae K. Oh, MD

Cardiology Co-Director, Integrated Cardiac Imaging
Consultant, Division of Cardiovascular Diseases
Professor of Medicine
Mayo Clinic
Rochester, Minnesota

Co-Director, Cardiac and Vascular Center
Samsung Medical Center
Seoul, South Korea

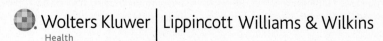

Wolters Kluwer | Lippincott Williams & Wilkins
Health

Philadelphia · Baltimore · New York · London
Buenos Aires · Hong Kong · Sydney · Tokyo

Acquisitions Editor: Frances DeStefano
Product Manager: Leanne Vandetty
Production Manager: Alicia Jackson
Senior Manufacturing Manager: Benjamin Rivera
Marketing Manager: Kimberly Schonberger
Design Coordinator: Holly Reid McLaughlin
Production Service: S4Carlisle

Printed in China

978-1-4511-0961-0
1-4511-0961-X
Library of Congress Cataloging-in-Publication Data

Kane, Garvan C.
Echocardiography : a case-based review / authors, Garvan C. Kane, Jae K. Oh.
 p. ; cm.
Complement to: Echo manual / Jae K. Oh, James B. Seward, A. Jamil Tajik. 3rd ed. c2006.
Includes bibliographical references and index.
ISBN 978-1-4511-0961-0 (alk. paper)—ISBN 1-4511-0961-X (alk. paper)
I. Oh, Jae K. II. Oh, Jae K. Echo manual. III. Title.
[DNLM: 1. Heart Diseases—ultrasonography—Case Reports. 2. Heart Diseases—ultrasonography—Examination Questions. 3. Echocardiography—methods—Case Reports. 4. Echocardiography—methods—Examination Questions. WG 18.2]

616.1'207543—dc23

2012015884

Care has been taken to confirm the accuracy of the information presented and to describe generally accepted practices. However, the authors, editors, and publisher are not responsible for errors or omissions or for any consequences from application of the information in this book and make no warranty, expressed or implied, with respect to the currency, completeness, or accuracy of the contents of the publication. Application of the information in a particular situation remains the professional responsibility of the practitioner.

The authors, editors, and publisher have exerted every effort to ensure that drug selection and dosage set forth in this text are in accordance with current recommendations and practice at the time of publication. However, in view of ongoing research, changes in government regulations, and the constant flow of information relating to drug therapy and drug reactions, the reader is urged to check the package insert for each drug for any change in indications and dosage and for added warnings and precautions. This is particularly important when the recommended agent is a new or infrequently employed drug.

Some drugs and medical devices presented in the publication have Food and Drug Administration (FDA) clearance for limited use in restricted research settings. It is the responsibility of the health care provider to ascertain the FDA status of each drug or device planned for use in their clinical practice.

To purchase additional copies of this book, call our customer service department at (800) 638-3030 or fax orders to (301) 223-2320. International customers should call (301) 223-2300.

Visit Lippincott Williams & Wilkins on the Internet: at LWW.com. Lippincott Williams & Wilkins customer service representatives are available from 8:30 am to 6 pm, EST.

10 9 8 7 6 5 4 3 2 1

In memory of

Mark J. Callahan, MD

Preface

Echocardiography has become an essential diagnostic tool across the spectrum of cardiovascular disease. In the era of rapid technology development and the increasing use of other imaging modalities, echocardiography remains the single most useful imaging technique which couples comprehensive hemodynamic data with information on cardiac structure and systolic and diastolic function. Strain-based imaging now provides sensitive incremental quantitation of myocardial function with 3-dimensional echocardiography allowing real-time views of detailed true cardiac anatomy.

We have been very gratified by the success of *The Echo Manual*, currently in its 3rd edition, which has aided the education of physicians and sonographers since its first publication in 1994. As its name indicates, the book is first and foremost a manual to provide instruction to the learner on the various aspects of echocardiography and their clinical applications, highlighting the strengths and limitations of the modality and providing the reader the necessary steps to accomplish a comprehensive, quantitative diagnostic examination.

Echocardiography is a dynamic modality and *The Echo Manual* has not had real-time moving images or actual clinical cases to utilize comprehensive echocardiographic data including hemodynamic calculation. In this new case-based echocardiography book, we hope to fill this void, highlighting the importance of interpreting echocardiographic images in the setting of the clinical scenario. This book is designed as a guide for learners in the use of echocardiography data in the evaluation of patients through review of 100 selected cases from the Mayo Clinic with a variety of clinical conditions, both commonly and uncommonly encountered. We have placed a particular emphasis on the assessment of systolic and diastolic function and

quantitative hemodynamics throughout. This book needs to be used in tandem with review of the moving images, available through the on-line site. We recommend each case be reviewed in isolation from start to finish following the order of the case questions. In many cases, further echocardiographic images play an important role as the clinical cases develops, whether transesophageal, intracardiac or supplemental or subsequent transthoracic imaging. While we have selected cases that hopefully are useful to the learner, whether new or old to the practice of clinical echocardiography, we have tried to keep the cases true to life. Images at times are 'presentation quality' while at other times challenging and we have chosen to portray the cases in a predominantly random order. The focus of this book is on the interpretation of the echocardiographic data to provide guidance in the management of the patient. While acting as a stand-alone educational tool, this case-book also serves as a companion to *The Echo Manual, 3rd Edition*. Here we provide an answer and explanation to each question asked and we also include the location of a more detailed discussion of the topic in *The Echo Manual, 3rd Edition*.

We have had and continue to have the good fortune to learn and practice echocardiography with a wonderful team of physicians and sonographers. We thank our colleagues for sharing their expertise and interesting cases with us. We would like to thank our families, time from whom was taken to help complete this project. Finally we thank our patients for their educational images and we hope that this book will provide the reader with the tools to better diagnose and manage their patients through high quality echocardiography.

Garvan C. Kane
Jae K. Oh

Contents

Contents by Subject

Congenital Heart Disease

Coronary Artery Disease, including Stress Echocardiography

Native and Prosthetic Valvular Disease, including Infective Endocarditis

Pericardial and Right-sided Disease, including Pulmonary Hypertension

Systemic Diseases

Echocardiography

A Case-Based Review

Normal Images and Values

*B*efore looking at abnormal studies, we need to be familiar with normal images and values from a comprehensive echocardiographic examination. Please review all moving (**Videos 1-1 to 1-23**) and still images (Figs. 1-1 to 1-18) obtained from an otherwise healthy normal individual who was referred for a transthoracic echocardiogram in the setting of palpitations. A comprehensive echocardiography study demonstrated no abnormal findings. Also shown are animations demonstrating four standard transthoracic echocardiographic views and representative images obtained from each view (Animations 1-1 to 1-4). After your review of all images, please answer the following questions. You should be able to answer and understand all the questions to be able to provide diagnostically helpful data to clinicians ordering an echocardiogram.

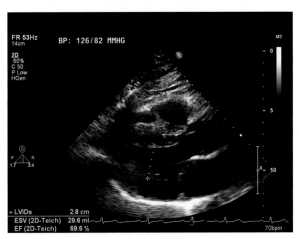

Figure 1-1

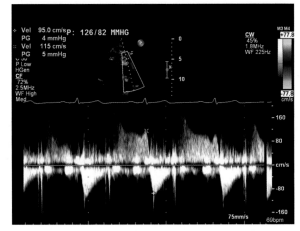

Figure 1-3

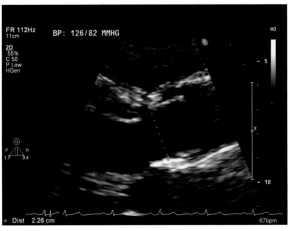

Figure 1-2

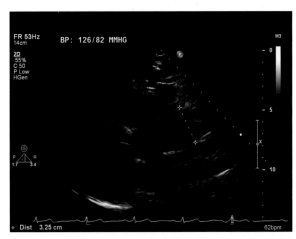

Figure 1-4

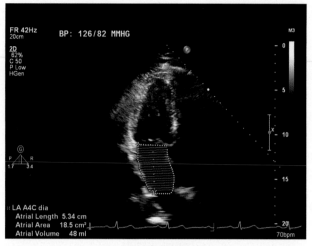

Figure 1-5

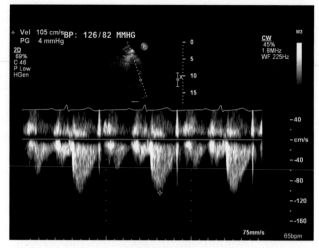

Figure 1-8

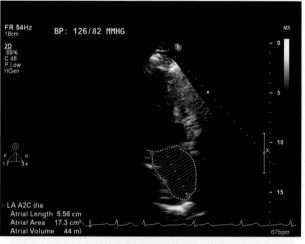

Figure 1-6

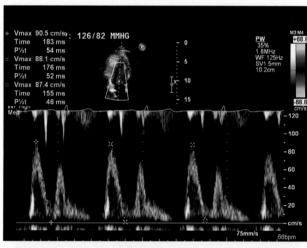

Figure 1-9

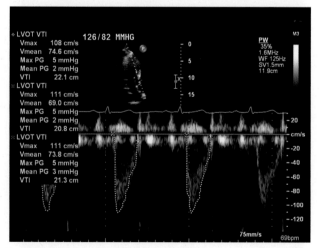

Figure 1-7

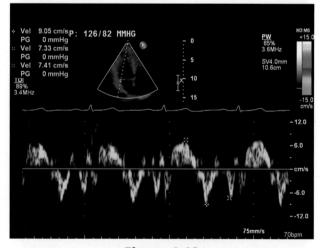

Figure 1-10

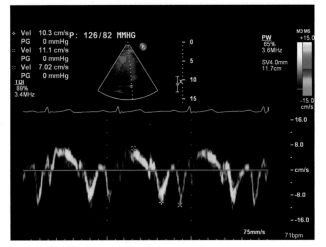

Figure 1-11

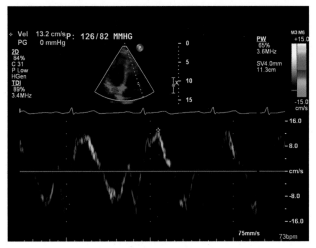

Figure 1-14

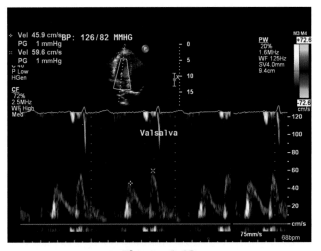

Figure 1-12

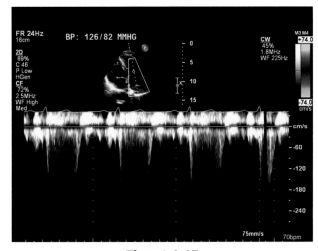

Figure 1-15

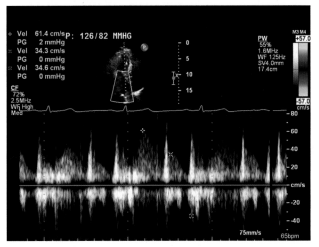

Figure 1-13

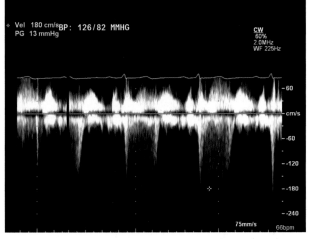

Figure 1-16

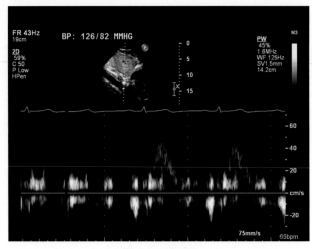

Figure 1-17

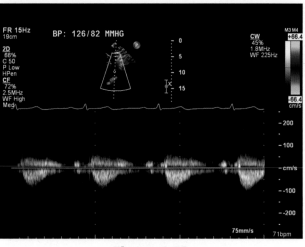

Figure 1-18

QUESTION 1. Please estimate left ventricular ejection fraction (LVEF) by your visual subjective reading. Write that ejection fraction (EF) down somewhere. Then, calculate LVEF from left ventricular (LV) end-diastolic dimension of 45 mm and end-systolic dimension of 28 mm. (This is a Quinones, simple method for calculating EF, which we still use in our clinical practice.) If you are not familiar with this equation, please see **pages 115 to 116, section on ejection fraction, in *The Echo Manual, 3rd Edition.*** Please compare your visual EF with the EF from Quinones method. You need to understand the apical factor.

QUESTION 2. Which of the following is the modified Bernoulli equation?

A. $(2 \times velocity)^2$
B. $4 \times velocity$
C. $4 + velocity^2$
D. $4^2 \times velocity$

QUESTION 3. From this case, calculate right ventricular systolic pressure (RVSP). How would you report this patient's RVSP?

A. Cannot calculate
B. 13 mm Hg
C. 18 mm Hg
D. Normal

QUESTION 4. Calculate cardiac output.

A. 4.4 L per minute
B. 5.5 L per minute
C. 6.6 L per minute
D. 7.7 L per minute
E. 8.8 L per minute

QUESTION 5. Which of the following parameters represents normal LV myocardial relaxation property?

A. E/A >1
B. Isovolumic relaxation time (IVRT) IVRT 70 to 100 milliseconds
C. Deceleration time 160 to 240 milliseconds
D. Mitral medial annulus e' 10 cm per second

QUESTION 6. Which of the following statements is correct regarding left atrial (LA) volume?

A. Enlarged LA volume does not always indicate increased LV filling pressure
B. Healthy individuals cannot have large LA volume
C. LA volume is always increased in patients with atrial fibrillation

QUESTION 7. Which of the following conditions can be correctly diagnosed from abdominal aortic pulsed wave Doppler examination?

A. Mild to moderate aortic regurgitation (AR)
B. Constrictive pericarditis
C. Aortic coarctation
D. Hypertrophic cardiomyopathy (HCM)

QUESTION 8. What value of diastolic reversal flow time velocity integral (TVI) in the proximal descending aorta indicates severe AR?

A. 5 cm
B. 10 cm
C. 15 cm
D. Depends on heart rate

QUESTION 9. Which of the following segments is not seen from apical three- or five-chamber (long-axis) view?

A. Inferobasal septum
B. Inferolateral wall
C. Anteroseptum
D. Apical septum

QUESTION 10. Pulmonary vein Doppler recording is useful in all of the following situations *except*:

A. Diastolic function assessment
B. Aortic stenosis
C. Mitral valve regurgitation
D. After atrial fibrillation ablation procedure

QUESTION 11. Which of the following situations is best to use Valsalva maneuver?

A. To differentiate Grade 2 from Grade 1 diastolic dysfunction
B. To differentiate aortic stenosis from HCM
C. To evaluate patent foramen ovale
D. To differentiate constriction from restriction

ANSWER 1: $(45^2 − 28^2)/45^2$ gives 0.62. Therefore, LVEF is 62% uncorrected.

As apical contractility is normal,

Corrected LVEF = 62% + [(100 − 62) × 15%]
$$= 60\% + 6\%$$
$$= 66\%$$

See *The Echo Manual, 3rd Edition*, discussion of ejection fraction on pages 115 to 116, and Figure 7-1 on page 110.

ANSWER 2: A. The Modified Bernoulli equation is 4 × velocity^2, which can be further simplified as (2 × velocity)^2.

The simplified method is more practical for velocities such as 3.5 m per second. Rather than squaring 3.5 m per second first before being multiplied by 4, (2 × 3.5) is 7, which can be squared to provide the value of 49.

See *The Echo Manual, 3rd Edition*, discussion of transvalvular gradients on pages 63 to 66, and Figure 4-8 on page 65.

ANSWER 3: D. Using the modified Bernoulli equation, the tricuspid regurgitation (TR) velocity of 1.8 m/s gives a transtricuspid valve gradient of 13 mm Hg. If you add a normal right atrial pressure estimate of 5 mm Hg, RVSP is 23 mm Hg. However, the TR velocity profile is incomplete and likely underestimated, and we may just say that pulmonary artery systolic pressure is normal rather than giving an actual value. Right ventricular outflow tract velocity also shows rapid onset of systolic velocity compatible with a normal RVSP.

ANSWER 4: D. Stroke volume (SV) is calculated from the left ventricular outflow tract (LVOT) as a product of the LVOT area (LVOT diameter × 0.785) and the LVOT TVI.

Cardiac output is the product of SV and heart rate.

Here SV = (2.3 cm)^2 × 21 cm = 111 ml at a heart rate of 69 beats per minute = 7.7 L per minute

See *The Echo Manual, 3rd Edition*, Figure 4-16 on page 71.

ANSWER 5: D. All other parameters could also be consistent with normal myocardial relaxation but not specific since a combination of high filling pressure and abnormal relaxation can give a similar value for E/A, IVRT, and deceleration time. Early diastolic velocity of the mitral annulus has been found to have a good correlation with tau which is the gold-standard measure of myocardial relaxation by cardiac catheterization. Almost if not all of myocardial diseases have abnormal myocardial relaxation.

ANSWER 6: A. Any chronic elevation in LA pressure will lead to LA dilatation over time. However, in the absence of elevation in LA pressure, modest degrees of LA dilatation may occur in the setting of atrial fibrillation. Chronic diastolic dysfunction also produces LA enlargement without an increase in filling pressure. Well trained healthy individuals can have increased LA volume. In that situation, you would expect an increased stroke volume.

ANSWER 7: C. Abdominal aortic velocity shows diastolic flow reversal in severe AR. Ascending aorta shows a notched velocity in patients with hypertrophic obstructive cardiomyopathy, but it is not usually seen in abdominal aorta. Nonobstructive HCM does not have characteristic flow velocity pattern in the aorta. Frequently, characteristic abdominal aorta pulse wave Doppler velocity gives an initial diagnostic clue for coarctation.

ANSWER 8: C. Descending aorta pulse wave Doppler is very helpful in determining the severity of aortic regurgitation especially when AR jet is eccentric. Although there are not many publications regarding the parameter, time velocity integral of diastolic reversal flow velocity from the descending aorta (by placing the sample volume away from the inner wall of the aorta at the level of the left subclavian artery) of 15 cm or greater indicates severe AR. There are however several other conditions which can give a similar diastolic reversal flow velocities.

ANSWER 9: A. The inferior septum is seen from the apical four-chamber view. Inferior wall is seen from apical 2 chamber view.

ANSWER 10: B. The pulmonary vein Doppler profile gives insights into the diastolic function (systolic blunting suggests elevated LA pressure), presence of severe mitral valve regurgitation (systolic flow reversals), or the presence of pulmonary vein stenosis (a complication after a pulmonary vein isolation procedure). There is no specific pulmonary vein Doppler finding that suggests aortic stenosis.

ANSWER 11: C. The Valsalva maneuver reduces venous return by increasing intrathoracic pressure. It is often helpful (but not always) to differentiate pseudo-normalized mitral inflow (grade 2) from true normal mitral inflow. However, the distinction can be done now easily by tissue Doppler imaging with the early diastolic velocity of the mitral annulus (e'). One of most valuable indications for the Valsalva maneuver is to assess right to left shunt via the patent foramen ovale. Upon release of the maneuver, venous return increases to the right atriium and augment or demonstrate right to left atrial shunt.

Syncopal Episode

*M*s. NE is a 19-year-old woman who is referred for a transthoracic echocardiogram after a syncopal episode. She was at college basketball practice and felt briefly light-headed and then passed out, striking her head and sustaining a scalp laceration. She has no known cardiac history and is on no medications. On physical examination, her blood pressure is 100/62 mm Hg and heart rate 50 beats per minute with a regular rhythm. Carotid pulses and jugular venous pulse were normal. Precordial examination was normal apart from a 1/6 systolic ejection murmur.

QUESTION 1. Concerning measurement of left ventricular (LV) dimensions (see **Video 2-1** and Figs. 2-1 and 2-2), which of the following statements is correct?

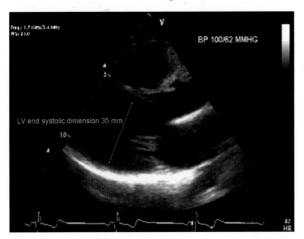

Figure 2-1

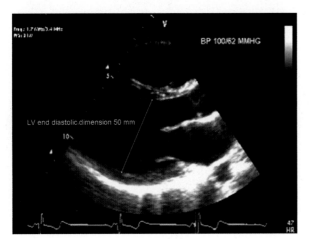

Figure 2-2

A. LV end-diastolic and end-systolic dimensions are measured at the level of the mitral valves tips

B. The timing of the LV end-diastolic dimension measurement is at the time of the largest dimension, typically at the onset of the QRS complex

C. Using the apical contractility correction factor (assuming it is normal), the calculated LV ejection fraction is 58%

D. All of the choices

QUESTION 2. The estimated pulmonary artery systolic (PASP) and diastolic pressures (PADP) (see **Video 2-2** and Figs. 2-3 and 2-4) are:

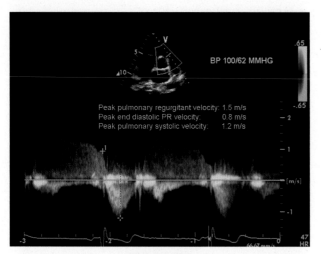

Peak pulmonary regurgitant velocity: 1.5 m/s
Peak end diastolic PR velocity: 0.8 m/s
Peak pulmonary systolic velocity: 1.2 m/s

Figure 2-3

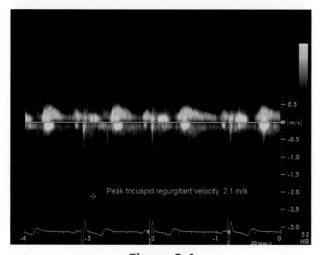

Peak tricuspid regurgitant velocity: 2.1 m/s

Figure 2-4

A. 18/3 mm Hg
B. 23/14 mm Hg
C. 23/8 mm Hg
D. 23/11 mm Hg
E. 18/8 mm Hg

QUESTION 3. The grade of diastolic (dys) function (see **Video 2-3** and Figs. 2-5 to 2-7) is:

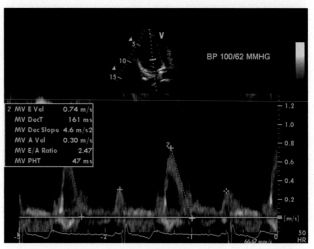

2 MV E Vel   0.74 m/s
MV DecT   161 ms
MV Dec Slope 4.6 m/s2
MV A Vel   0.30 m/s
MV E/A Ratio 2.47
MV PHT   47 ms

Figure 2-5

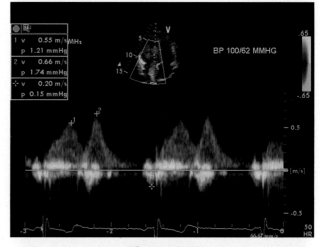

1 v 0.55 m/s
  p 1.21 mmHg
2 v 0.66 m/s
  p 1.74 mmHg
  v 0.20 m/s
  p 0.15 mmHg

Figure 2-6

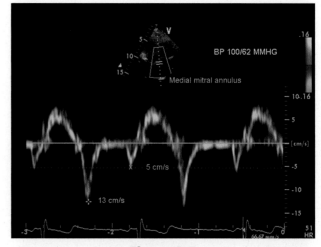

Medial mitral annulus

5 cm/s

13 cm/s

Figure 2-7

A. Normal diastolic function
B. Grade 1 (impaired diastolic dysfunction)
C. Grade 2 (delayed relaxation diastolic dysfunction)
D. Grade 3 (restrictive diastolic dysfunction)

QUESTION 4. This pulsed wave flow pattern taken in the abdominal aorta (see Fig. 2-8) would be compatible with:

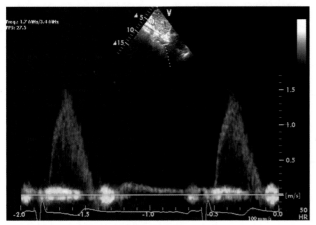

Figure 2-8

A. Coarctation of the descending thoracic aorta
B. What is seen in the majority of patients with a bicuspid aortic valve
C. Patent ductus arteriosus
D. Severe congenital aortic stenosis

QUESTION 5. Transthoracic echocardiography can exclude the following potential causes for syncope in a young women except:

A. Critical congenital aortic stenosis
B. Dilated cardiomyopathy with reduced ejection fraction
C. Pulmonary arterial hypertension
D. Aortic dissection
E. Hypertrophic cardiomyopathy

ANSWER 1: D. As recommended by the American Society of Echocardiography, the long- and short-axis dimensions can be obtained directly from the end-systolic and end-diastolic dimensions (ESd and EDd), measured at the level of the mitral tips as the smallest and largest diameters, respectively. If there are no regional wall motion abnormalities, the LV dimensions measured from the level of the papillary muscles can be used to calculate the left ventricular ejection fraction (LVEF) as follows:

Uncorrected LVEF = $[(EDd)^2 - (ESd)^2] / (EDd)^2 \times 100$

Corrected LVEF = uLVEF + [(100 − uLVEF) × 15%]

uLVEF = uncorrected LVEF

Here,

Uncorrected LVEF = $[(50)^2 - (35)^2] / (50)^2$ × 100 = 51%

Corrected LVEF = 51 + [(100 − 51) × 15%] = 58%

See *The Echo Manual, 3rd Edition,* page 109.

ANSWER 2: C. In the absence of pulmonary stenosis, demonstrated here by a pulmonary valve that opens normally on two-dimensional (2D) imaging without turbulence on color flow imaging and a peak velocity of only 1.2 m per second, the right ventricular (RV) systolic pressure is equivalent to the PASP. RV systolic (and therefore PA systolic) pressure can reliably be estimated on the basis of Doppler interrogation of tricuspid valve regurgitation. RV systolic pressure is calculated by adding an estimate of right atrial pressure to the peak gradient between the RV and the RA (i.e., four times [the peak tricuspid regurgitant velocity]^2).

Here RV systolic pressure = 4 (2.1)^2 + right atrial pressure

= 18 + RA pressure

See *The Echo Manual, 3rd Edition,* **Figure 9-2 on page 145, and pages 144 to 146.**

The diastolic PA pressure can be estimated by adding an estimate of right atrial pressure to the gradient between the PA and the RV in end diastole (i.e., four times [the end pulmonary regurgitant velocity]^2).

See *The Echo Manual, 3rd Edition,* **text and Figure 9-7 on page 147.**

Here PADP = 4 (0.8)^2 + right atrial pressure

= 3 + RA pressure

When the diameter of the inferior vena cava is small (<17 to 20 mm) and decreases by 50% or more on inspiration, the RA pressure is normal (approximately 5 mm Hg).

So here RV systolic pressure = PASP = 18 + 5 mm Hg

= 23 mm Hg

And PADP = 3 + 5 mm Hg

= 8 mm Hg

See *The Echo Manual, 3rd Edition,* **pages 143 to 147.**

ANSWER 3: A. The mitral inflow pattern (Fig. 2-5) demonstrates that most of LV filling occurs early in diastole with an E velocity of 0.7 m per second with a relatively short deceleration time of 161 millisecond and a diminutive A velocity of 0.3 m per second (E/A ratio of 2.5). Doppler interrogation of the pulmonary veins (Fig. 2-6) demonstrates a diastolic predominant pattern. This combination of findings would point toward a restrictive, Grade 3, severe diastolic dysfunction pattern.

However, one also notes that 2D images demonstrate normal LV size and ejection fraction and the left atrium is also of normal size. Figure 2-7 demonstrates the medial mitral annulus tissue Doppler with evidence of excellent myocardial relaxation with an e prime (e') velocity of 13 cm per second.

In normal young people, LV relaxation is so vigorous that the negative pressures generated in the left ventricle lead to almost all filling to occur early in diastole, leaving little for atrial contraction to contribute. It is not uncommon to see dominant diastolic forward flow velocity in pulmonary vein in healthy young individual. Again, the most important parameter for assessing diastolic function is the status of myocardial relaxation assessed by e'. If e' velocity is normal, diastolic function is usually normal. An important disease condition with normal e' velocity (from medial mitral annulus) is constrictive pericarditis.

See *The Echo Manual, 3rd Edition,* **Figure 8-22 on page 133, and text on pages 132 to 136.**

ANSWER 4: B. Here shown is an example of a normal pulse wave Doppler assessment of the abdominal aorta taken from the subcostal longitudinal plane. This should be part of the standard echocardiographic examination especially in young patients with cardiovascular symptoms and/or hypertension. Shown here are a brisk systolic upstroke, brisk systolic downstroke, and a small early diastolic flow reversal (seen below the baseline). Note also the lack of forward flow. The typical findings in coarctation of the aorta are a prolonged time to peak velocity and persistent forward diastolic flow. Large diastolic flow reversals are a feature of a patent ductus arteriosus or severe aortic regurgitation. Severe aortic stenosis typically will have a blunted peak systolic velocity with a decreased time to peak. Although a patient with a bicuspid aortic valve is at risk for coarctation, aortic valve stenosis, and regurgitation—any of which if severe may give rise to abnormalities on pulse wave interrogation of the abdominal aorta—the vast majority of patients with a bicuspid valve will have a normal finding as seen here.

See *The Echo Manual, 3rd Edition,* **Figure 20-29 on page 354.**

ANSWER 5: D. All of the options in the question stem are potential cardiovascular causes for syncope. A normal transthoracic echocardiogram can reliably exclude all of these as a cause for syncope except for an aortic dissection. Should an aortic dissection be suspected clinically, a transesophageal echocardiogram or a contrast CT angiogram of the aorta is required. Another potential cause for syncope in a young person is an arrhythmia triggered by myocardial ischemia in the setting of an anomalous coronary artery. Although anomalous coronary ostia may be seen on transthoracic imaging, an alternative imaging modality is often needed to exclude this also. It is also often difficult to exclude arrhythmogenic right ventricular dysplasia which may require cardiac computed tomography or magnetic resonance imaging.

See *The Echo Manual, 3rd Edition,* **discussion of goal directed echo exam of syncope on pages 396 and 397.**

CASE 3

Progressive Exertional Shortness of Breath

Mr. HM is a 42-year-old man with a 7-month history of progressive exertional shortness of breath (NYHA functional class III). He is a prior smoker, but has no other known cardiovascular disease. His family history is notable for sudden unexplained death of his mother at the age of 40. His only sibling who is 55 years of age recently underwent a normal cardiovascular comprehensive examination with echocardiography.

On examination, his blood pressure is 125/70 mm Hg and heart rate 60 bpm. His carotid pulses have brisk upstrokes, and his central venous pressure is normal. He has a sustained and localized left ventricular (LV) apical impulse. There is a 2/6 systolic ejection murmur that increases when the patient goes from a squat position to standing.

He is referred for transthoracic echocardiography (see **Video 3-1**).

QUESTION 1. Which of the following factors is *not* associated with an increased risk of sudden cardiac death in this case?

A. Septal wall thickness
B. Sudden death of his mother at the age of 40
C. Severe central mitral valve regurgitation
D. Nonsustained ventricular tachycardia on a Holter

QUESTION 2. Calculate the maximal instantaneous intracavitatory gradient (see Fig. 3-1).

A. 16 mm Hg
B. 49 mm Hg
C. 64 mm Hg
D. 136 mm Hg
E. 196 mm Hg

QUESTION 3. In this setting, the overall LV hemodynamics in this case would be consistent with which of the following aortic systolic blood pressures, assuming the left atrial pressure is 20 mm Hg (see Fig. 3-1)?

A. 90 mm Hg
B. 120 mm Hg
C. 150 mm Hg
D. 200 mm Hg

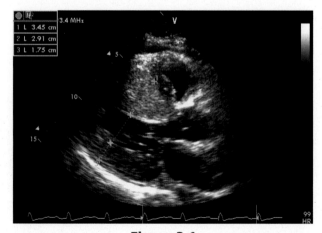

Figure 3-1

QUESTION 4. In hypertrophic cardiomyopathy (HCM), what happens to the left ventricular outflow tract (LVOT) gradient after a PVC (see Fig. 3-2)?

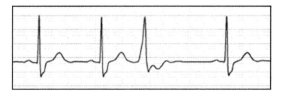

Figure 3-2

A. It goes up
B. It goes down

QUESTION 5. With regard to the management of this patient, which of the following is true?

A. The overall complication rate is greater with surgical myectomy than with alcohol septal ablation
B. The risk of sudden cardiac death would be lower after septal alcohol ablation than after surgical myectomy
C. Complete heart block is more likely with alcohol ablation than with surgical myectomy
D. Alcohol septal ablation would obviate the need for defibrillator to reduce the risk of sudden cardiac death

QUESTION 6. Following surgical myectomy, what abnormal finding is present (see **Video 3-2** and Fig. 3-3)?

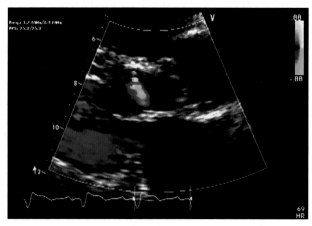

Figure 3-3

A. Ventricular septal defect
B. Significant aortic valve regurgitation
C. Coronary-ventricular fistula
D. Residual systolic anterior motion of the mitral valve with mitral valve regurgitation

ANSWER 1: C. Echocardiography in this case demonstrates severe increase in circumferential LV wall thickness with massive thickening of the intraventricular septum (septal dimension of 43 mm). LV ejection fraction is normal. In HCM, several clinical and echocardiographic factors have been associated with an increased risk of sudden cardiac death. The five most frequently cited factors are as follows:

Sudden Cardiac Death Risk Stratification in HCM

  I. LV wall thickness ≥30 mm (typically septum—but any wall)
  II. Abnormal blood pressure response to exercise
  III. Nonsustained ventricular tachycardia
  IV. Family history of SCD
  V. Recurrent syncope[1–3]

See *The Echo Manual, 3rd Edition,* **page 257, last sentence in the right column.**

ANSWER 2: C. 64 mm Hg. This continuous wave Doppler obtained from the apex illustrates two signals: the LVOT (*right*) obstruction and superimposed incomplete signal of mitral regurgitation (*left*). It can be sometimes difficult to distinguish between them. In HCM, mitral regurgitation usually begins at midsystole when there is systolic anterior motion of the mitral valve. Therefore, the Doppler spectrum of mitral regurgitation is often incomplete and may superficially resemble the LVOT flow velocity spectrum. However, the rising slope at midsystole is usually perpendicular to the baseline in mitral regurgitation, whereas it is curvilinear until it reaches the highest velocity in the LVOT signal. Furthermore, the mitral regurgitation velocity signal extends beyond ejection and culminates in mitral forward flow during the onset of diastole. Remember that the mitral regurgitation velocity will always be more (7 m per second) than that of the LVOT jet velocity (4 m per second). Using the modified Bernoulli equation, the peak pressure gradient may be calculated from the late-peaking dagger-shaped LVOT Doppler signal as follows $4v^2 = 4(4)^2 = 64$ mm Hg.

See *The Echo Manual, 3rd Edition,* **pages 259 to 261, and Figures 15-14 to 15-17 on page 261.**

ANSWER 3: C. 150 mm Hg. With the available data, LV systolic pressure can be calculated in two ways. In the hemodynamic echocardiographic assessment of a patient with HCM, it is good practice to derive both measures to ensure internal consistency. LV systolic pressure equals the peak gradient across the mitral valve ($4v^2$; where *v* is the peak mitral regurgitant velocity) plus an estimate of left atrial pressure. In this case, $4(7)^2 + 20 = 216$ mm Hg.

LV pressure = systolic blood pressure + intracavitatory gradient

Systolic blood pressure = LV pressure – intracavitatory gradient

Systolic blood pressure = 216 – 64 = 152 mm Hg

Alternatively (in the absence of aortic valve disease), LV pressure also equals systolic blood pressure plus the intracavitatory gradient.

Hence, using this strategy, one can estimate the LVOT gradient in two separate ways in HCM patients in the echo laboratory: the first through directly measuring the peak velocity of the LVOT continuous wave Doppler signal and the second using the peak velocity of the mitral regurgitant continuous wave Doppler signal and the brachial systolic blood pressure. It is advisable to ensure the consistency of these two strategies wherever possible.

See *The Echo Manual, 3rd Edition,* **first paragraph on page 261.**

ANSWER 4: A. It goes up. During the prolonged phase of LV filling associated with a premature ventricular complex, there is an increase in LV volume that in turn potentiates an increase in LV pressure. In this setting, there is a differential physiologic response in the setting of fixed (e.g., aortic stenosis) or dynamic (e.g., hypertrophic obstructive cardiomyopathy) LV obstruction. The intensity of the systolic flow increases in aortic stenosis and HCM. The aortic pressure increases in fixed obstruction, but decreases or remains unchanged in dynamic obstruction. These findings in patients with HCM reflect the Brockenbrough–Braunwald–Morrow sign where postextrasystolic potentiation results in an increased LVOT gradient with decreased or unchanged aortic pulse pressure.

See *The Echo Manual, 3rd Edition,* **Figure 15-15 on page 261.**

ANSWER 5: C. Patients with hypertrophic obstructive cardiomyopathy, who remain symptomatic (NYHA class III to IV) despite medical therapy, are candidates for invasive therapy with either surgical myectomy or septal ablation. The goal of either therapy is to relief the outflow tract obstruction through physical removal (myectomy) or through therapeutic infarction of the excess septal muscle mass. In experienced centers, the inhospital mortality rates with surgical myectomy are low and the overall success rates high. Patients with concomitant organic mitral valve disease or obstructive coronary disease are candidates for combined surgical corrective procedures. Mitral regurgitation related to systolic anterior motion of the mitral valve is usually corrected by myectomy without a mitral valve procedure. Both surgical septal myectomy and septal alcohol ablation reduce LVOT obstruction and improve symptom grade. To date, there has been no randomized comparison trial of myectomy versus ablation. A recent meta-analysis indicates a similar in hospital mortality (0.6% for myectomy and 1.6% for ablation). Septal myectomy appears to have a lower rate of permanent pacemaker implantation for complete heart block (3.3% vs. 18.4%), a higher success rate (required repeat procedure 0.6% in myectomy patients vs. 5.5% in ablation patients). Published data point to a possible reduction in sudden cardiac death and rates of appropriate defibrillator discharges following myectomy. This does not appear to be the case following septal ablation.[4–9]

ANSWER 6: C. A complication that is relatively unique to surgical myectomy is the unroofing of an intramural septal coronary artery at the myectomy site, thus creating a coronary to LVOT fistula. Seen here is a Doppler flow signal, below the aortic valve, arising from within the septal myocardium into the LVOT. Two distinct characteristics separating a coronary fistula from a ventricular septal defect are direction (into the left ventricle as opposed to typically into the right ventricle) and timing (diastolic as opposed to systolic). Postmyectomy septal coronary to LV fistula is very rarely of any clinical significance.[10]

References

1. Spirito P, Bellone P, Harris KM, et al. Magnitude of left ventricular hypertrophy and risk of sudden death in hypertrophic cardiomyopathy. *New Engl J Med.* 2000;342:1778–1785.

2. McKenna WJ, Behr ER. Hypertrophic cardiomyopathy: management, risk stratification, and prevention of sudden death. *Heart.* 2002;87:169.

3. Maron BJ, McKenna WJ, Danielson GK, et al. American College of Cardiology/European Society of Cardiology clinical expert consensus document on hypertrophic cardiomyopathy. A report of the American College of Cardiology Foundation Task Force on Clinical Expert Consensus Documents and the European Society of Cardiology Committee for Practice Guidelines. *J Am Coll Cardiol.* 2003;42:1687.

4. McLeod CJ, Ommen SR, Ackerman MJ, et al. Surgical septal myectomy decreases the risk for appropriate implantable cardioverter defibrillator discharge in obstructive hypertrophic cardiomyopathy. *Eur Heart J.* 2007;28:2583–2588.

5. Ommen SR, Maron BJ, Olivotto I, et al. Long-term effects of surgical septal myectomy on survival in patients with obstructive hypertrophic cardiomyopathy. *J Am Coll Cardiol.* 2005;46:470–476.

6. Qin JX, Shiota T, Lever HM, et al. Outcome of patients with hypertrophic obstructive cardiomyopathy after percutaneous transluminal septal myocardial ablation and septal myectomy surgery. *J Am Coll Cardiol.* 2001;38:1994–2000.

7. Sorajja P, Valeti U, Nishimura RA, et al. Outcome of alcohol septal ablation for obstructive hypertrophic cardiomyopathy. *Circulation.* 2008;118:131–139.

8. Talreja DR, Nishimura RA, Edwards WD, et al. Alcohol septal ablation versus surgical septal myectomy: comparison of effects on atrioventricular conduction tissue. *J Am Coll Cardiol.* 2004;44:2329–2332.

9. Woo A, Williams WG, Choi R, et al. Clinical and echocardiographic determinants of long-term survival after surgical myectomy in obstructive hypertrophic cardiomyopathy. *Circulation.* 2005;111:2033–2038.

10. Bax JJ, Raphael D, Bernard X, et al. Echocardiographic detection and long-term outcome of coronary artery-left ventricle fistula after septal myectomy in hypertrophic obstructive cardiomyopathy. *J Am Soc Echocardiogr.* 2001;14:308–310.

CASE 4

Heart Murmur

A 70-year-old woman presents with a heart murmur. She has a history of a systolic ejection murmur for the past 15 years. Over the past 2 years, she describes mildly increasing exertional shortness of breath. She now gets shortness of breath walking a 500 yards. On examination, her blood pressure is 130/80 mm Hg and her heart rate 65 beats per minute. Her central venous pressure is normal. Her carotid upstroke is delayed. She has a 3/6 ejection systolic murmur and a single second heart sound.

She is referred for transthoracic echocardiography (**Videos 4-1 to 4-6** and Figs. 4-1 to 4-5).

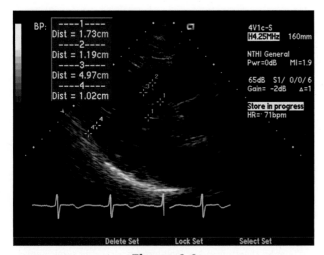

Figure 4-1

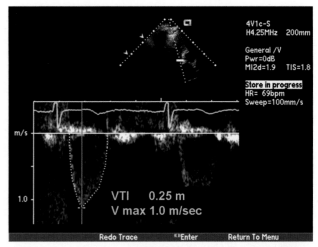

Figure 4-3

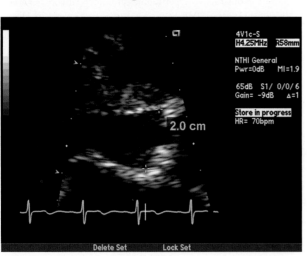

Figure 4-2

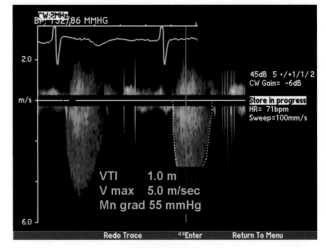

Figure 4-4

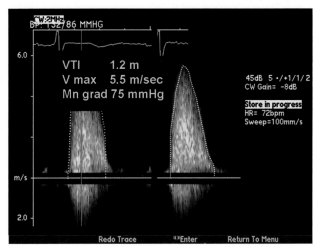

Figure 4-5

QUESTION 1. What is the calculated aortic valve area?

A. 0.65 cm²
B. 0.80 cm²
C. 0.85 cm²
D. 1.0 cm²

QUESTION 2. What is the peak transaortic pressure gradient?

A. 75 mm Hg
B. 95 mm Hg
C. 100 mm Hg
D. 121 mm Hg

QUESTION 3. Doppler-derived aortic valve pressure gradients are typically slightly lower than that of the catheter-derived aortic valve pressure gradients.

A. True
B. False

QUESTION 4. Which of the following factors may lead to a disproportionately elevated aortic mean gradient for a given aortic valve area?

A. An increase in left ventricular (LV) contractility
B. Anemia
C. Aortic valve regurgitation
D. All of the choices

QUESTION 5. Which of the following is the next best management step?

A. Aortic valve replacement
B. Coronary angiography and then aortic valve replacement
C. Treadmill exercise testing
D. Hemodynamic catheterization to assess the aortic valve area

QUESTION 6. Which of the following statements is *not* correct regarding left ventricular outflow tract (LVOT) time velocity integral (TVI) and aortic valve TVI ratio?

A. It is inversely proportional to aortic valve area and LVOT area ratio
B. When multiplied by LVOT area, aortic valve area is calculated
C. Aortic valve area is larger when the ratio is smaller
D. It is useful when LVOT diameter cannot be determined

ANSWER 1: A. Aortic valve area = [(LVOT TVI) × (LVOT area)]/Ao TVI

$$= [(LVOT\ TVI) \times (0.785\ (LVOT\ D)^2]/Ao\ TVI$$
$$= [(25) \times (3.14)]/120$$
$$= 78.5/120$$
$$= 0.65\ cm^2$$

Here two continuous wave Doppler signals are shown, one from the apex (Fig. 4-4) and one from the right parasternal area (Fig. 4-5). In a comprehensive examination of a patient with aortic stenosis, it is critical to perform a Doppler evaluation from all available transducer windows. Fifteen to twenty percent of the time, the peak signal will be obtained from a window other than the apex.

See *The Echo Manual, 3rd Edition*, **discussion of Doppler echocardiography in aortic stenosis on pages 190 and 191.**

ANSWER 2: D. Blood flow velocity *(v)* measured with Doppler echocardiography reliably reflects the pressure gradient according to the modified Bernoulli equation. According to the equation, pressure gradient = $4v^2$. Here the peak transaortic flow velocity is 5.5 m per second, which corresponds to a peak transaortic pressure gradient of 121 mm Hg.

ANSWER 3: B. False. There typically is a small difference between the Doppler-derived and catheter-derived aortic valve pressure gradients because of the pressure recovery phenomenon. Part of the kinetic energy lost during flow passage through a small orifice is recovered. Therefore, this pressure recovery results in a higher absolute pressure in the ascending aorta away from the stenotic aortic valve, explaining why the catheter-derived pressure gradient is lower than the Doppler-derived pressure gradient (Doppler echocardiography measures the highest value). Pressure recovery is smaller when the aorta is dilated. However, pressure recovery may be an important factor in causing a discrepancy between echo-derived aortic valve area and catheter-derived aortic valve area.

ANSWER 4: D. When LV systolic function and cardiac output are abnormally high, the following point should be considered: peak velocity and mean aortic gradient vary with changes in stroke volume. In patients with increased cardiac output across the aortic valve (as in aortic regurgitation or anemia), aortic stenosis may not be severe even when the peak velocity is 4.5 m per second or greater and the mean gradient is 50 mm Hg or higher. Aortic valve area should be more helpful in determining the severity of aortic stenosis in those situations.

ANSWER 5: B. This woman has symptoms and signs of severe aortic valve stenosis. The echocardiogram demonstrates a mean systolic gradient over 50 mm Hg and a valve area <0.75 cm². The diagnosis is clear, and no further assessment is required. Given the patients age, a coronary angiogram is appropriate to assess for concomitant coronary artery disease. However, a hemodynamic left heart catheterization is in most cases unnecessary and should be avoided. A substantial portion of patients develop subclinical as well as clinical embolic lesion after a hemodynamic cardiac catheterization for aortic stenosis.[1]

ANSWER 6: C. The ratio of the TVI of the LVOT to that of the aortic valve is a useful parameter that does not require the measurement of the LVOT diameter. This "dimensionless index" is helpful particularly in cases of a very heavily calcified valve where an accurate measurement of the LVOT diameter is not feasible. As the severity of the aortic stenosis increases (decreasing aortic valve area), the ratio will decrease. A cutoff of <0.25 corresponds with a severely stenotic aortic valve.

Reference

1. Omran H, Schmidt H, Hackenbroch M, et al. Silent and apparent cerebral embolism after retrograde catheterization of aortic valve in valvular stenosis: a prospective, randomized study. *Lancet*. 2003;361:1241–1246.

CASE 5

Systemic Hypertension

*A*21-year-old man with systemic hypertension is referred for transthoracic echocardiogram.

QUESTION 1. Which of the following factors is not associated with this aortic valve finding (see **Video 5-1**)?

A. Aortic valve stenosis
B. A similar long-term survival to those with a normal aortic valve anatomy
C. Thoracic aortic dissection
D. 2:1 Female:male incidence

QUESTION 2. Which of the following cusps is fused (**Video 5-1** and Fig. 5-1)?

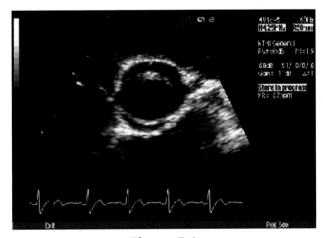

Figure 5-1

A. Right and left cusps
B. Right and noncoronary cusps
C. Noncoronary and left cusps

QUESTION 3. Which of the following patients with bicuspid aortic valve disease requires endocarditis prophylaxis?

A. Bicuspid aortic valve without stenosis or regurgitation
B. Bicuspid aortic valve with severe aortic valve regurgitation
C. Bicuspid aortic valve with severe aortic valve stenosis
D. Bicuspid aortic valve with healed endocarditis and trivial regurgitation
E. All of the choices
F. B, C, and D only

QUESTION 4. This pulsed wave Doppler signal taken from the abdominal aorta (Fig. 5-2) indicates:

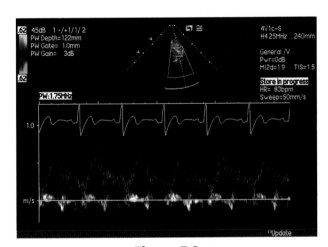

Figure 5-2

A. Normal flow
B. Contamination of the signal from a mesenteric artery
C. Coarctation of the descending thoracic aorta
D. Severe aortic valve regurgitation

QUESTION 5. Which of the following findings is *unlikely* to be present on clinical examination?

A. Radiofemoral pulse delay

B. An elevated femoral arterial pressure

C. A midsystolic murmur heard over the back

D. Rib notching on chest roentography

QUESTION 6. Which of the following statements concerning bicuspid aortic valve and coarctation of the descending thoracic aorta is true?

A. Coarctation of the aorta is present in 15% to 20% of patients with bicuspid aortic valve

B. Bicuspid aortic valve is present in 5% to 10% of patients with coarctation of the aorta

C. Bicuspid aortic valve is present in 50% to 75% of patients with coarctation of the aorta

D. Coarctation and bicuspid valve are present together only in female patients

ANSWER 1: D. Present in approximately 1% to 2% of the general population a bicuspid aortic valve is the most common congenital heart defect occurring with a male to female ratio of approximately 3:1. Common resulting pathologies are the development of aortic valve stenosis, regurgitation, and/or dilation of the ascending aorta with a concomitant risk of dissection. A longitudinal analysis of asymptomatic community patients with bicuspid aortic valve disease showed a similar long-term survival to peers, but incurred frequent cardiac events especially progressive valve dysfunction over time.

ANSWER 2: A. Seen here is a raphe at 12 to 1 o'clock owing to fusion on the left and right commissures.

The most common configuration of a bicuspid aortic valve is where there is fusion of two cusps resulting in a raphe or ridge resulting in an asymmetrical valve with two functioning leaflets. There are two common patterns. The first involves a raphe between the right and left sinuses resulting in an anterior cusp giving rise to both coronary ostia and a posterior cusp. The second is when there is a raphe between the right sinus and the noncoronary cusp resulting in a left and right cusp (with the right coronary artery originating from the right cusp and the left main coronary artery from the left cusp). Fusion of the left and noncoronary cusps is rare. It is important to recognize that the raphe may make the valve appear tricuspid during diastole, and therefore, attention to the valve opening during systole is critical. Very rarely the valve will be configured with two symmetrical cusps and no raphe (a "pure bicuspid valve").[1,2]

ANSWER 3: D. Because of a low incidence of endocarditis and limited data supporting the routine use of antibiotic prophylaxis, the updated American College of Cardiology / American Heart Association ACC/AHA guidelines in 2008 no longer recommend bacterial prophylaxis for patients with bicuspid aortic disease in the absence of prior endocarditis reference 3.

ANSWER 4: C. Pulsed wave Doppler signal recorded from the abdominal aorta demonstrates characteristics seen with a patient with severe coarctation of the aorta. Note the delayed upstroke and prolonged time to peak velocity, reduced pulsatility (difference between the maximal and minimal velocities), and the continuation of forward flow throughout diastole. This is in contrast to the normal abdominal

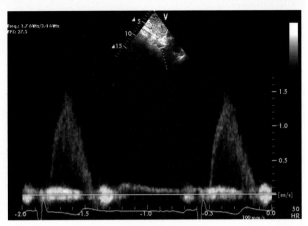

Figure 5-3

aorta Doppler flow (Fig. 5-3) with a brisk upstroke (short time to peak velocity) and rapid downstroke as well as the early diastolic reversal of flow and lack of notable forward flow in diastole or that seen with severe aortic valve regurgitation with holodiastolic flow reversals.

See *The Echo Manual, 3rd Edition,* **Figure 12-24B on page 209.**

Pulsed wave Doppler of abdominal branch vessels will demonstrate diastolic persistent diastolic forward flow; however, the differences in initial systolic upstroke, peak systolic velocity, and time to peak velocity seen here will not be present in the absence of obstruction to flow.

See *The Echo Manual, 3rd Edition,* **Figure 20-29 on page 354.**

ANSWER 5: B. The coarctation leads to hypertension in the upper extremities and relatively low pressure in the lower extremities. The femoral pulses tend to be weak, with a delay between the radial and femoral pulses. Flow in large collateral thoracic vessels may be heard as a systolic murmur over the thorax and back and may lead to rib notching seen on chest roentography.

ANSWER 6: C. Approximately 50% to 75% of patients with coarctation of the aorta will have a concomitant bicuspid valve, and this should always be evaluated for. Fusion of the right and left cusps (as in the case) is the variant of bicuspid valve disease that is most commonly associated with coarctation. Approximately 5% of patients with a bicuspid valve will have coarctation of the aorta.

References

1. Sievers HH, Schmidtke C. A classification system for the bicuspid aortic valve from 304 surgical specimens. *J Thoracic Cardiovasc Surg.* 2007;133:1226–1233.

2. Siu S, Silversides CK. Bicuspid aortic valve disease. *J Am Coll Cardiol.* 2010;55:2789–2800.

3. Nishimura RA, Carabello BA, Faxon DP, et al. ACC/AHA 2008 Guideline update on valvular heart disease: focused update on infective endocarditis: a report of the American College of Cardiology/American Heart Association Task Force on Practice Guidelines endorsed by the Society of Cardiovascular Anesthesiologists, Society for Cardiovascular Angiography and Interventions, and Society of Thoracic Surgeons. *J Am Coll Cardiol.* 2008;52:676–685.

CASE 6

Myocardial Infarction

A 56-year-old woman presents for transthoracic echocardiogram 4 weeks following a myocardial infarction (**Video 6-1**). She is asymptomatic.

QUESTION 1. The diastolic function grade in this patient is (Fig. 6-1):

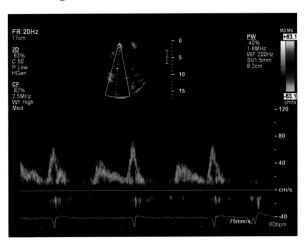

Figure 6-1

A. Normal
B. Grade 1
C. Grade 2
D. Grade 3

QUESTION 2. Assuming the left ventricular outflow tract (LVOT) diameter is 2 cm, what is the Doppler-derived cardiac output (CO) (Fig. 6-2)?

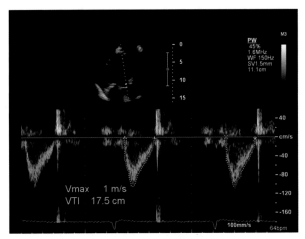

Figure 6-2

A. 2.5 L per minute
B. 3.5 L per minute
C. 4.5 L per minute
D. 5.5 L per minute

QUESTION 3. The echocardiogram demonstrates which of the following complications?

A. A left ventricular pseudoaneurysm
B. A left ventricular aneurysm
C. A left ventricular diverticulum

QUESTION 4. Management should include:

A. General medical management without anticoagulation
B. General medical management with anticoagulation
C. Urgent/emergent surgical consultation

QUESTION 5. Following an ST elevation myocardial infarction, each of the following factors is associated with adverse prognosis *except*:

A. A left ventricular ejection fraction (LVEF) <35%
B. Trans-mitral E/e' ratio >15
C. An early mitral inflow deceleration time >140 milliseconds
D. A left ventricular wall motion core index >2

ANSWER 1: B. The diastolic filling pattern demonstrates a low peak early (E) velocity compared with the late filling wave with atrial contraction (A) with a prolonged E-wave deceleration time. This is a pattern that defines group 1 or mild diastolic dysfunction. This typically is associated with normal or low left ventricular filling pressures, which would correlate with the absence of symptomatic dyspnea.

ANSWER 2: B. Stroke volume (SV) is calculated as the product of the cross-sectional area of the LVOT and the time velocity integral (TVI) of a pulse wave sample from the LVOT.

$$SV \ (ml) = [(D/2)^2 \times \pi] \times [LVOT \ TVI]$$
$$= [(2/2)^2 \times \pi] \times [17.5]$$
$$= 55 \ ml = 0.055 \ L$$

CO is calculated as the product of SV and heart rate
$$CO \ (L \ per \ minute) = 0.055 \times 64$$
$$= 3.5 \ L \ per \ minute$$

See *The Echo Manual, 3rd Edition*, Figure 4-16 on page 71.

ANSWER 3: B. A left ventricular pseudoaneurysm that may occur post myocardial infarction develops when a left ventricular free wall rupture is contained by overlying, adherent pericardium. A pseudoaneurysm is characterized on echocardiography as a small necked communication between the cavity and the sac, which is lined by pericardium rather than thinned muscle. The ratio of the maximum cavity to the diameter of the neck is >2. A left ventricular aneurysm that occurs following a myocardial infarction is caused by formation of a scar that leads to thinning and expansion of the myocardium. A diverticulum is a very rare cardiac abnormality characterized by a local embryologic development failure of the ventricular muscle.[1,2]

See *The Echo Manual, 3rd Edition*, section on true ventricular aneurysm and thrombus on page 166, and Figure 10-15 on page 168.

ANSWER 4: B. The usual treatment of ventricular aneurysms that occur after myocardial infarction is conservative unless the patient develops refractory angina, heart failure, or ventricular arrhythmias. In the early phase following of a myocardial infarction that leads to the development of an aneurysm, a reasonable consideration is systemic anticoagulation. However, long-term anticoagulation is not necessary in patients with ventricular aneurysms unless the patient develops a thrombus. Seen here is a large inferolateral aneurysm with thrombus. Aneurysms have a low risk of rupture. However, pseudoaneurysms are at a high risk for rupture, and the general recommendation for pseudoaneurysms is urgent surgical repair.

ANSWER 5: C. Many factors on echocardiography performed following a myocardial infarction provide useful prognostic information for patients. One of the strongest predictors of mortality is the LVEF with mortality greatly increasing as LVEF falls below 35%. A restrictive mitral inflow pattern (deceleration time ≤140 milliseconds) is a strong predictor of mortality following a myocardial infarction. Similarly, there are data demonstrating that using E/e' ratio as a surrogate for an estimation of left ventricular filling pressure at a cutoff of 15 is associated with a 5-fold increased risk of death post infarct, which has independent prognostic power over LVEF. Wall motion score index may have a better predictive power than LVEF after acute myocardial infarction. Other prognostic factors include LV volume, the degree of mitral valve regurgitation, left atrial enlargement, and right ventricular enlargement and dysfunction.[3–7]

References

1. Brown SL, Gropler RJ, Harris KM. Distinguishing left ventricular aneurysm from pseudoaneurysm. A review of the literature. *Chest.* 1997;111:1403–1409.

2. Ohlow MA. Congenital left ventricular aneurysms and diverticula: definition, pathophysiology, clinical relevance and treatment. *Cardiology.* 2006;106:63–72.

3. Brodie BR, Stuckey TD, Hansen CJ, et al. Importance of a patent infarct-related artery for hospital and late survival after direct coronary angioplasty for acute myocardial infarction. *Am J Cardiol.* 1992;69:1113–1119.

4. Nijland F, Kamp O, Karreman AJ, et al. Prognostic implications of restrictive left ventricular filling in acute myocardial infarction:

a serial Doppler echocardiographic study. *J Am Coll Cardiol.* 1997;30:1618.

5. Hillis GS, Møller JE, Pellikka PA, et al. Noninvasive estimation of left ventricular filling pressure by E/e' is a powerful predictor of survival after acute myocardial infarction. *J Am Coll Cardiol.* 2004;43:360–367.

6. Møller JE, Hillis GS, Oh JK, et al. Wall motion score index and ejection fraction for risk stratification after myocardial infarction. *Am Heart J.* 2006;151:419–425.

7. Møller JE, Hillis GS, Oh JK, et al. Left atrial volume: a powerful predictor of survival after acute myocardial infarction. *Circulation.* 2003;107:2207–2212.

CASE 7

Acute Severe Dyspnea

A 54-year-old previously well man presents with acute severe dyspnea. He was unable to lie flat. He denied chest pain. On examination, his systolic blood pressure was 80 mm Hg. He had a left-sided third heart sound without a murmur. He had inspiratory crackles bilaterally in the lung fields. His oxygen saturation was 85% on continuous flow oxygen by mask. A 12-lead ECG demonstrated sinus tachycardia without ST segment change. A chest radiograph is shown (Fig. 7-1). He was intubated. He undergoes transthoracic echocardiogram (**Videos 7-1 to 7-10**).

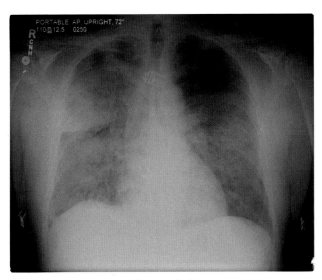

Figure 7-1

QUESTION 1. The next appropriate diagnostic step should be:

A. Admit to the intensive care unit for the management of presumed septic shock

B. Transfer to cardiac catheterization laboratory for diagnostic coronary angiography

C. Obtain chest CT iodinated contrast scan

QUESTION 2. After this study, the patient has placement of a pulmonary artery catheter. The mean right atrial pressure was 20 mm Hg, pulmonary artery pressure 55/30 mm Hg with a V-wave, and mean pulmonary capillary wedge pressure 34 and 24 mm Hg. The next step should include:

A. Transesophageal echocardiography

B. Contrast left ventriculography

C. Ventilation perfusion scan

D. Cardiac magnetic resonance scan

QUESTION 3. On the basis of **Videos 7-11 to 7-20**, the likely diagnosis is:

A. Ischemic (functional) mitral valve regurgitation

B. Myxomatous mitral valve disease with a flail segment

C. Infective endocarditis of the mitral valve

D. Ruptured papillary muscle

QUESTION 4. The flail scallop of the mitral valve is:

A. A1

B. A2

C. A3

D. P1

E. P2

F. P3

QUESTION 5. In this setting, if the expertise is available, the procedure associated with the best outcome is:

A. Medical management and elective mitral valve replacement
B. Emergent mitral valve replacement
C. Emergent mitral valve repair

QUESTION 6. On the basis of **Video 7-21**, obtained immediately coming off bypass, what is the appropriate next step?

A. Emergent exploration of left anterior descending artery with possible need for coronary bypass
B. Surgical manipulation of the heart
C. Removal of aortic vent

QUESTION 7. On the basis of **Videos 7-22 and 7-23**, the appropriate next step might include:

A. Satisfactory surgical result, no further intervention required
B. Intravenous phenylephrine and increasing the intravascular volume
C. Putting the patient back on bypass for re-repair of the mitral valve
D. Intra-aortic balloon pump

ANSWER 1: B. The clinical presentation is consistent with acute pulmonary edema and shock. Transthoracic echocardiography demonstrates hyperdynamic left ventricular systolic function. Left ventricular wall motion assessment is suboptimal because of image quality; however, no obvious left ventricular wall motion abnormalities are present. The right ventricle is enlarged and dysfunction with some flattening of the interventricular septum. The mitral valve, particularly the posterior leaflet, is thickened, and there is mitral valve regurgitation. The likely cause of the patient's presentation is acute severe mitral valve regurgitation. The next appropriate steps include placement of an intra-aortic balloon pump to provide hemodynamic support and perform diagnostic angiography (which was normal) before the consideration of mitral valve surgery. A heart murmur may not be heard in acute mitral regurgitation.

ANSWER 2: A. The right heart catheterization findings are consistent with mitral valve regurgitation (high V-wave) and associated pulmonary capillary wedge and pulmonary hypertension. It is important to confirm the severity of mitral regurgitation and importantly characterize the likely pathology. High pulmonary capillary wedge V-wave velocities can also be seen in other clinical situations. TEE could have been performed even before coronary angiography if he was more stable hemodynamically. In the acute unstable setting, cardiac MRI is not appropriate because the ability to monitor the patient is suboptimal and the balloon pump will not be compatible. Although contrast left ventriculography would confirm the presence of severe mitral regurgitation and often provide some insight into the mechanism in the setting of acute mitral regurgitation and high left atrial pressure, it comes with an increased risk. Moreover, the actual mechanism for severe mitral regurgitation cannot be assessed by left ventriculography. Transesophageal echocardiography is an ideal study because of easy availability and ability to be performed in the catheterization laboratory or in the coronary care unit. It will also allow the rapid characterization of the etiology.

ANSWER 3: B. Transesophageal echocardiography demonstrates a hyperdynamic left ventricle without wall motion abnormalities. The papillary muscles are intact; however, there is disruption of a number of chords resulting in a large segment of the mitral valve that is flail. This gives rise to severe mitral valve regurgitation. Although the mitral valve leaflets are myxomatous, there is no evidence of vegetation or other finding to suggest endocarditis.

ANSWER 4: E. Each of the mitral valve leaflets can be divided in three scallops namely lateral (1), middle (2), and medial (3). Identification of which scallop is involved by the pathology is best performed in a two-step process by transesophageal echocardiography. Step 1: at 0° with a multiplane TEE, one can easily identify whether the involved leaflet is anterior, posterior, or bileaflet (**Video 7-24**). On **Videos 7-11, 7-12, or 7-13**, the flail segment clearly involves the posterior leaflet. However, at 0°, because you are cutting across the valve from anterior to posterior, it is difficult to determine which part of the leaflet is involved. To decide which of the three scallops is affected, the probe needs to be rotated to about 60° to 75° (the commissural view). Here all three scallops are seen: the lateral scallop (1) (closest to left atrial appendage), the medial scallop (2), and the medial scallop (3) (**Video 7-25**). On **Video 7-15**, it is clear that it on the middle (P2) scallop that is flail (**Video 7-26**).

See *The Echo Manual, 3rd Edition,* **Figures 21-11 and 21-12 on pages 374 and 375, respectively.**

ANSWER 5: C. The patient presents with acute left ventricular failure and cardiogenic shock because of a large flail mitral valve segment and severe mitral regurgitation. Presumably, the patient previously did not have significant mitral valve regurgitation because the left ventricle is not dilated and is unable to cope with the degree of volume loading. Although intra-aortic balloon pump helps in stabilizing the patient, the patient needs to be considered for emergent mitral valve surgery. If the surgical expertise is available, this lesion should be quite amenable to repair with better long-term outcomes.

ANSWER 6: B. An important role for intraoperative TEE immediately coming off bypass includes ensuring that all the air has left the heart. Air frequently collects along the ventricular septum that appears echo-bright. This collection of air is dislodged by the surgeon by gentle shaking of the heart before removing the vent.

See *The Echo Manual, 3rd Edition,* **Figure 12-24 on page 381.**

ANSWER 7: B. TEE demonstrates systolic anterior motion of the anterior mitral valve leaflet. This is not an uncommon finding in the acute postbypass setting where the intravascular volume may be low. Increasing the intravascular volume and increasing the afterload with vasoactive agents with vasopressor (e.g., phenylephrine) rather than inotropic actions are appropriate. With these steps, the degree of SAM is reduced (**Video 7-27**). It should be noted that, even with this degree of SAM, the mitral valve does not leak and the surgical result is satisfactory. Intra-aortic balloon pump (by reducing left ventricular afterload) will, if anything, make SAM worse in this setting.

CASE 8

Exertional Shortness of Breath and Lower Extremity Edema

A 60-year-old woman presents with exertional shortness of breath and lower extremity edema. She has an enlarged cardiac size on chest x-ray.

QUESTION 1. Transthoracic images (**Videos 8-1 to 8-7** and Figs. 8-1 to 8-3) demonstrate evidence of:

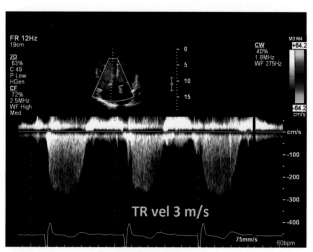

Figure 8-1

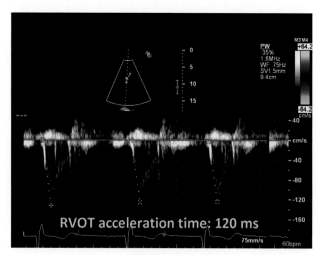

Figure 8-2

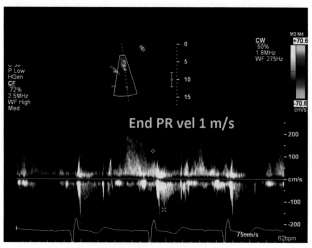

Figure 8-3

A. A normal right ventricle (RV)
B. RV pressure overload
C. RV volume overload

QUESTION 2. The estimated mean pulmonary artery (PA) pressure based on the RV outflow tract (RVOT) acceleration time (Fig. 8-2) is:

A. 10 mm Hg
B. 25 mm Hg
C. 40 mm Hg
D. 55 mm Hg

QUESTION 3. On the basis of the echocardiographic images, the underlying cause of the RV enlargement is:

A. Pulmonary hypertension
B. Atrial septal defect (ASD)
C. Tricuspid valve regurgitation (TR)
D. RV infarction

QUESTION 4. Which of the following facts is true concerning sinus venosus ASDs?

A. They comprise 20% of ASDs in adults
B. They are associated with mitral valve disease
C. When significant, they typically can be treated with a percutaneous closure device
D. They are typically located in the superior aspect of the intra-atrial septum

QUESTION 5. On auscultation, which of the following characteristics of the second heart sound is expected?

A. A split S_2 heard only during expiration
B. A split S_2 heard only during inspiration
C. A similarly split S_2 throughout the respiratory cycle

QUESTION 6. Which of the following is frequently associated with this condition?

A. Cleft mitral valve
B. "tear drop" sign
C. Anomalous left pulmonary venous connection
D. LBBB

ANSWER 1: C. There is 2D echocardiographic evidence of RV volume overload with a severely enlarged RV with flattening of the septum only during diastole. This is in contrast to the flattening of the ventricular septum throughout the cardiac cycle that is seen in pressure overload. This impression is supported by the absence of sufficient elevation in PA pressures to explain this degree of RV enlargement. On the basis of a right atrial (RA) pressure of 10 mm Hg, the estimate of the RV systolic pressure is 4 (TR vel)^2 + RA pressure = $4(3)^2$ + 10 = 34 mm Hg and the PA diastolic pressure is 4 (end pulmonary regurgitation [PR] vel)^2 + RA pressure = $4(1)^2$ +10 = 14 mm Hg.

ANSWER 2: B. The RVOT flow velocity has a characteristic pattern as PA pressure increases with shortening of the acceleration phase with increasing PA pressure.

See *The Echo Manual, 3rd Edition*, **Figure 9-8 on page 148.**

The simplest regression equation to estimate mean PA pressure (MPAP) MPAP from the RVOT acceleration time (AcT) is:

MPAP = 79 − 0.45 (AcT) = 25 mm Hg

Although this comes very close to the estimated PA pressures derived by the standard Doppler method based on the TR and PR velocities in this case, the acceleration time method is less accurate and more prone to error. Factors that may lead to erroneous values include variations in cardiac output and heart rate. With increased output through the cardiac chambers on the right side (as may be the case with an ASD), acceleration time may be normal even when PA pressure is increased. If the heart rate is <60 beats per minute or >100 beats per minute, acceleration time needs to be corrected for heart rate.

ANSWER 3: B. Here there is evidence of a sinus venosus ASD. To see this on subcostal imaging, the transducer is tilted superiorly and rotated clockwise to bring the intra-atrial septum near the SVC RA junction into view.

ANSWER 4: D. Sinus venosus defects occur in <5% of adults with ASDs. These defects are usually located in the superior and posterior aspects of the atrial septum, near the superior vena cava. They are frequently associated with anomalous connections of the right pulmonary veins, typically the right upper or middle veins (or both) to either the superior vena cava (SVC) the SVC or the RA. In older patients, Transesophageal echocardiography (TEE) TEE is often required to confidently visualize these posteriorly positioned abnormalities.

See *The Echo Manual, 3rd Edition*, **Figure 20-7 on page 339.**

It is the primum defect that is associated with atrioventricular valve abnormalities, typically a cleft of the anterior mitral valve leaflet. Although secundum defects can usually be closed satisfactorily with a percutaneous device, the sinus venosus defects frequently require surgical closure because of the absence of a circumferential rim of tissue and the common concomitant anomalous pulmonary vein connection.

ANSWER 5: C. The classic sound of an ASD is the "fixed" split of the S$_2$ owing to the reciprocal relationship between the caval flow and the transseptal flow. When the patient inspires, the effects of the increase in volume of venous return to the RA from the SVC are balanced by a reciprocal decrease in the degree of shunting across the ASD.

On the basis of the presence of symptoms and the degree of right heart enlargement, the patient was referred to a cardiac surgeon for primary closure of the ASD.

ANSWER 6: B. Sinus venosus ASD is associated with anomalous right pulmonary venous connection which is seen as "tear-drop" created by the pulmonary vein connection to the superior vena cava.

CASE 9

Systolic Murmur

A 45-year-old man is referred for a transthoracic echocardiogram to evaluate a systolic murmur. He is asymptomatic (see **Video 9-1**).

QUESTION 1. The aortic valve cusp marked by the arrow (Fig. 9-1) is:

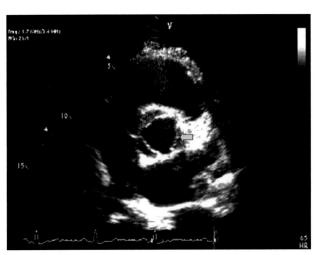

Figure 9-1

A. The left coronary cusp
B. The noncoronary cusp
C. The right coronary cusp

QUESTION 2. What is the diagnosis of the mitral valve (MV) pathology?

A. Mitral stenosis
B. MV prolapse
C. Mitral leaflet flail
D. Functional mitral regurgitation (MR)

QUESTION 3. The calculated regurgitant volume by the proximal isovelocity surface area (PISA) method (see Figs. 9-2 and 9-3) is:

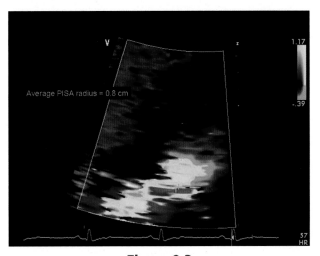

Figure 9-2

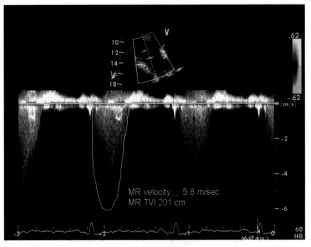

Figure 9-3

A. 40 cc
B. 45 cc
C. 52 cc
D. 57 cc
E. 63 cc

QUESTION 4. The calculated effective regurgitant orifice (ERO) by the continuity/volumetric method (see Figs. 9-4 to 9-7) is:

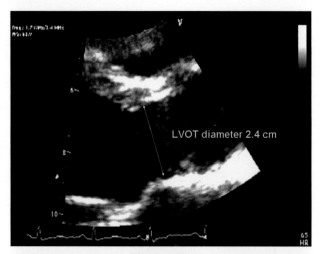

LVOT diameter 2.4 cm

Figure 9-4

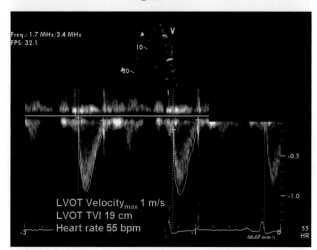

LVOT Velocity$_{max}$ 1 m/s
LVOT TVI 19 cm
Heart rate 55 bpm

Figure 9-5

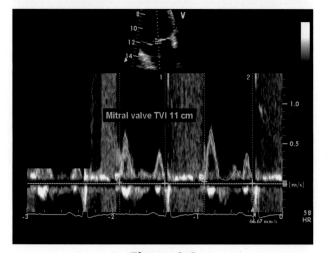

Mitral valve TVI 11 cm

Figure 9-6

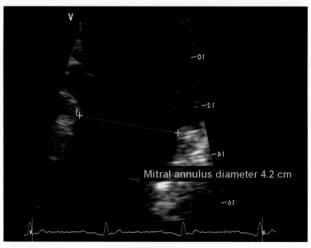

Mitral annulus diameter 4.2 cm

Figure 9-7

A. 0.22
B. 0.33
C. 0.27
D. 0.42

QUESTION 5. When is the best timing for measuring PISA radius?

A. Early systole
B. Midsystole
C. Late systole
D. Anytime during systole

QUESTION 6. The degree of MV regurgitation is:

A. Mild
B. Moderate
C. Moderately severe
D. Severe

ANSWER 1: A. The left coronary cusp lies opposite to the left atrial appendage. The noncoronary cusp lies opposite to the intra-atrial septum (7 o'clock in Fig. 9-1). The right coronary cusp faces the right ventricular outflow tract (12 o'clock in Fig. 9-1).

ANSWER 2: B. Here, best evaluated in the parasternal long-axis view, there is bileaflet prolapse resulting in anteriorly directed MV regurgitation. MV prolapse is defined as systolic displacement (>2 mm) of one or both mitral leaflets into the left atrium, below the plane of the mitral anulus. The diagnosis is more certain when the mitral leaflets are thickened (>5 mm) or myxomatous.

See *The Echo Manual, 3rd Edition,* **pages 210 and 211.**

ANSWER 3: C. 52 cc

The regurgitant flow can be calculated as follows:

Flow rate = $(r)^2 \times 6.28 \times$ aliasing velocity
$$= (0.8 \text{ cm})^2 \times 6.28 \times 39 \text{ cm per second}$$
$$= 157 \text{ cc per second}$$
ERO = Flow rate/Peak MR velocity
$$= 157 \text{ cc per second}/610 \text{ cm per second}$$
$$= 0.26 \text{ cm}^2$$

Regurgitant volume = ERO × regurgitant TVI
$$= 0.26 \text{ cm}^2 \times 201 \text{ cm}$$
$$= 52 \text{ cc}$$

See *The Echo Manual, 3rd Edition,* **page 215.**

ANSWER 4: B. Without notable aortic regurgitation, the difference between the flow across the MV and the left ventricular outflow tract (LVOT) is the mitral regurgitant volume. Flow across the MV is calculated by the product of the area of the mitral anulus and the TVI of flow obtained by placing the sample volume at the mitral anulus.

Flow across the LVOT is calculated by the product of the area of the aortic anulus and the TVI of flow obtained by placing the sample volume at the aortic anulus.

The regurgitant fraction is calculated by dividing regurgitant volume (RegV) by flow across the MV and multiplying by 100:

$$MV_{RegV} = MV \text{ flow} - LVOT \text{ flow}$$
$$= (\text{Anulus } D^2 \times 0.785 \times TVI)_{MV} - (D^2 \times 0.785 \times TVI)_{LVOT}$$
$$= [(4.2)^2 \times 0.785 \times 11] - [(2.4)^2 \times 0.785 \times 19]$$
$$= 152 \text{ cc} - 86 \text{ cc}$$
$$= 66 \text{ cc}$$

The ERO area is estimated by dividing the RegV by the TVI of MR velocity recorded with continuous wave Doppler echocardiography:

$$ERO_{MV} = \frac{MV_{RegV}}{MR_{TVI}} = 66/201 = \mathbf{0.33cm^2}$$

See *The Echo Manual, 3rd Edition,* **discussion of volumetric method on page 213.**

ANSWER 5: B. The optimal timing for the measurement of the PISA radius is in midsystole.

See *The Echo Manual, 3rd Edition,* **discussion of PISA on page 215.**

ANSWER 6: C. The quantitative data collectively indicate moderately severe , but not severe, MV regurgitation supported by a dilated left ventricle with LVEF of 60%. Although MR regurgitant volume was calculated to be greater than 60 cc by the volumetric method, it was less than 60 cc by PISA method, and ERO was less than 0.4 cm^2

See *The Echo Manual, 3rd Edition,* **Appendix 19 on page 412.**

Increasing Dyspnea and Orthopnea

A 63-year-old farmer with a history of coronary artery bypass grafting, chronic obstructive pulmonary disease, atrial fibrillation, and heart failure presents with increasing dyspnea and orthopnea. He denies chest pain. He recently discontinued coumadin, a β-blocker, and digoxin because of his concerns for their side effects. He is on furosemide 40 mg twice daily and lisinopril 5 mg once a day. An echocardiogram was obtained for further evaluation.

QUESTION 1. On the basis of wall motion analysis (**Videos 10-1 to 10-8**), which of the following coronary artery distributions has the most abnormalities?

A. Left main coronary artery
B. Left anterior descending coronary artery (LAD)
C. Left circumflex coronary artery
D. Right coronary artery (RCA)

QUESTION 2. Which of the following parameters is most closely related to the severity of mitral regurgitation in patients with ischemic cardiomyopathy?

A. Mitral valve tenting area
B. Mitral annulus diameter
C. Left ventricular (LV) volume
D. Wall motion score index

QUESTION 3. What is the round structure in the left atrioventricular (AV) groove?

A. Left circumflex coronary artery
B. RCA
C. Coronary sinus
D. Azygo vein

QUESTION 4. Mitral regurgitation severity is:

A. Mild
B. Moderate
C. Severe
D. Indeterminate

QUESTION 5. Based on 2-D findings and Figures 10-1 to 10-3, LV filling pressure is:

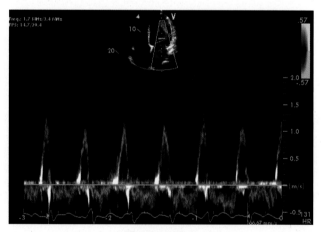

Figure 10-1

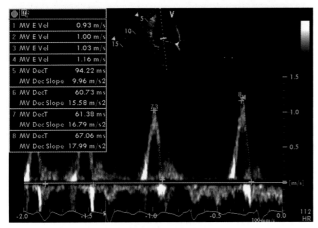

Figure 10-2

A. Increased
B. Reduced
C. Normal
D. Indeterminate

QUESTION 6. What do the velocities labeled as 4 and 5 represent in Figure 10-3?

A. S wave
B. Atrial relaxation
C. Isovolumic contraction
D. L wave

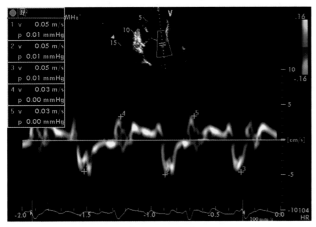

Figure 10-3

ANSWER 1: D. The inferior and inferolateral walls are akinetic. Although the other walls are not entirely normal, they have preserved contractility (i.e., they are not akinetic). This patient has a patent left internal mammary graft to the LAD, but the venous graft to the RCA is occluded as well as the native RCA.

ANSWER 2: A. Mitral valve tenting area has been most closely related to the severity of functional mitral regurgitation. It is the area enclosed by both mitral leaflets and the mitral annulus.

See *The Echo Manual, 3rd Edition*, **discussion of functional mitral regurgitation and Figure 12-31 on pages 211 and 212, respectively.**

ANSWER 3: C. The coronary sinus is a smaller structure present in the posterior AV grove present within the pericardium.

See *The Echo Manual, 3rd Edition*, **page 8, and Figure 2-4 on page 11.**

ANSWER 4: C. Color Doppler demonstrates a broad mitral regurgitant jet that extends the full length of a severely enlarged left atrium extending into the pulmonary vein consistent with severe mitral valve regurgitation.

ANSWER 5: A. There are several features in this patient indicating that LV filling pressure is markedly elevated even in the presence of mitral valve regurgitation and atrial fibrillation. Mitral inflow E velocity deceleration time is extremely short that indicated poor compliance or increased filling pressure even in the setting of severe mitral regurgitation. E velocity is increased mainly because of severe mitral regurgitation, and hence, increased E/e' only may not suggest increased filling pressure. There is very little variation in mitral E velocity in the setting of atrial fibrillation that suggests increased left atrial pressure.

If LA pressure is not high in atrial fibrillation, peak mitral E velocities vary with the cardiac cycle length. Another feature for increased filling pressure is a short isovolumic relaxation time which is shown in Figure 10-3. Each cardiac cycle has 3 velocities above the baseline. One close to the QRS is isovolumic contraction velocity (marked and 4 and 5), the second velocity is S wave, and the third is isovolumic relaxation velocity whose duration is very short.

ANSWER 6: C. I believe the first velocity above the baseline in Figure 10-3 was measured (marked as 4 and 5) as S wave, but it is isovolumic contraction velocity which is very prominent in patients with LBBB. The second velocity is S wave, and the third one is isovolumic relaxation velocity. You can also see in Figure 10-1 that LVOT velocity below the baseline begins at the end of QRS as the beginning of S wave in Figure 10-3.

CASE 11

Severe Chest Pain

A 52-year-old man presents to the emergency department with 1 hour of severe chest pain. A transthoracic echocardiogram is performed (**Videos 11-1 to 11-13**).

QUESTION 1. Potential findings on clinical evaluation may include all of the following *except*:

A. Holodiastolic murmur
B. Absent left radial pulse
C. Low blood pressure
D. Hypertension

QUESTION 2. Risk factors for this complication include all of the following *except*:

A. Bicuspid aortic valve
B. Systemic hypertension
C. Female sex
D. Pregnancy
E. Turner syndrome

QUESTION 3. An appropriate treatment for hypotension in this setting in addition to intravenous fluids is:

A. Dopamine
B. Phenylephrine
C. Epinephrine
D. Intra-aortic balloon pump

QUESTION 4. The appropriate next step in this patient's management is:

A. CT
B. Bedside transesophageal echocardiography
C. Surgical consultation
D. Coronary angiography

ANSWER 1: A. Hypertension is commonly seen in patients with acute aortic dissection, although hypotension (because of severe aortic regurgitation, rupture, or hemopericardium) or pseudohypotension (because of dissection into a branch vessel) may be seen. Acute aortic regurgitation occurs in 20% to 50% of cases and denotes proximal root involvement. When present, aortic regurgitation tends to be present in the earlier part of diastole only with a rapid equilibration of aortic diastolic and left ventricular diastolic pressures. The resulting aortic regurgitant murmur will often be soft and in early diastole.

ANSWER 2: C. Conditions that are associated with an increased risk of aortic dissection include male sex, advancing age, systemic hypertension, pregnancy, congenital unicuspid or bicuspid aortic valve, previous cardiac surgery, and the following syndromes: Ehlers–Danlos, Marfan, Noonan, or Turner.

ANSWER 3: B. If vasopressors are required for hemodynamic stabilization before definitive therapy, agents that increase left ventricular contractility should be avoided. Pure vasopressor agents such as phenylephrine are preferred. Intra-aortic balloon pumps are contraindicated.

ANSWER 4: C. Although transthoracic echocardiography has only a sensitivity of approximately 75% for the diagnosis of an ascending aortic dissection, if seen no other imaging study is required and the patient should proceed directly to the operating room for definitive repair. An intraoperative transesophageal echocardiogram may be performed to delineate extent of aortic involvement and better define the degree of aortic valve regurgitation; however, definitive treatment should not be delayed by further investigations.

Systolic Murmur, Asymptomatic

A 56-year-old man is referred for a transthoracic echocardiogram (**Videos 12-1 to 12-5** and Figs. 12-1 to 12-5) to evaluate a systolic murmur. He is asymptomatic.

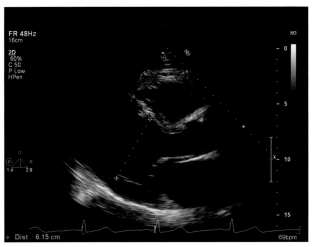

Figure 12-1

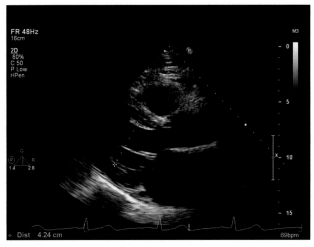

Figure 12-2

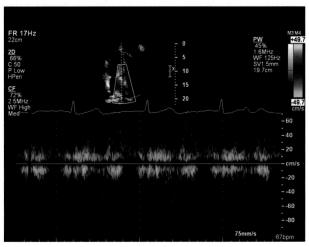

Figure 12-3

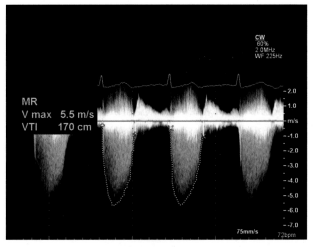

Figure 12-4

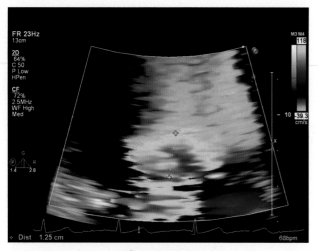

Figure 12-5

QUESTION 1. The calculated effective regurgitant orifice (ERO) by the proximal isovelocity surface area (PISA) method (Figs. 12-4 and 12-5) is:

A. 0.5cm^2
B. 0.6 cm^2
C. 0.7 cm^2
D. 0.8 cm^2

QUESTION 2. The calculated regurgitant volume by the PISA method (Figs. 12-4 and 12-5) is:

A. 80 cc
B. 100 cc
C. 120 cc
D. 140 cc

QUESTION 3. With the aliasing velocity of 39 cm per second and the PISA radius of 1.25 cm, which of the following can calculate ERO as a simplified method?

A. $39 \times 1.25/100$
B. $1.25/39$
C. $1.25/2$
D. $(1.25)^2/2$

QUESTION 4. Regarding the mitral valve, there is evidence of:

A. Anterior leaflet prolapse with mild to moderate mitral valve regurgitation (MR)
B. Anterior leaflet prolapse with severe MR
C. Posterior leaflet prolapse with mild to moderate MR
D. Posterior leaflet prolapse with severe MR

QUESTION 5. Regarding the management of this patient, based on the absence of symptoms and the echocardiographic findings, the patient should be counseled to:

A. Initiate an angiotensin converting enzyme inhibitor and have a repeat echocardiogram in 1 year or be evaluated sooner if he develops symptoms
B. Referral for mitral valve surgery
C. Consider mitral valve repair if surgical expertise of a high likelihood of repair is available, alternatively have a repeat echocardiogram in 1 year or be evaluated sooner if he develops symptoms

QUESTION 6. Concerning pulsed wave Doppler assessment of pulmonary vein flow (Fig. 12-3):

A. Is a sensitive finding for severe MR
B. May be seen in mitral stenosis

QUESTION 7. Transesophageal echocardiography (**Videos 12-6 to 12-10**) confirms evidence of:

A. Prolapse of the anterior mitral valve leaflet with a flail middle scallop
B. Prolapse of the anterior mitral valve leaflet with a flail lateral scallop
C. Prolapse of the anterior mitral valve leaflet without unsupported segments

ANSWER 1: C.

$$ERO = 6.28\ (r)^2 \times \text{aliasing velocity/Peak MR velocity}$$
$$= 6.28\ (1.25)^2 \times 39/550$$
$$= 0.70\ cm^2$$

Figure 12-5 shows beautifully that PISA radius was measured at mid-systole along the same direction as the ultrasound beam.

See *The Echo Manual, 3rd Edition*, discussion of PISA method on page 215.

ANSWER 2: C.

$$\text{Regurgitant volume} = ERO \times \text{regurgitant TVI}$$
$$= 0.7\ cm^2 \times 170\ cm$$
$$= 119\ cc$$

See *The Echo Manual, 3rd Edition*, discussion of PISA method on page 215.

ANSWER 3: D. See *The Echo Manual, 3rd Edition*, discussion of simplification of the PISA method on page 216.

The PISA method can be simplified, which is especially helpful when the peak velocity of the MR jet cannot be obtained. Also, simplification is helpful in determining the severity of MR intraoperatively when a surgical decision needs to be made without delay.

If the aliasing velocity is about 40 cm per second and the MR velocity is assumed to be 500 cm per second, then

$$ERO = \frac{6.28 \times r^2 \times 40 \text{ cm per second}}{500 \text{ cm per second}}$$
$$= \frac{251 \times r^2}{500}$$
$$= \frac{r^2}{2}$$

ERO becomes half of the r^2 value.

ANSWER 4: B.

Here, best demonstrated in the parasternal long-axis view, there is prolapse of the anterior mitral valve resulting in posteriorly directed MR. Mitral valve prolapse is defined as systolic displacement (>2 mm) of one or both mitral leaflets into the left atrium, below the plane of the mitral annulus. The diagnosis is more certain when the mitral leaflets are thickened (>5 mm) or myxomatous. On the basis of visual assessment and PISA-based quantification, the severity of the MR is severe.

ANSWER 5: B.

Even in the absence of symptoms, mitral valve surgery is beneficial for asymptomatic patients with chronic severe MR and mild to moderate LV dysfunction, that is, a left ventricular ejection fraction between 35% and 60% and/or an end-systolic dimension between 40 and 55 mm. Repair of the mitral valve is preferable and in this case has a high likelihood of success with the appropriate surgical expertise. However, regardless of repairability, the setting of mild to moderate left ventricular systolic dysfunction is a class I indication for mitral valve surgery. There is no proven role for vasodilator therapy to prevent/attenuate left ventricular remodeling with MR in the absence of systemic hypertension.

ANSWER 6: B.

Systolic flow reversals in the pulmonary veins are a useful indicator of severity with a high specificity for severe regurgitation (80% to 90%) but a relatively low specificity. Both early and late systolic flow reversals, though, may be seen in patients with very high left atrial pressure and poor left atrial compliance (such as mitral stenosis) in the absence of significant MR.[1,2]

ANSWER 7: A.

Transesophageal echocardiography confirms evidence of anterior mitral valve leaflet prolapse with a flail middle scallop. The patient underwent successful mitral valve repair.

References

1. Enriquez-Sarano M, Dujardin KS, Tribouilloy CM, et al. Determinants of pulmonary venous flow reversal in mitral regurgitation and its usefulness in determining the severity of regurgitation. *Am J Cardiol.* 1999;83:535–541.

2. Tice FD, Heinle SK, Harrison JK, et al. Transesophageal echocardiographic assessment of reversal of systolic pulmonary venous flow in mitral stenosis. *Am J Cardiol.* 1995;75:58–60.

Exertional Shortness of Breath and Systolic Murmur

A 55-year-old man is referred for an echocardiogram for the evaluation of exertional shortness of breath and a systolic murmur. Systemic blood pressure is 120/45 mm Hg (**Videos 13-1 to 13-7** and Figs. 13-1 to 13-7).

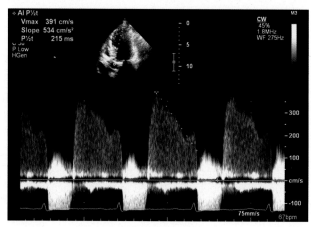

Figure 13-1

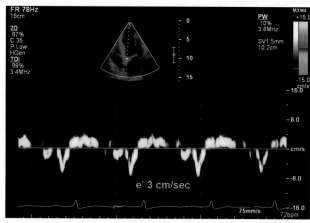

Figure 13-3

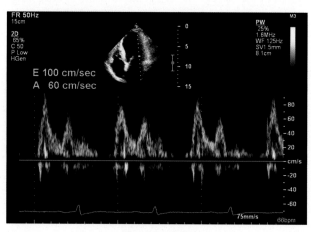

Figure 13-2

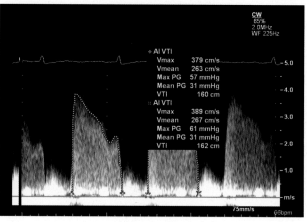

Figure 13-4

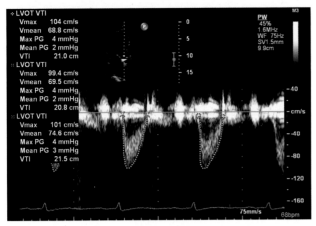

Figure 13-5

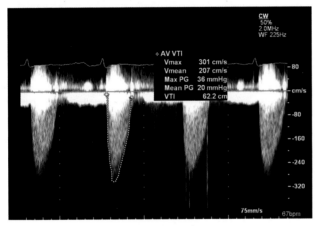

Figure 13-6

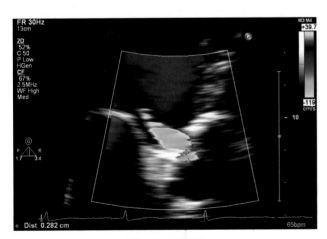

Figure 13-7

QUESTION 1. What is the severity of aortic regurgitation?

   A. Mild
   B. Moderate
   C. Severe
   D. Cannot be determined

QUESTION 2. The brevity of the aortic valve diastolic pressure halftime is related to:

   A. Severe aortic valve regurgitation
   B. Elevated left ventricular (LV) diastolic pressure
   C. Concomitant aortic valve stenosis

QUESTION 3. What is estimated LV end-diastolic pressure (LVEDP)?

   A. 15 mm Hg
   B. 20 mm Hg
   C. 25 mm Hg
   D. 30 mm Hg

QUESTION 4. The quantified effective regurgitant orifice (ERO) of the aortic valve by the proximal isovelocity surface area method is:

   A. 0.05 cm^2
   B. 0.10 cm^2
   C. 0.15 cm^2
   D. 0.20 cm^2
   E. 0.25 cm^2

QUESTION 5. On the basis of a LV outflow tract (LVOT) diameter of 24 mm, calculate the Doppler derived aortic valve area.

   A. 1.0 cm^2
   B. 1.25 cm^2
   C. 1.5 cm^2
   D. 1.75 cm^2
   E. 2.0 cm^2

QUESTION 6. There is evidence of:

A. Wall motion abnormalities in the distribution of the left anterior descending coronary artery
B. Wall motion abnormalities in the distribution of the left circumflex coronary artery
C. Wall motion abnormalities in the distribution of the right coronary artery
D. No regional wall motion abnormalities

ANSWER 1: A. Mild aortic valve regurgitation (see Answer 2).

ANSWER 2: B. The aortic regurgitant pressure half-time is short at 215 milliseconds, which typically is an indicator of severe aortic valve regurgitation. In severe aortic valve regurgitation, the systemic diastolic blood pressure decreases significantly, so that the aortic regurgitant signal (which corresponds to the pressure difference between the LV and the aorta) has a shortened deceleration time and thereby a shortened pressure halftime. However, the gradient between the LV and the aorta may also be reduced during diastole if there is a progressive and marked rise in LV diastolic pressure because of LV dysfunction. Here there is evidence of a marked relaxation abnormality, with an e' of 3 cm per second, and a marked elevation of LV filling pressures, with an E/e ratio of >30. This is a good example of a "falsely reduced" aortic regurgitant pressure halftime because of high LV diastolic pressure rather than severe aortic valve regurgitation.

See *the Echo Manual, 3rd Edition*, page 208.

ANSWER 3: D. End-diastolic AR velocity is 2 m per second corresponding to 16 mm Hg pressure difference between aortic diastolic pressure and LV end-diastolic pressure. Hence,

LVEDP = 45 − 16 = 29 mm Hg.

ANSWER 4: A. The regurgitant flow rate across the aortic valve is obtained from the flow rate of a proximal surface area with a known flow velocity as follows:

$$
\begin{aligned}
\text{Flow rate} &= 2\pi(r)^2 \times \text{aliasing velocity} \\
&= 6.28\,(r)^2 \times \text{aliasing velocity} \\
&= 6.28\,(0.28)^2 \times 40 \\
&= 19.7\ \text{cm}^3\ \text{per second} \\
\text{ERO} &= \text{Flow rate/Peak AR velocity} \\
&= 19.7\ (\text{cm}^3\ \text{per second})/385\ (\text{cm per second}) \\
&= 0.05\ \text{cm}^2
\end{aligned}
$$

See *The Echo Manual, 3rd Edition*, page 209.

ANSWER 5: C.

$$
\begin{aligned}
\text{Aortic valve area} &= [(\text{LVOT TVI}) \times (\text{LVOT area})]/\text{Ao TVI} \\
&= [(21) \times (\pi(1)^2)]/62 \\
&= 95/62 \\
&= 1.5\ \text{cm}^2
\end{aligned}
$$

See *The Echo Manual, 3rd Edition*, discussion of Doppler echocardiography (in aortic stenosis) on pages 190 and 191.

ANSWER 6: A. There is evidence of severe hypokinesis of the mid- and apical septum and anterior walls, areas of the LV myocardium supplied by the left anterior coronary artery.

CASE 14

Cardiac Murmur during Pregnancy

A 25-year-old woman 24 weeks pregnant with twins is noted to have a cardiac murmur by her obstetrician. She describes mild fatigue and denies a history of cardiovascular disease. This is her first pregnancy.

On examination, her blood pressure was 110/60 mm Hg and heart rate 90 beats per minute. First and second heart sounds are normal with a 2/6 midpeaking systolic ejection murmur with an audible third heart sound. There is mild edema of the lower extremities (**Videos 14-1 to 14-7**).

QUESTION 1. What is the most likely etiology of the murmur?

- A. Mitral valve regurgitation secondary to mitral valve prolapse
- B. Aortic stenosis secondary to a bicuspid aortic valve
- C. Benign flow murmur
- D. Atrial septal defect

QUESTION 2. What is most likely time velocity integral (TVI) of the left ventricular outflow tract (LVOT) in this patient?

- A. 15 cm
- B. 20 cm
- C. 30 cm
- D. 40 cm

QUESTION 3. Pregnancy is complicated by gestational diabetes that is managed with dietary control. At 38 weeks, she undergoes a planned uncomplicated cesarean section with delivery of healthy twin girls. One day later, she becomes acutely dyspneic and hypotensive. On the basis of the emergent transthoracic echocardiogram performed, the most likely complication is:

- A. Acute pulmonary embolism
- B. Primary pulmonary hypertension complicating pregnancy

- C. Spontaneous dissection of the left anterior descending coronary artery with acute myocardial infarction
- D. Acute peripartum cardiomyopathy

QUESTION 4. The patient required intubation and mechanical ventilation. Owing to hemodynamic instability and poor oxygenation, a veno-venous extracorporeal membrane oxygenation ECMO catheter was placed in the right internal jugular vein. However, despite this, the patient failed to improve. A transesophageal echocardiogram (TEE) was performed (**Videos 14-8 to 14-11**).

Left ventricular ejection fraction (LVEF) is:

- A. 30%
- B. 40%
- C. 50%
- D. 60%
- E. 75%

QUESTION 5. On the basis of the TEE images (**Videos 14-11 to 14-14**), the appropriate next step should be:

- A. Advance the ECMO catheter
- B. Redraw the ECMO catheter
- C. Remove the ECMO catheter
- D. Continue the ECMO catheter and place an intra-aortic balloon pump

ANSWERS 1 AND 2: *C and C.* During pregnancy, there is an increase in intravascular volume with an overall increase in systemic cardiac output of 60% to 75%. This is brought about by an increase in stroke volume and heart rate. Hence, there is an expected increase in the TVI through the LVOT. These hyperdynamic changes are typically associated with a benign early to midpeaking systolic crescendo-decrescendo murmur secondary to increased flow through the LVOT (increased LVOT and aortic flow velocities). Rapid early left ventricular filling (increased E velocities) on mitral inflow Doppler is often associated with an audible third heart sound.

ANSWER 3: *A.* Transthoracic echocardiography demonstrates normal left ventricular size with LVEF 75% to 80%, hence making either acute myocardial infarction or peripartum cardiomyopathy unlikely. The right ventricle (RV) is enlarged and dysfunctional. Primary pulmonary hypertension may occur with pregnancy and is associated with high maternal mortality. The early peripartum period is particularly high risk in a patient with pulmonary hypertension. However, antecedent symptoms of dyspnea, chest pain, and/or right heart failure would have been expected in the recent days to weeks. In the setting of the early peripartum period, particularly after cesarean section, the finding of dyspnea, hypotension, and acute RV dysfunction is very concerning for an acute pulmonary embolus. Chest CT angiography demonstrated no evidence of thromboembolic disease, and the presumed diagnosis was amniotic fluid embolism syndrome.

ANSWER 4: *E.* Both ventricles appear small with a LVEF of 75% to 80%, and a RV that has reduced systolic function.

ANSWER 5: *B.* TEE imaging demonstrates a dilated inferior vena cava and hepatic vein. The ECMO catheter is situated in the IVC with continuous flow present at the level of the hepatic vein. The appropriate step is to withdraw the ECMO catheter until the output port is situated at the level of the right atrium (RA), yet leaving the input port (at the tip of the catheter) in the IVC. If the catheter is placed too deep as in this case, the blood is drawn in through from the IVC but then returned through the output (side port) back into the IVC leading to the oxygenated blood circling in the IVC without any benefit to the patient. Under guidance by dynamic TEE imaging, the catheter was withdrawn by 4 to 5 cm until the output port was located at the level of the RA (**Videos 14-15 to 14-17**). The patient's oxygenation and hemodynamics improved promptly.

Progressive Dyspnea with Asthma, Rhinosinusitis, Weight Loss, and Peripheral Neuropathy

A 30-year-old woman with asthma, rhinosinusitis, weight loss, and peripheral neuropathy is referred for an echocardiogram to evaluate progressive dyspnea.

QUESTION 1. Concerning left ventricular (LV) function, which of the following is true (**Videos 15-1 to 15-8**)?

A. Normal LV size and systolic function

B. Inferior wall akinesia with preserved LV ejection fraction

C. Hyperdynamic LV basal function with apical dysfunction (apical ballooning)

D. Multiple regional wall motion abnormalities including severe anterior hypokinesis with reduced LV ejection fraction

QUESTION 2. Concerning pulmonary arterial flow (Fig. 15-1), which of the following is true?

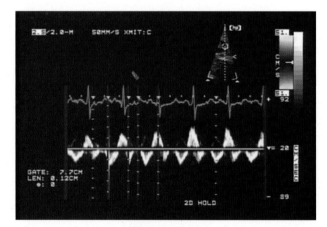

Figure 15-1

A. Findings consistent with severe pulmonary valve regurgitation

B. Narrowed right ventricular (RV) outflow tract with minimal impairment of pulmonary flow

C. Severe RV outflow tract obstruction

QUESTION 3. The best unifying diagnosis is:

A. Sarcoidosis

B. Churg–Strauss syndrome

C. Carcinoid heart disease

D. Glycogen storage disease

E. Amyloidosis

ANSWER 1: D. Although the most striking findings are in the RV, the LV is also quite abnormal. There are inferoseptal, anterior, lateral, and apical wall motion abnormalities with an associated overall reduction in LV ejection fraction.

ANSWER 2: C. The RV outflow tract is dilated with a significant mass (likely thrombotic material) that leads to outflow tract obstruction. Doppler examination demonstrates complete cessation of flow in mid to late systole because of outflow tract obstruction.

ANSWER 3: B. Churg–Strauss syndrome is characterized by asthma, peripheral and tissue eosinophilia, and systemic small vessel vasculitis. The heart can be involved in up to 20% of patients. Myocardial involvement in Chug-Strauss syndrome includes classic cardiac findings seen in other eosinophilic disorders with endocardial thickening, thrombus often with involvement of the papillary muscles and our valve leaflets. Regional wall motion abnormalities and ventricular systolic dysfunction may also occur. Alternatively, patients may display pericardial disease or rarely ischemic changes because of coronary artery vasculitis. Myocardial involvement in Churg–Strauss syndrome appears to negatively correlate with antineutrophilic cytoplasmic antibodies implicating an eosinophilic or granulomatous rather than vasculitic pathogenesis.[1,2]

References

1. Keogh KA, Specks U. Churg–Strauss syndrome: clinical presentation, antineutrophil cytoplasmic antibodies, and leukotriene receptor antagonists. *Am J Med.* 2003;115:284–290.

2. Kane GC, Keogh KA. Involvement of the heart by small and medium vasculitis. *Curr Opin Rheumatol.* 2009;21:29–34.

CASE 16

Liver Function Test Abnormalities, Ascites, and Dyspnea

A 55-year-old woman with a known history of hereditary hemorrhagic telangiectasia (Osler–Weber–Rendu syndrome) presents with liver function test abnormalities, ascites, and dyspnea. (**Videos 16-1 to 16-6** and Figs. 16-1 to 16-10)

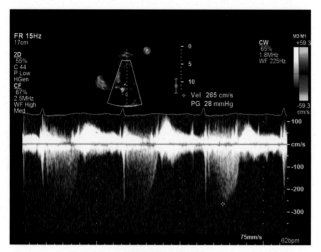

Figure 16-1

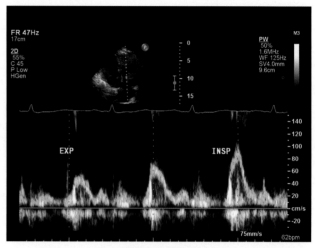

Figure 16-3

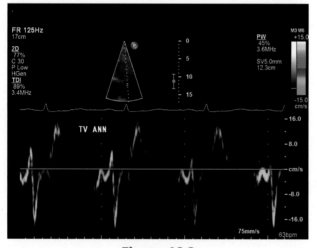

Figure 16-2

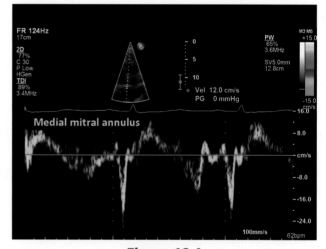

Figure 16-4

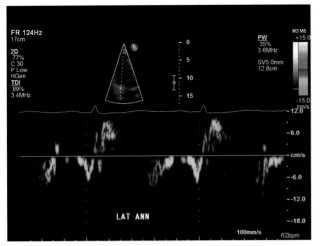

Figure 16-5

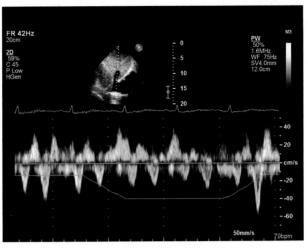

Figure 16-8

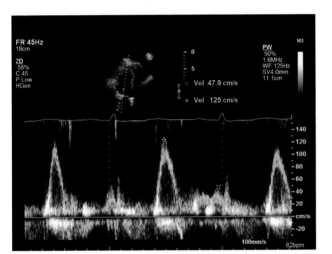

Figure 16-6

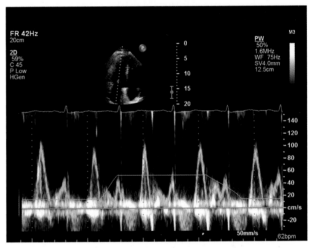

Figure 16-9

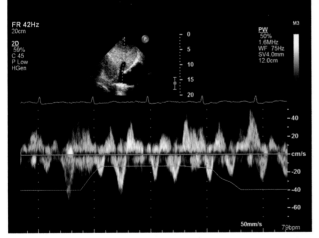

Figure 16-7

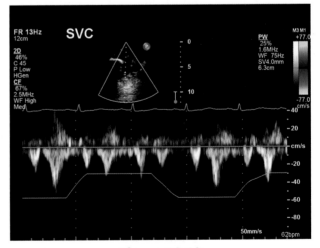

Figure 16-10

QUESTION 1. What echocardiographic findings are associated with hereditary hemorrhagic telangiectasia (Osler–Weber–Rendu syndrome)?

A. Biventricular systolic dysfunction
B. Intrapulmonary shunting, increased cardiac output, pulmonary hypertension
C. Right-sided valve thickening and dysfunction
D. Ebstein anomaly
E. Anomalous pulmonary veins

QUESTION 2. The likely cause for the patient's ascites is:

A. Noncardiac disease
B. Restrictive cardiomyopathy
C. Constriction
D. Pulmonary hypertension and right heart dysfunction

QUESTION 3. There is echocardiographic evidence of intrapulmonary shunting.

A. True
B. False

QUESTION 4. With regard to the mitral inflow pattern seen in this case, which of the following statements is true?

A. The absence of variation with respiration in the mitral inflow pattern suggests localized right-sided constriction
B. The absence of variation in the mitral inflow pattern suggests concomitant pulmonary obstructive disease
C. Variation in the mitral inflow pattern with respiration may be seen if the patient was imaged sitting up

QUESTION 5. What early diastolic medial annular peak tissue velocity (e') separates constriction from restriction?

A. 4 cm per second
B. 6 cm per second
C. 8 cm per second
D. 10 cm per second
E. 12 cm per second

QUESTION 6. With regard to mitral annular early diastolic velocities (e'), which of the following statements is true?

A. Lateral e' is lower than medial e' in constriction
B. Lateral e' is lower than medial e' in restriction
C. The ratio of lateral e' to medial e' is variable and is not helpful

QUESTION 7. Which of the following statements is true with regard to pericardial thickening in constriction?

A. CT is better than MRI in separating pericardial thickening from fluid
B. Pericardial thickening is present in 95% of cases of constrictive pericarditis
C. Transesophageal echocardiography is not useful for the diagnosis of pericardial thickening
D. Pericardial calcification is present on chest x-ray in approximately 25% of patients with constriction

QUESTION 8. Which of the following Doppler profiles taken from patients with right heart failure is consistent with the diagnosis of constriction?

A.

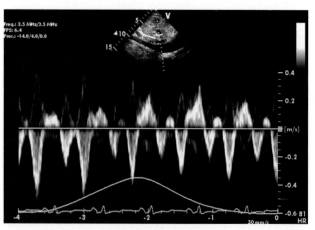

Figure 16-11

B.

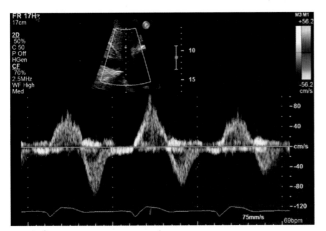

Figure 16-12

C.

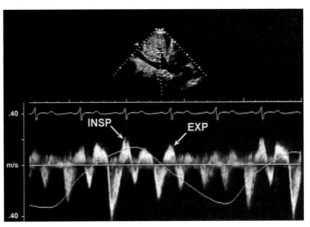

Figure 16-13

ANSWER 1: B. The Osler–Weber–Rendu syndrome is a disorder of arterial-venous malformations, which involve the skin (telangiectasias), gastrointestinal tract, liver, and lungs. These may give rise to high-output states, right-to-left shunting (particularly intrapulmonary), and/or pulmonary arterial hypertension with associated right heart dysfunction.

ANSWER 2: C. Echocardiography demonstrates a constellation of findings that indicate the presence of constrictive pericarditis. There is a prominent septal bounce seen on **Videos 16-1 to 16-3**. There is dilated inferior vena cava and hepatic veins with diastolic flow reversals with expiration. The medial mitral annular early diastolic tissue velocity is elevated. Of note on subcostal imaging, there is absence of the normal sliding of the right ventricle along the hepatic border (**Video 16-5**).[1]

ANSWER 3: A. **Video 16-6** demonstrates evidence of right-to-left shunting that is delayed occurring approximately five to six beats after agitated saline is seen in the right atrium. This suggests that the shunt occurs not at the atrial level but rather in the lungs.

ANSWER 4: C. Respiratory variation of >25% in mitral E velocity is a characteristic Doppler feature in constrictive pericarditis. If left atrial pressure is markedly increased, mitral valve opening occurs on a steep part of the left ventricular (LV) pressure curve, when the respiratory change has little effect on the transmitral pressure gradient and typical respiratory changes in mitral inflow are absent. Maneuvers to lower LV preload such as diuresis, imaging in the sitting position, or with head-up tilt are recommended to unmask the respiratory variation in mitral inflow E velocity. In any event, the lack of respiratory variation in mitral inflow velocities does not—and should not—exclude the diagnosis of constrictive pericarditis.

In chronic obstructive lung disease, individual mitral inflow velocities usually are not restrictive because the LV filling pressure is not increased; however, mitral inflow variation with respiration may be seen in lung disease with the highest mitral E velocity occurring toward the end of expiration, although it occurs immediately after the onset of expiration in constrictive pericarditis. In distinguishing between chronic obstructive lung disease and constrictive pericarditis, Doppler interrogation of the superior vena cava flow velocities is very helpful (Fig. 16-10). In chronic obstructive lung disease, superior vena cava flow is markedly increased with inspiration because the underlying mechanism for respiratory variation in chronic obstructive lung disease is a greater decrease in intrathoracic pressure with inspiration, which generates greater negative pressure changes in the thorax. This enhances flow to the RA from the superior vena cava with inspiration. In constrictive pericarditis, superior vena cava systolic flow velocities do not change markedly with respiration; the difference in systolic forward flow velocity between inspiration and expiration is rarely 20 cm per second in constrictive pericarditis. It needs to be emphasized that systolic, not diastolic, flow velocities of the superior vena cava should be compared with respiration (Fig. 16-10).[2]

ANSWER 5: C. In patients with heart failure, an e' of >8 cm per second has a high diagnostic accuracy for separating constriction from restriction. In restriction, the medial e' is reduced, typically significantly, because of a marked reduction in myocardial relaxation (often in the 3 to 6 cm per second range). In contrast, in constriction, myocardial relaxation is normal and e' is normal or even increased. The explanation for this is that ventricular filling is limited by the lateral expansion of the heart because of the constrictive pericardium, and most ventricular filling is accomplished by an exaggerated longitudinal motion of the heart. Myocardial relaxation is relatively well preserved in constriction unless the myocardium is also involved, as in radiation injury to the heart. Still e' in patients with constriction because of radiation or previous cardiac surgery is lower than e' in patients with constriction because of previous pericarditis or collagen vascular diseases.[3]

ANSWER 6: A. As discussed in the answer to Question 4, myocardial relaxation is normal in constriction. In fact, because radial motion of the myocardium maybe restricted by the scarred pericardium, the medial e' velocity is often higher than would be expected for the patient's age. In almost all cardiac conditions, the lateral e' is 20% greater than the medial e'. However, in constriction, the lateral e', although typically of normal velocity, is often lower than the medial e' in 80% of cases leading to an "annulus reversus." This reversed lateral and medial e' ratio returns to normal after pericardiectomy.[4-6]

ANSWER 7: D. Although most patients with constrictive pericarditis have evidence of pericardial thickening, approximately 20% will have normal thickness. Useful measures of pericardial thickness include cardiac MR, TEE, and cardiac CT. However, it may be difficult to distinguish small amounts of pericardial fluid from thickening by CT. The presence of pericardial calcification, best appreciated by CT, is highly specific for constriction, although it is present infrequently.[7,8]

ANSWER 8: A. All clips demonstrate blunted systolic forward flow consistent with an elevation in right atrial pressure. There is evidence of diastolic flow reversals that increase with expiration in (Fig. 16-11) that is consistent with constriction. In contrast, diastolic flow reversals that increase with inspiration (Fig.16-13) are consistent with restrictive cardiomyopathy. Mid to late peaking systolic flow reversals (Fig. 16-12) are characteristic of severe tricuspid valve regurgitation.

References

1. Oh JK, Hatle LK, Seward JB, et al. Diagnostic role of Doppler echocardiography in constrictive pericarditis. *J Am Coll Cardiol.* 1994;23(1):154–162.

2. Oh JK, Tajik AJ, Appleton CP, et al. Preload reduction to unmask the characteristic Doppler features of constrictive pericarditis. A new observation. *Circulation.* 1997;95(4):796–799.

3. Ha JW, Ommen SR, Tajik AJ, et al. Differentiation of constrictive pericarditis from restrictive cardiomyopathy using mitral annular velocity by tissue Doppler echocardiography. *Am J Cardiol.* 2004;94(3):316–319.

4. Reuss CS, Wilansky SM, Lester SJ, et al. Using mitral "annulus reversus" to diagnose constrictive pericarditis. *Eur J Echocardiogr.* 2009;10(30):372–375.

5. Veress G, Ling LH, Kim KH, et al. Mitral and tricuspid annular velocities before and after pericardiectomy in patients with constrictive pericarditis. *Circ Cardiovasc Imaging.* 2011;4(4):399–407. Epub 2011 May 4.

6. Choi JH, Choi JO, Ryu DR, et al. Mitral and tricuspid annular velocities in constrictive pericarditis and restrictive cardiomyopathy: correlation with pericardial thickness on computed tomography. *JACC Cardiovasc Imaging.* 2011;4(6):567–575.

7. Ling LH, Oh JK, Tei C, et al. Pericardial thickness measured with transesophageal echocardiography: feasibility and potential clinical usefulness. *J Am Coll Cardiol.* 1997;29:1317.

8. Talreja DR, Edwards WD, Danielson GK, et al. Constrictive pericarditis in 26 patients with histologically normal pericardial thickness. *Circulation.* 2003;108:1852–1857.

CASE 17

Right Heart Failure

A 74-year-old woman was referred for a possible pericardiectomy to manage constrictive pericarditis. She was well until 2 years ago when she began having fluid retention with leg edema and abdominal bloating. She was treated initially with a diuretic and had some improvement. However, her symptoms became gradually worse and underwent comprehensive evaluation. Cardiac catheterization showed normal coronaries, but equalization of diastolic pressures with right atrial pressure of 20 mm Hg, right ventricular (RV) end-diastolic pressure of 21 mm Hg, and left ventricular end-diastolic pressure of 19 mm Hg. A presumptive diagnosis of constrictive pericarditis was made, and the patient was recommended to have pericardiectomy. The following echocardiogram images were obtained (Figs. 17-1 to 17-6 and **Videos 17-1 to 17-7**).

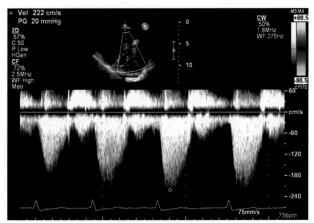

Figure 17-1

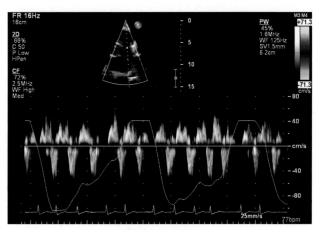

Figure 17-3

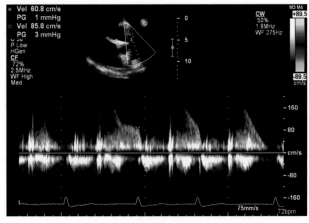

Figure 17-2

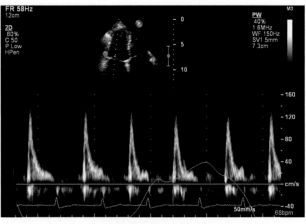

Figure 17-4

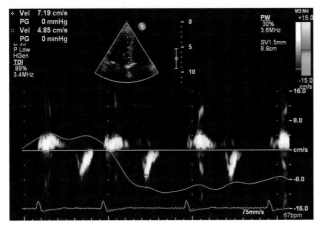

Figure 17-5

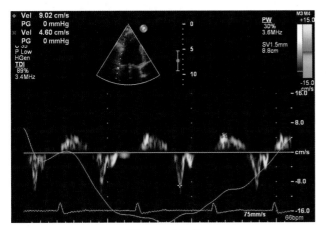

Figure 17-6

QUESTION 1. What is the diagnosis of this patient?

A. Constrictive pericarditis
B. Restrictive cardiomyopathy
C. Severe tricuspid regurgitation
D. RV cardiomyopathy
E. B and C

QUESTION 2. Which of the following statements is correct regarding pulmonary artery systolic pressure based on the shown tricuspid regurgitant velocity (Fig. 17-1) in this patient?

A. Pulmonary artery systolic pressure is normal
B. Pulmonary artery systolic pressure cannot be reliably obtained
C. Pulmonary artery systolic pressure is severely elevated

QUESTION 3. Figure 17-2 shows pulmonary regurgitation (PR) velocity obtained by continuous wave Doppler echocardiography. Which of the following is related to the Doppler finding?

A. Normal RV diastolic pressure because PR diastolic velocity is <1 m per second
B. This is a normal PR pattern with respiratory variation
C. Patient has severe PR
D. Pulmonary artery end-diastolic pressure is high

QUESTION 4. What does the following hepatic vein Doppler with respirometer indicate (Fig. 17-3)?

A. Severe tricuspid regurgitation
B. Constrictive pericarditis
C. RV dysfunction
D. RV cardiomyopathy

QUESTION 5. Mitral inflow (Fig. 17-4) and mitral annulus velocity (Figs. 17-5 and 17-6) recordings are shown. Which of the following is correct regarding these recordings?

A. Typical for constrictive pericarditis
B. Left ventricular cardiomyopathy with increased filling pressure
C. Not able to assess diastolic function because of atrial fibrillation

ANSWER 1: C. The primary finding is one of torrential tricuspid valve regurgitations. 2D echocardiography demonstrates an enlarged RV with tricuspid annular dilation, incomplete tricuspid valve leaflet coaptation, and severe tricuspid valve regurgitation, demonstrated on color Doppler and characterized on continuous wave Doppler by a dense, early peaking, "Dagger-shaped" signal. There is also evidence of a left ventricular myopathic process with restrictive physiology. Although in the setting of atrial fibrillation, there is an elevated early left ventricular diastolic filling velocity (E) with reduced diastolic tissue Doppler velocities, with a medial E/e' ratio of 17. This correlates with the elevated left ventricular filling pressures found at hemodynamic catheterization.

ANSWER 2: B. There are three necessary components to the estimation of pulmonary artery systolic pressure. The first is exclusion of RV outflow tract (RVOT) obstruction, the second a properly aligned tricuspid regurgitant velocity, and the third estimation of right atrial pressure. In this case, a peak systolic velocity through the RVOT of 0.6 m per second excludes significant outflow tract obstruction indicating that the derived RV systolic pressure should equate to the pulmonary artery systolic pressure. On the basis of on the modified Bernoulli equation, the trans-tricuspid gradient is equal to four times the (peak tricuspid regurgitant velocity),[2] which in this case is $4 (2.2)^2 = 18$ mm Hg. On the basis of the dilated coronary sinus on the parasternal long-axis view, the dilated inferior vena cava and hepatic veins, and the marked systolic flow reversals in the hepatic veins, the right atrial pressure likely is markedly elevated, ≥20 mm Hg. Often right atrial pressure will exceed 20 mm Hg, which is, generally, the recommended upper limit of noninvasively estimated right atrial pressure. Therefore, the RV systolic pressure may be underestimated in this setting. Finally, in severe tricuspid valve regurgitation there can be ventricularization of the atrial pressures. This renders the simplified Bernoulli equation unsuitable because the proximal velocity is no longer significantly less than the distal velocity and therefore cannot be discounted. Therefore, in torrential tricuspid valve regurgitation,

the classic estimation of RV systolic pressure cannot be relied on and an alternative method should be considered.

ANSWER 3: D. The end-diastolic velocity of PR reflects the end-diastolic pressure gradient between the pulmonary artery and the RV. At end diastole, RV pressure should be equal to RA pressure. Therefore,

$$PAEDP = 4 \times End\text{-}PRvel^2 + RAP,$$

where PAEDP is pulmonary artery end-diastolic pressure, End-PRvel is PR end-diastolic velocity and RAP is right atrial pressure. A normal PAEDP is ≤15 mm Hg.

See **The Echo Manual, 3rd Edition**, Figure 9-7 on page 147.

ANSWER 4: A. Throughout the respiratory cycle, there is evidence of consistent systolic flow reversals in the hepatic veins, which tend to be late peaking in severe tricuspid valve regurgitation and early peaking if related to severe RV dysfunction. The typical findings of constriction that are present on interrogation of the hepatic veins are diastolic flow reversals that increase with expiration.

ANSWER 5: B. The typical findings in constrictive pericarditis are normal or elevated myocardial relaxation velocities often with reversal of the peak velocities between the medial and lateral annuluses. In the normal setting, the lateral mitral annulus has an early relaxation velocity of 1 to 5 cm per second higher than that of the medial annulus. In constriction where there the lateral annulus has some constraint and a greater proportion of myocardial relaxation is driven through the septum, the medial annulus tends to be higher. Although the mitral inflow profile may appear similarly restrictive (early peaking, short deceleration times) in both constrictive and restrictive physiologies, integration with the myocardial relaxation velocities allows easy separation of these two phenomena. Here the high ratio of early filling blood velocity (E) to the early myocardial relaxation velocity (e') indicates the presence of elevated left ventricular filling pressures as opposed to constrictive physiology.

CASE 18

Harsh Systolic Murmur

A 55-year-old asymptomatic woman is referred for transthoracic echocardiography to evaluate a harsh systolic murmur.

On examination, her blood pressure is 110/60 mm Hg. Heart rate regular at 68 beats per minute. Carotid pulses are reduced in intensity. The apex beat is forceful and nondisplaced. There is a 3/6 systolic ejection murmur throughout the precordium with a single second heart sound.

QUESTION 1. On the basis of the echocardiogram (**Videos 18-1 to 18-4** and Figs. 18-1 to 18-5), which of the following is true?

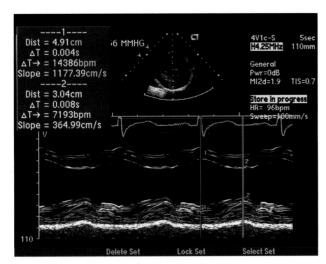

Figure 18-1

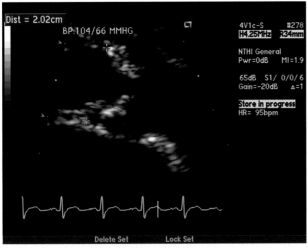

Figure 18-2

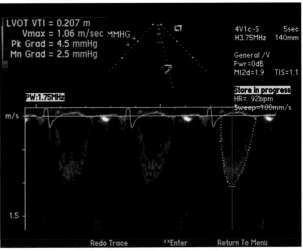

Figure 18-3

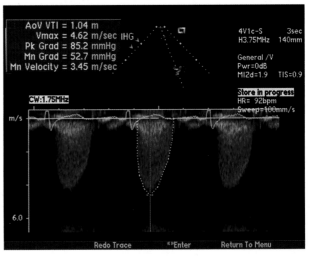

Figure 18-4

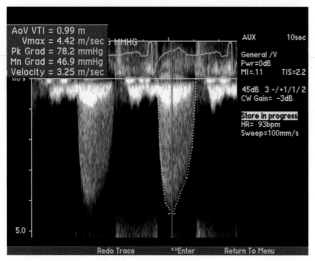

Figure 18-5

A. The echocardiographic findings are discordant from the physical examination
B. There is severe aortic valve (AV) stenosis with an aortic valve area (AVA) <0.5 cm²
C. There is concordance between the left ventricular outflow tract (LVOT)/AV time velocity integral (TVI) ratio and the calculated AVA
D. There is evidence of severe supravalvular stenosis

QUESTION 2. Appropriate management includes:

A. Repeat transthoracic echocardiogram in 2 years or sooner if symptoms develop
B. Transesophageal echocardiography
C. Hemodynamic cardiac catheterization
D. Treadmill exercise stress test
E. AV replacement

QUESTION 3. With regard to transthoracic echocardiography after an aortic valve replacement, which of the following is true?

A. A routine transthoracic echocardiogram should be performed in all patients within the first 3 months after valve surgery
B. Serial echocardiography performed every 2 years following valve replacement is appropriate
C. Echocardiography within the first 3 years after replacement should not be considered in the absence of known or suspected valve dysfunction

QUESTION 4. Two years later, she became acutely unwell. She presented to the emergency department with 3 days of fever (temperature, 40°C), fatigue, and nausea. Renal function is normal. Blood cultures were drawn and grew out *Streptococcus viridans* relatively resistant to penicillin G. She is referred for transesophageal echocardiography (**Videos 18-12 to 18-18**). On the basis of the images, which is the appropriate management?

A. AV re-replacement
B. Combination antibiotic therapy with a β-lactam and an aminoglycoside for 6 weeks
C. Combination antibiotic therapy with a β-lactam and an aminoglycoside for 2 weeks followed by β-lactam antibiotic therapy for an additional 4 weeks
D. β-Lactam antibiotic therapy for 6 weeks
E. Vancomycin for 4 weeks

QUESTION 5. After 9 days of appropriate therapy, the patient is noted to have a PR interval of 230 milliseconds. She is asymptomatic. Which of the following management steps is correct?

A. Continue antibiotic course unless symptoms develop
B. Obtain transthoracic echocardiography
C. Obtain transesophageal echocardiography

QUESTION 6. On the basis of the echocardiographic images (**Videos 18-5 to 18-11**), which of the following findings is true?

A. There is a new mitral valve vegetation
B. There has been an interim ascending aortic dissection
C. There is evidence of AV leaflet perforation
D. The findings suggest an interim change in organism resistance
E. The findings occur in the setting of AV endocarditis in >25% of cases

QUESTION 7. The correct appropriate next step is:

A. Complete the course of antibiotics, then probable elective AV replacement, based on the results of a repeat TEE
B. Urgent AV replacement without further testing
C. Diagnostic coronary angiography followed by urgent AV replacement
D. Permanent pacemaker placement followed by urgent AV replacement

ANSWER 1: C. There is clinical and echocardiographic evidence of severe AV stenosis. The calculated AVA (see below) is 0.66 cm². The LVOT/AV TVI ratio (dimensionless index) is 0.21. Both of these parameters are in the severe range.

AVA = [(LVOT TVI) × (LVOT area)]/Ao TVI
= [(LVOT TVI) × (0.785 (LVOT D)²]/Ao TVI
= [(21) × (3.14)]/100
= 66/100
= 0.66 cm²

ANSWER 2: D. The diagnosis of severe AV stenosis is clear, and no further anatomical or hemodynamic evaluation is required. A TEE of hemodynamic catheterization should only be considered in the setting if there is discordance between the clinical and transthoracic data. The only treatment option of symptomatic aortic stenosis is valve replacement, and this should be considered because the outcome of symptomatic patients otherwise is poor. Even in the setting of truly asymptomatic AV stenosis, most patients will develop symptoms within a few years. A treadmill exercise stress test, to ascertain functional limitation or an abnormal blood pressure response to exercise, is a useful test to guide management in the patient with apparent asymptomatic AV stenosis because many of these patients when tested have functional limitation. At our institution, we typically perform an oxygen consumption treadmill exercise stress test for this purpose. If a patient has severe truly asymptomatic AV stenosis with an excellent functional capacity, a strategy of careful observation is reasonable although a repeat transthoracic echocardiographic evaluation at least on an annual basis is required.

Here the patient went only 65% of predicted functional capacity and was referred for valve replacement.[1,2]

The patient underwent elective AV replacement with a 21-mm bioprosthesis.

ANSWER 3: A. An initial postoperative transthoracic echocardiogram should be performed in all patients following valve replacement to serve as an individual "fingerprint" to establish a baseline for future assessment. This should be performed immediately before hospital discharge or within the first few months after surgery. After that, any further echocardiogram in the next 3 years to assess prosthetic valve function is inappropriate in the absence of known or suspected valve dysfunction. Routine surveillance after 3 years is reasonable.[3]

ANSWER 4: B. TEE demonstrates a small mobile lesion on the anterior AV prosthetic leaflet without valvular dysfunction. Initial management in this setting of *Streptococcus* prosthetic valve endocarditis requires 6 weeks of either combination of a β-lactam and aminoglycoside antibiotic or 6 weeks of vancomycin. If the *Streptococcus* was sensitive to penicillin G, 6 weeks of penicillin ± 2 weeks of an aminoglycoside would be appropriate. Surgery is not indicated at this time.[4]

ANSWER 5: C. The development of any degree of heart block in a patient with known or suspected endocarditis is very concerning for the development of an aortic root abscess involving the upper intraventricular septum, which houses the conduction system. In this setting, a transesophageal, rather than transthoracic, echocardiogram is indicated.

ANSWER 6: E. Despite the absence of significant valvular vegetation, the TEE confirms the suspicion of interim abscess development in the aortic root extending down into the mitral-aortic intervalvular fibrosa with a rupture of the aneurysm of the mitral-aortic intervalvular fibrosa into the left atrium. This is a marked difference to the study from 9 days earlier. Prosthetic aortic regurgitation is now also present. This is a recognized complication of AV endocarditis (native and prosthetic) occurring in 30% to 50% of patients with AV endocarditis.[5,6]

ANSWER 7: B. The patient is at very high risk and should be considered for urgent AV replacement. Surgery will include debridement of the intervalvular fibrosa and repair or replacement of the mitral valve. Coronary angiography is contraindicated in a patient with known or suspected aortic root abscess. Although the patient is at very high risk for progressive heart block, there is no immediate indication for pacemaker placement and the determination would be made after surgery.

References

1. Pellikka PA, Sarano ME, Nishimura RA, et al. Outcome of 622 adults with asymptomatic, hemodynamically significant aortic stenosis during prolonged follow-up. *Circulation.* 2005;111:3290–3295.

2. Rosenhek R, Binder T, Porenta G, et al. Predictors of outcome in severe asymptomatic aortic valve stenosis. *N Engl J Med.* 2000;343:611–617.

3. Douglas P, Garcia MJ, Haines DE, et al. ACCF/ASE/AHA/ASNC/HFSA/HRS/SCAI/SCCM/SCCT/SCMR 2011 appropriate use criteria for echocardiography. A report of the American College of Cardiology Foundation Appropriate Use Criteria Task Force, American Society of Echocardiography, American Heart Association, American Society of Nuclear Cardiology, Heart Failure Society of America, Heart Rhythm Society, Society for Cardiovascular Angiography and Interventions, Society of Critical Care Medicine, Society of Cardiovascular Computed Tomography, Society for Cardiovascular Magnetic Resonance American College of Chest Physicians. *J Am Soc Echocardiogr.* 2011;24:229–267.

4. Baddour LM, Wilsom WR, Bayer AS, et al. AHA Scientific Statement. Infective endocarditis: diagnosis, antimicrobial therapy, and management of complications: a statement for healthcare professionals from the Committee on Rheumatic Fever, Endocarditis, and Kawasaki Disease, Council on Cardiovascular Disease in the Young, and the Councils on Clinical Cardiology, Stroke, and Cardiovascular Surgery and Anesthesia, American Heart Association—Executive Summary: Endorsed by the Infectious Diseases Society of America. *Circulation.* 2005;111:3167.

5. Karalis DG, Bansal RC, Hauck AJ, et al. Transesophageal echocardiographic recognition of subaortic complications in aortic valve endocarditis. Clinical and surgical implications. *Circulation.* 1992;86;353–362.

6. Daniel WG, Mügge A, Martin RP, et al. Improvement in the diagnosis of abscesses associated with endocarditis by transesophageal echocardiography. *N Engl J Med.* 1991;324:795–800.

CASE 19

Harsh Systolic Murmur in Nursery Examination

A 1-day-old newborn undergoes a nursery examination. She has a harsh systolic murmur. She is feeding well and of normal weight, and her mother had an uncomplicated 40-week pregnancy. She is referred for transthoracic echocardiography (**Videos 19-1 to 19-13** and Figs. 19-1 to 19-4).

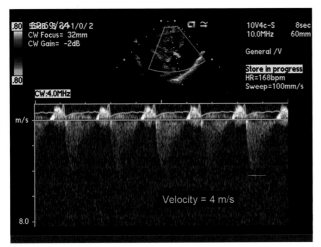

Figure 19-1

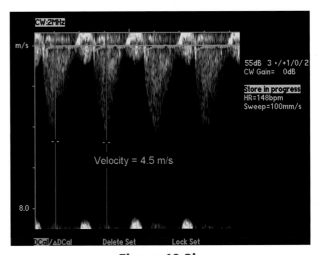

Figure 19-2b

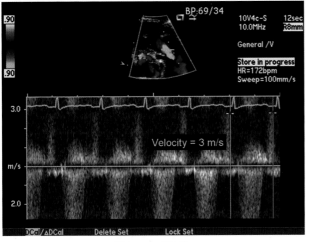

Figure 19-2a

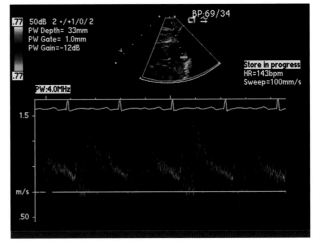

Figure 19-3

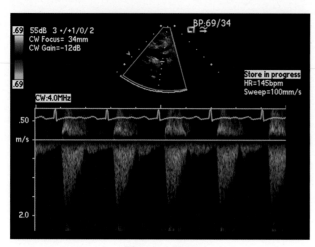

Figure 19-4

QUESTION 1. What is the defect?
  A. Secundum atrial septal defect
  B. Tetralogy of Fallot
  C. Congenital pulmonary valve stenosis
  D. Membranous ventricular septal defect
  E. Congenital aortic valve stenosis

QUESTION 2. The maximum instantaneous systolic gradient across the pulmonary valve is:
  A. 17 mm Hg
  B. 36 mm Hg
  C. 64 mm Hg
  D. 81 mm Hg

QUESTION 3. There is evidence of concomitant:
  A. Coarctation of the aorta
  B. Patent ductus arteriosus
  C. Atrial septal defect
  D. None of the choices

QUESTION 4. Acute management might include:
  A. Oxygen
  B. Prostaglandin infusion
  C. Referral for pulmonary balloon valvuloplasty
  D. Oxygen and prostaglandin infusion
  E. Oxygen, prostaglandin infusion, and referral for pulmonary balloon valvuloplasty

QUESTION 5. Signs of severe pulmonary valve stenosis may include all *except:*
  A. A pan-systolic murmur
  B. A widened split S_2
  C. Marked right ventricular hypertrophy
  D. Cyanosis
  E. Ejection click maximal on inspiration

ANSWER 1: C. There is evidence of a dysplastic pulmonary valve with severe stenosis.

See *The Echo Manual, 3rd Edition*, pages 353 to 356 and Figure 20-32 on page 356.

ANSWER 2: D. The peak velocity across the pulmonary valve is 4.5 m per second. We can calculate the peak instantaneous gradient as $4(v)^2 = 4(4.5)^2 = 81$ mm Hg.

ANSWER 3: B. Seen on **Video 19-10** and Figure 19-3, there is continuous flow seen coming from the aorta toward the pulmonary artery consistent with flow through the ductus arteriosus.

See *The Echo Manual, 3rd Edition*, page 347, and Figure 20–25 on page 351.

ANSWER 4: E. The treatment of valvular pulmonic stenosis is straightforward. If the right ventricular systolic pressure is >50 to 60 mm Hg, patients should undergo balloon valvuloplasty, which has a very high success rate and a low risk (**Video 19-13**). In the setting of systemic right sided pressures and severe pulmonic stenosis, pulmonary blood flow is being maintained in the early neonatal period through the ductus arteriosus. Maintenance of ductal patency as a bridge to definitive therapy is critical and can be obtained through peripheral infusion of prostaglandins. Oxygen should also be given to promote pulmonary arterial dilation.

ANSWER 5: E. Valvular pulmonic stenosis is suggested by a pulmonary ejection click that is maximal on expiration, followed by an ejection systolic murmur and a widely split second heart sound. The more severe the stenosis, the longer the murmur and the wider the second heart sound is split. The right ventricular response is hypertrophic, although right ventricular failure may occur in critical stenosis. In some severe cases of pulmonary stenosis, the elevated right atrial pressure will lead to patency of the foramen ovale leading to a significant right-left shunt and cyanosis.

CASE 20

Progressive NYHA Class III Dyspnea

A 75-year-old man presents for the evaluation of progressive, New York Heart Association class III dyspnea. He denies chest pain, presyncope, or syncope. His medical history is significant for paroxysmal atrial fibrillation and chronic kidney disease secondary to hypertensive nephrosclerosis, with estimated glomerular filtration rate of 15 to 20 cc per minute.

On examination, his systemic blood pressure is 100/60 mm Hg. He has a diminished pulse volume, a third heart sound, and a 2/6 systolic ejection murmur. His ECG is shown in Figure 20-1.

He is referred for transthoracic echocardiogram (**Video 20-1** and Figs. 20-2 to 20-7).

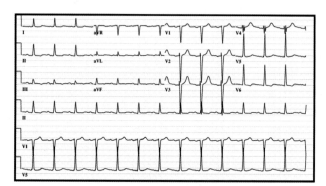

Figure 20-1

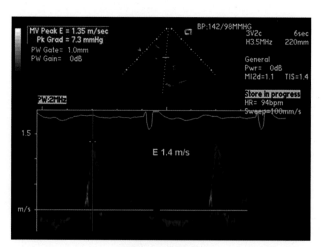

Figure 20-3

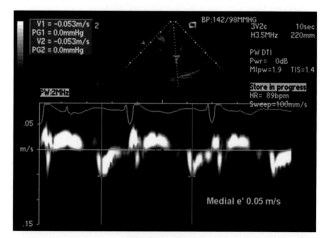

Figure 20-2

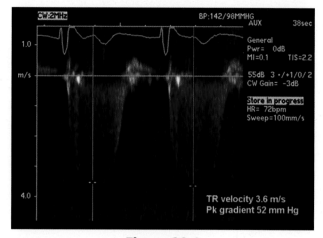

Figure 20-4

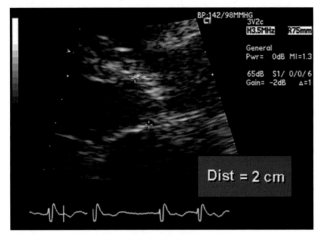

Figure 20-5

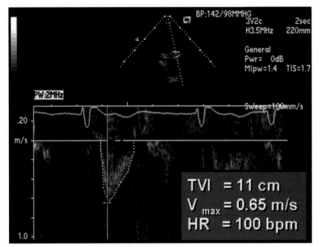

Figure 20-6

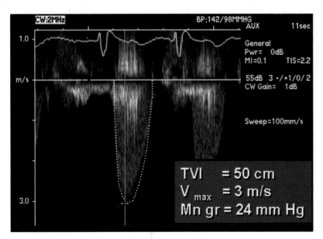

Figure 20-7

QUESTION 1. On the basis of the available data, calculate the Doppler-derived left ventricular stroke volume (SV).

    A. 25cc

    B. 35cc

    C. 50cc

    D. 70cc

QUESTION 2. On the basis of the available data (Figs. 20-2 to 20-7), calculate the Doppler-derived aortic valve area.

    A. 0.6 cm^2

    B. 0.7 cm^2

    C. 0.8 cm^2

    D. 0.9 cm^2

    E. 1.0 cm^2

QUESTION 3. How would you grade this patient's diastolic function?

    A. Normal

    B. Grade 1

    C. Grade 2

    D. Grade 3

QUESTION 4. His left ventricular diastolic filling pressure is:

    A. Normal

    B. Increased

    C. Reduced

    D. Not able to be determined

QUESTION 5. His lateral mitral e′ velocity is most likely:

    A. 4 cm per second

    B. 5 cm per second

    C. 6 cm per second

    D. 15 cm per second

QUESTION 6. A reasonable next step may include:

A. Aortic valve replacement after diagnostic coronary angiography

B. Contrast cardiac CT to assess aortic valve and left ventricular systolic function

C. Cardiac hemodynamic catheterization with dobutamine infusion

D. Transesophageal echocardiography

QUESTION 7. The patient was referred for stress echocardiogram to assess aortic valve hemodynamics and contractile reserve in response to dobutamine (**Videos 20-2 and 20-3** and Fig. 20-8). (In both the videos, image orientation is as follows: top left parasternal long axis, top right parasternal short axis, bottom left apical four-chamber view with left ventricle on the left, and bottom right apical two-chamber view with inferior wall on the left and anterior wall on the right.) The next appropriate step is:

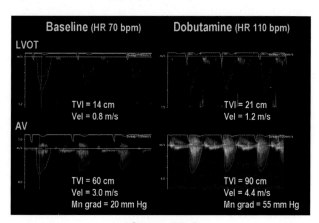

Figure 20-8

A. Aortic valve replacement after diagnostic coronary angiography

B. Cardiac hemodynamic catheterization with dobutamine infusion

C. Transesophageal echocardiography

D. Initiation of medical management of dilated cardiomyopathy with angiotensin-converting inhibitors and β-blockers

QUESTION 8. Contractile reserve is defined as:

A. An increase in SV of >10% with dobutamine

B. An increase in SV of >20% with dobutamine

C. An increase in SV of >30% with dobutamine

D. An increase in SV of >50% with dobutamine

ANSWER 1: B. SV is calculated as the product of the cross-sectional area of the left ventricular outflow tract (LVOT) and the time velocity integral (TVI) of a pulse wave sample from the LVOT:

$$SV \; (ml) = [(D/2)^2 \times \pi] \times [LVOT \; TVI]$$
$$= [(2/2)^2 \times \pi] \times [11]$$
$$= 34.5 \; ml$$

See *The Echo Manual, 3rd Edition*, **Figure 4-16 on page 71.**

ANSWER 2: B.

$$Aortic \; valve \; area = [(LVOT \; TVI) \times (LVOT \; area)]/Ao \; TVI$$
$$= [(11) \times (\pi \; (1)^2)]/50$$
$$= 34.5/50$$
$$= 0.7 \; cm^2$$

See *The Echo Manual, 3rd Edition*, **discussion of Doppler echocardiography (in aortic stenosis) on pages 190 and 191.**

ANSWER 3: D. Mitral early filling peak velocity is elevated at 1.4 m per second with a diminutive A wave and visually short deceleration time. A similar pattern can be seen in a healthy young well conditioned individuals, it is not a normal pattern in an elderly patient. Moreover, medial mitral annulus velocity of 5 cm/sec shows that the underlying myocardium has a profound diastolic dysfunction. This describes a restrictive filling pattern in keeping with Grade 3 or severe diastolic dysfunction.

ANSWER 4: B. Left ventricular filling pressure can be estimated by the ratio of the early mitral peak velocity (E) to the early diastolic relaxation tissue velocity of the mitral annulus (e′), with a ratio >15 correlating with an elevation in left ventricular diastolic filling pressure. Here the E/e′ ratio is 1.4/0.05 that is very high at 28.

ANSWER 5: C. The mitral lateral annulus e′ velocity is typically 10% to 20% higher than that of the medial annulus. Conditions which produce lower lateral e′ than medial e′ are constrictive pericarditis and lateral wall myocardial infarction.

ANSWER 6: C. When LV systolic function is abnormal and cardiac output is reduced, aortic stenosis is probably severe if (1) the aortic valve area by the continuity equation is 0.75 cm² or less and (2) the LVOT:AoV TVI (or velocity) is 0.25 or less. In this situation, however, there are two diagnostic possibilities: one, true anatomically severe aortic stenosis and, two, functionally severe aortic stenosis, because an aortic valve with mild or moderately severe stenosis may not open fully if the SV is low. Gradual infusion of dobutamine (up to 20 μg/kg/minute) to increase SV may be helpful in differentiating morphologically severe aortic stenosis from a decreased effective stenotic orifice area caused by low cardiac output (pseudo-severe aortic stenosis). This can be accomplished by echocardiography or catheterization. Dobutamine stress echocardiography affords the diagnostic capabilities while avoiding the potential embolic risks of transverses a potentially severely stenotic aortic valve with a hemodynamic catheter.[1–3]

ANSWER 7: A. In the setting of low-output, low-gradient aortic stenosis, dobutamine stress echocardiography has two distinct roles. The first is with regard to distinguishing severe stenosis from pseudo-severe (functional) stenosis of the valve. The secondary role is with regard to assessing for the presence or absence of inotropic left ventricular reserve.

Here gradual infusion of dobutamine led to a progressive normalization of LVOT velocity and TVI. At this level, there was a parallel increase in transvalvular velocity and TVI with a preservation of LVOT/aortic valve ratios, thus confirming true severe aortic valve stenosis (Fig. 20-9). Aortic stenosis should be considered severe, warranting aortic valve replacement, if the aortic valve area is 1.0 cm² or less and the mitral gradient 30 mm Hg or more with dobutamine.

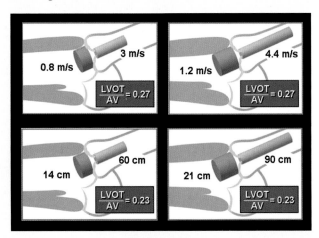

Figure 20-9

ANSWER 8: B. Beyond diagnosis, dobutamine plays a critical role in assessing the presence or absence of inotropic reserve, defined as an increase in SV (or LVOT TVI) of >20% with dobutamine. Although valve replacement remains a better option than conservative therapy, the absence of inotropic reserve with dobutamine portends a poor perioperative mortality (50% vs. 7%) if aortic valve replacement is attempted.

Consideration of percutaneous aortic valve replacement in this setting is prudent.

In patients with aortic valve areas <1 cm^2 and tricuspid regurgitant velocities >4 m per second, operative mortality is high, but still better than conservative (nonoperative) management.[4-7]

See *The Echo Manual, 3rd Edition*, pages 186 and 192 to 196.

References

1. deFilippi CR, Willet DL, Brickner ME, et al. Usefulness of dobutamine echocardiography in distinguishing severe from nonsevere valvular aortic stenosis in patients with depressed left ventricular function and low transvalvular gradients. *Am J Cardiol.* 1995;75:191–194.

2. Nishimura RA, Grantham JA, Connolly HM, Schaff HV, Higano ST, Holmes DR Jr. Low-output, low-gradient aortic stenosis in patients with depressed left ventricular systolic function: the clinical utility of the dobutamine challenge in the catheterization laboratory. *Circulation.* 2002;106:809–813.

3. Omran H, Schmidt H, Hackenbroch M, et al. Silent and apparent cerebral embolism after retrograde catheterisation of the aortic valve in valvular stenosis: a prospective, randomized study. *Lancet.* 2003;361:1241–1246.

4. Monin JL, Quéré JP, Monchi M, et al. Low-gradient aortic stenosis: operative risk stratification and predictors for long-term outcome: a multicenter study using dobutamine stress hemodynamics. *Circulation.* 2003;108:319–324. Epub 2003 Jun 30.

5. Schwammenthal E, Vered Z, Moshkowitz Y, et al. Dobutamine echocardiography in patients with aortic stenosis and left ventricular dysfunction: predicting outcome as a function of management strategy. *Chest.* 2001;119:1766–1777.

6. Pereira JJ, Lauer MS, Bashir M, et al. Survival after aortic valve replacement for severe aortic stenosis with low transvalvular gradients and severe left ventricular dysfunction. *J Am Coll Cardiol.* 2002;39:1356–1363.

7. Malouf JF, Enriquez-Sarano M, Pellikka PA, et al. Severe pulmonary hypertension in patients with severe aortic valve stenosis: clinical profile and prognostic implications. *J Am Coll Cardiol.* 2002;40:789–795.

8. Hachicha Z, Dumesnil JG, Bogaty P, Pibarot P. Paradoxical low-flow, low-gradient severe aortic stenosis despite preserved ejection fraction is associated with higher afterload and reduced survival. Circulation. 2007 Jun 5;115(22):2856-64.

CASE 21

Systemic Sclerosis

A 60-year-old man with a history of systemic sclerosis is referred to estimate pulmonary pressures (**Videos 21-1 to 21-6** and Figs. 21-1 to 21-11).

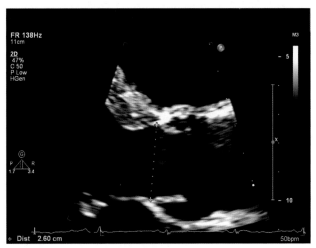

Figure 21-1

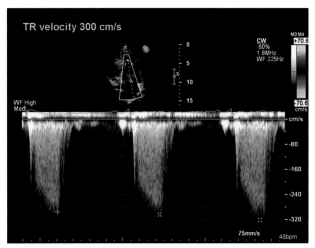

Figure 21-3

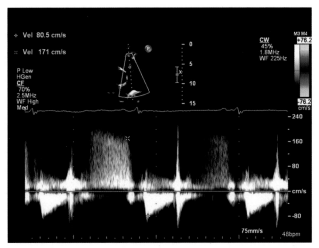

Figure 21-2

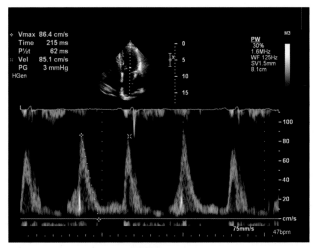

Figure 21-4

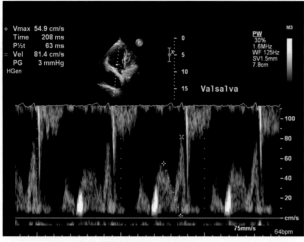

Figure 21-5

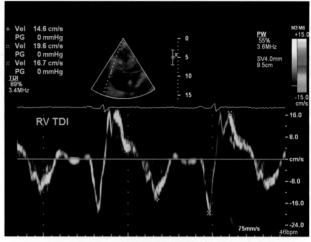

Figure 21-8

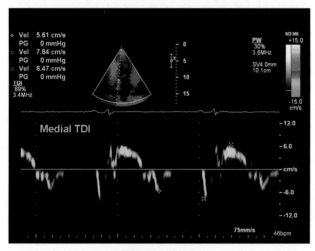

Figure 21-6

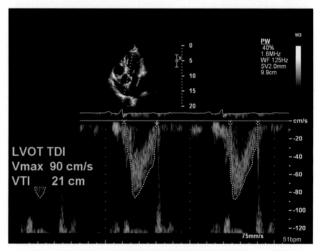

Figure 21-9

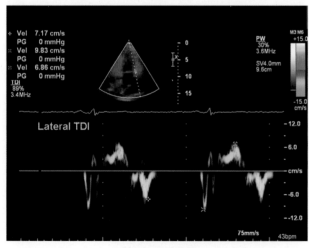

Figure 21-7

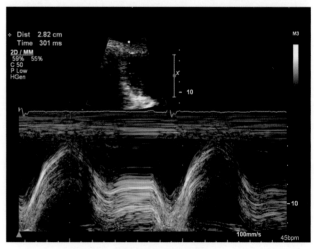

Figure 21-10

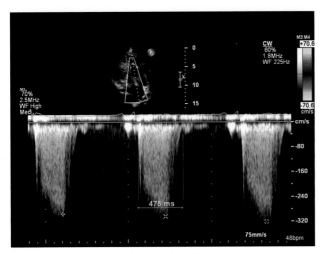

Figure 21-11

QUESTION 1. What are the estimated pulmonary artery systolic and diastolic pressures?

A. 41/17 mm Hg
B. 36/12 mm Hg
C. 13/8 mm Hg
D. 17/12 mm Hg

QUESTION 2. Pulmonary artery capacitance is:

A. 3.6
B. 4.6
C. 4.9
D. 5.5

QUESTION 3. Diastolic function is:

A. Normal
B. Grade 1 (mildly abnormal)
C. Grade 2 (moderately abnormal)
D. Grade 3 (severely abnormal)

QUESTION 4. The right index of myocardial performance (Tei index) is:

A. 0.34
B. 0.41
C. 0.52
D. 0.60

QUESTION 5. Which of the following contrast agents would be useful to identify the structure marked by a circle in **Video 21-6** and Figure 21-12?

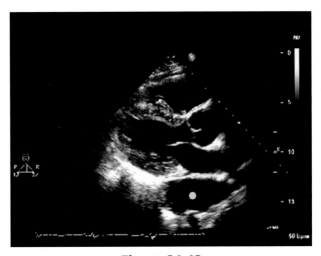

Figure 21-12

A. Agitated saline
B. Echo contrast
C. Carbonated beverage
D. Iodinated contrast

ANSWER 1: A. Pulmonary artery systolic pressure is estimated as four times the peak (tricuspid regurgitant velocity)^2 plus an estimate of right atrial pressure. Pulmonary artery diastolic pressure is estimated as four times the (end pulmonary regurgitant velocity)^2 plus an estimate of right atrial pressure. Here the inferior vena cava is of normal size and collapses normally with respiration, and hence, the right atrial pressure is normal (5 mm Hg). Here pulmonary artery systolic and diastolic pressures are estimated as $4(3)^2 + 5 = 41$ mm Hg and $4(1.7)^2 + 5 = 17$ mm Hg, respectively.

ANSWER 2: B. Incorporating the pulsatile component of right ventricular afterload, the pulmonary artery capacitance (PA CAP) as measured by catheterization or echocardiography[1] has been found to be highly predictive of outcome in patients with pulmonary hypertension. It is expressed as the ratio of stroke volume (SV) to pulmonary artery pulse pressure (PA PP).

PA CAP. = SV/PA PP

= 5.3 × 21/24 = 111 cc/24 mm Hg = 4.6 cc/mm Hgt

ANSWER 3: C. The mitral inflow pattern demonstrates a pseudonormal pattern with early (E) and atrial (A) velocities of similar magnitude. Medial and lateral mitral annular early velocities are depressed consistent with myocardial relaxation abnormalities. With a drop in preload by Valsalva, there was a change in the mitral inflow pattern to a delayed relaxation (Grade 1) pattern.

ANSWER 4: A. The right ventricular index of myocardial performance (RIMP) is a relatively load independent parameter of global function, which is a ratio of the sum of the isovolumic relaxation and contraction times to the right ventricular ejection time. It can be easily calculated by the following equation:

$$\text{RIMP} = \text{(Tricuspid valve closure to opening time)} - \text{(RV ejection time)/(RV ejection time)}$$
$$= 475 - 355/355 = 0.34$$

ANSWER 5: C. Parasternal long-axis imaging demonstrates a large esophageal structure (**Video 21-6** and Fig. 21-12) outside the pericardial space anterior to the descending thoracic aorta. Administration of a carbonated beverage (**Videos 21-6 and 21-7** and Fig. 21-12) identifies the structure as part of the gastrointestinal tract.

Reference

1. Mahapatra S, Nishimura RA, Oh JK, et al. The prognostic value of pulmonary vascular capacitance determined by Doppler echocardiography in patients with pulmonary arterial hypertension. *J Am Soc Echocardiogr.* 2006;19:1045–1050.

CASE 22

Progressive Dyspnea

An 85-year-old man presents to the emergency department with 4 days of progressive dyspnea.

He does not report any chest pain, but has cough and shortness of breath. He was treated for pneumonia with an antibiotic that did not help his dyspnea and cough. Examination showed heart rate of 100 beats per minute and blood pressure of 90/50 mm Hg. He has diffuse crackles on his lung fields. There was no audible murmur.

Chest x-ray showed pulmonary venous congestions, and ECG showed nonspecific ST-T changes and mild ST segment depression in V1 and V2. Transthoracic echocardiogram showed the following (see **Videos 22-1 to 22-9**).

QUESTION 1. On the basis of mitral inflow (Fig. 22-1), which of the following statements is *correct*?

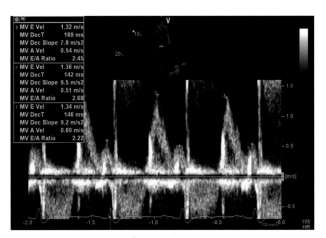

Figure 22-1

A. Most likely normal for this age
B. E velocity of 1.3 m per second indicates increased flow across the mitral valve
C. Mitral valve obstruction
D. Normal filling pressure

QUESTION 2. On the basis of the mitral inflow pattern and the tissue Doppler velocity of medial mitral annulus (Fig. 22-2), diastolic function is graded as which of the following?

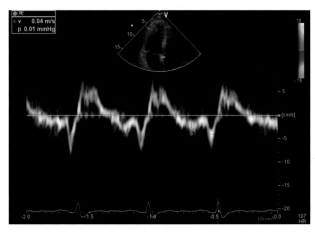

Figure 22-2

A. Grade 1
B. Grade 2
C. Grade 3

QUESTION 3. From this pulmonary vein Doppler tracing (Fig. 22-3), we obtained atrial flow reversal velocity duration of 108 milliseconds. What is the most likely duration of mitral inflow A wave duration?

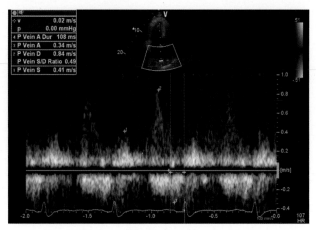

Figure 22-3

A. 70 milliseconds
B. 108 milliseconds
C. 150 milliseconds

QUESTION 4. Calculate effective regurgitant orifice (ERO) and regurgitant volume in this patient (Figs. 22-4 and 22-5).

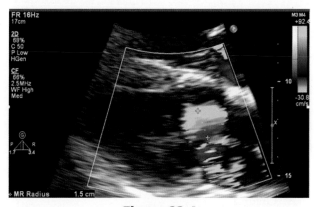

Figure 22-4

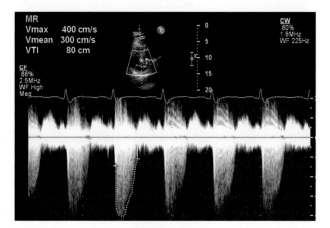

Figure 22-5

A. 1.1 cm² and 88 cc
B. 0.75 cm² and 64 cc
C. 0.6 cm² and 57 cc
D. 0.4 cm² and 45 cc

QUESTION 5. How would you grade the severity of mitral regurgitation?

A. Mild
B. Moderate
C. Severe
D. Falsely high because of poor quality proximal isovelocity surface area

QUESTION 6. What is the etiology for this patient's dyspnea?

A. Papillary muscle rupture
B. Flail mitral valve
C. Mitral valve endocarditis
D. Rheumatic mitral valve stenosis/regurgitation

QUESTION 7. What is your next step for this patient's management?

A. Triple antibiotic treatment
B. Surgery after intra-aortic balloon pump
C. Optimize medical therapy
D. Percutaneous valve procedure

ANSWER 1: B. Pulsed wave Doppler demonstrates a "restrictive" filling pattern with an early diastolic filling (E) velocity that is elevated with a shortened deceleration time and a diminutive late or atrial filling (A) wave. This pattern is seen in settings of increased transvalvular flow with a significant left atrial (LA) to left ventricular (LV) gradient, typically when the LA pressure is high and a high volume of blood rushes into the LV early in diastole. Occasionally, this can be observed in a young individual in the setting of a normal LA pressure with "super" normal relaxation of the heart. This generates a negative LV pressure at early diastole. Blood is "sucked" in by the low LV pressure rather than "pushed" in by the high LA pressure.

ANSWER 2: C. Pulsed wave tissue Doppler of the medial mitral annulus demonstrates a very low early diastolic relaxation tissue (e') velocity indicating a marked LV relaxation abnormality. Coupled with the mitral inflow pattern, this would be compatible with a severe degree of diastolic dysfunction (Grade 3).

ANSWER 3: A. Because LV pressure increases very rapidly with atrial contraction, there is a shortening of atrial filling time (mitral inflow A wave duration) that is less than pulmonary vein atrial flow reversals.

ANSWER 4: A.

The regurgitant flow can be calculated as follows:
Flow rate = $(r)^2 \times 6.28 \times$ aliasing velocity
$= (1.5 \text{ cm})^2 \times 6.28 \times 31 \text{ cm per second}$
$= 438 \text{ cc per second}$
ERO = Flow rate/Peak mitral regurgitant velocity
ERO = 438 cc per second/400 cm per second
$= 1.1 \text{ cm}^2$

Regurgitant volume = ERO × regurgitant time velocity integral
$= 1.1 \text{ cm}^2 \times 80 \text{ cm}$
$= 88 \text{ cc}$

ANSWER 5: C. There is torrential mitral valve regurgitation.

ANSWER 6: A. Best seen in **Videos 22-2**, **22-4**, and **22-8**, the lateral papillary muscle is detached from the ventricular surface and freely mobile. This leads to eccentric severe posteriorly directed mitral valve regurgitation. The presumed mechanism is a recent relatively asymptomatic myocardial infarction with secondary papillary muscle rupture. As is often the case, patients are hypotensive with pulmonary edema and little if any audible systolic murmur.

ANSWER 7: B. The treatment of choice is urgent surgical repair. Vasodilator therapy and intra-aortic balloon pump can be helpful temporizing measures; however, mortality is high short of corrective surgical procedure. There is no role for conservative medical management or at this time a percutaneous repair.

An intraoperative transesophageal echocardiogram (**Videos 22-10 and 22-11**) confirms a papillary muscle rupture, and the patient underwent successful repair.

CASE 23

Exertional Shortness of Breath, Bilateral Lower Extremity Edema, and Systolic Murmur after Coronary Artery Grafting

A 68-year-old man with a history of coronary artery grafting 10 years previously presents with exertional shortness of breath, bilateral lower extremity edema, and a systolic murmur.

QUESTION 1. On the basis of his transthoracic images (**Videos 23-1 and 23-2** and Figs. 23-1 and 23-2), his calculated mitral effective regurgitant orifice (ERO) area by the proximal isovelocity surface area (PISA) method is:

A. 0.36 cm²
B. 0.42 cm²
C. 0.58 cm²
D. 0.60 cm²

QUESTION 2. Which of the following provides a simplified method to calculate ERO when aliasing velocity is close to 40 cm per second?

A. Radius²/2
B. Radius/2
C. Radius × 4

QUESTION 3. On the basis of his transthoracic images (**Videos 23-3 and 23-4** and Figs. 23-3 and 23-4), his calculated tricuspid regurgitant volume by the PISA method is:

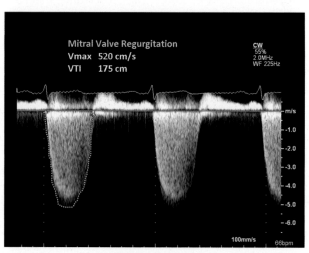

Figure 23-1

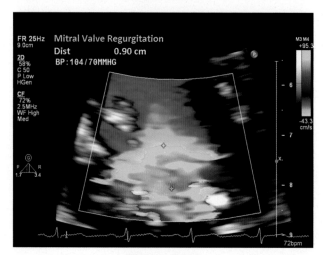

Figure 23-2

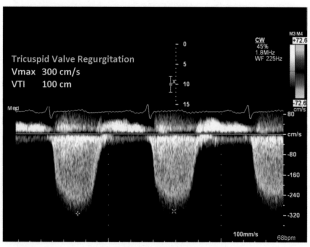

Figure 23-3

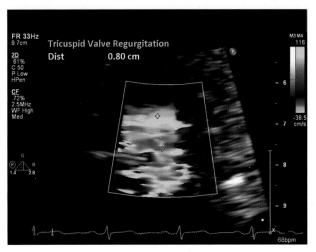

Figure 23-4

A. 40 cc
B. 45 cc
C. 52 cc
D. 57 cc
E. 63 cc

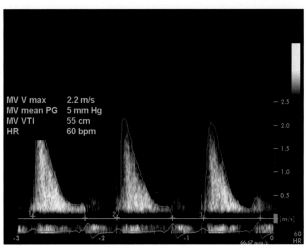

Figure 23-6

A. 1.6 cm²
B. 1.75 cm²
C. 1.9 cm²
D. 2.1 cm²
E. 2.5 cm²

QUESTION 4. For a similar ERO area, tricuspid regurgitation is associated with a smaller regurgitant volume than mitral valve regurgitation (MR).

A. True
B. False

QUESTION 5. The patient proceeds with surgical mitral valve replacement with a 31-mm St. Jude tissue prosthesis and tricuspid valve annuloplasty. On the basis of the predismissal echocardiogram (Video 23-5 and Figs. 23-5 and 23-6), calculate the effective mitral valve prosthetic orifice area by the continuity method (assume that the left ventricular outflow tract [LVOT] diameter is 22 mm).

QUESTION 6. The patient returns 3 months later after his physician heard a continuous murmur on examination. On the basis of the transthoracic (Videos 23-6 to 23-9) and transesophageal (Videos 23-10 to 23-13, Fig. 23-7) images, there is an abnormal communication between the right atrium and:

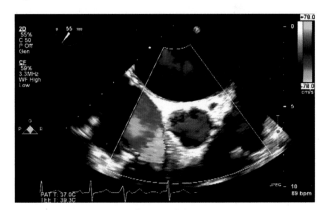

Figure 23-7

A. Right coronary cusp to right ventricle
B. Noncoronary cusp to right atrium
C. Noncoronary cusp to right ventricle
D. Right coronary cusp to right atrium

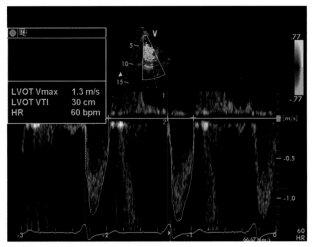

Figure 23-5

ANSWER 1: B. 0.42 cm²

The regurgitant flow can be calculated as follows:

Flow rate = $(r)^2$ × 6.28 × aliasing velocity
= $(0.90 \text{ cm})^2$ × 6.28 × 43 cm per second
= 219 cc per second
ERO = Flow rate/Peak MR velocity
ERO = 219 cc per second/520 cm per second
= 0.42 cm²

ANSWER 2: A. When aliasing velocity is 40 cm per second, 6.28 × 40 = 251. Because MR velocity is close to 500 cm per second, ERO is radius²/2.

See *The Echo Manual, 3rd Edition,* **PISA method on page 215.**

ANSWER 3: C. 52 cc

The regurgitant flow can be calculated as follows:

Flow rate = $(r)^2$ × 6.28 × aliasing velocity
= $(0.8 \text{ cm})^2$ × 6.28 × 39 cm per second
= 157 cc per second
ERO = Flow rate/Peak MR velocity
ERO = 157 cc per second/300 cm per second
= 0.52 cm²

Regurgitant volume = ERO × regurgitant time velocity integral (TVI)
= 0.52 cm² × 100 cm
= 52 cc

See *The Echo Manual, 3rd Edition,* **PISA method on page 215.**

ANSWER 4: A. True. The ERO and regurgitant volume of the tricuspid valve are calculated with the PISA method, as for the mitral valve. For a similar ERO area, however, tricuspid regurgitation is associated with a *smaller* regurgitant volume than MR. Patients with systolic venous flow reversal (the hepatic vein for tricuspid regurgitation and the pulmonary vein for MR) had a smaller regurgitant volume but similar ERO area in tricuspid regurgitation than those with MR. Therefore, the optimal diagnostic thresholds for severe tricuspid regurgitation and MR are different for regurgitant volume (45 and 60 ml, respectively) but similar for an ERO of 40 mm² or more.

ANSWER 5: D. The pressure half-time method overestimates the area of the mitral valve prosthesis. In the absence of significant aortic and MR, the continuity method is a better way to determine prosthetic valve areas.

Mitral valve prosthesis area = LVOT area × (LVOT TVI/ Mitral prosthesis TVI)
Mitral valve prosthesis area = (LVOT D² × 0.785) × (LVOT TVI/Mitral prosthesis TVI)
Mitral valve prosthesis area = (2.2² × 0.785) × (30/55)
Mitral valve prosthesis area = 2.1 cm²

See *The Echo Manual, 3rd Edition,* **PISA method on page 215.**

ANSWER 6: B. Transthoracic imaging demonstrates continuous flow between the proximal ascending aorta and an area either just proximal or just distal to the tricuspid valve. Transesophageal imaging is required to better localize the defect as arising in the noncoronary cusp and entering the right atrium (Fig. 23-7).

The patient proceeded to successful uncomplicated percutaneous device closure guided by intracardiac imaging (**Videos 23-14 to 23-17**).

CASE 24

Symptomatic Paroxysmal Atrial Fibrillation

*A*60-year-old woman is referred for the management of symptomatic paroxysmal atrial fibrillation. She has failed treatment trials of propafenone and sotalol. She is considered for a left atrial ablation procedure. She is referred for transesophageal echocardiography (**Videos 24-1 to 24-5** and Fig. 24-1).

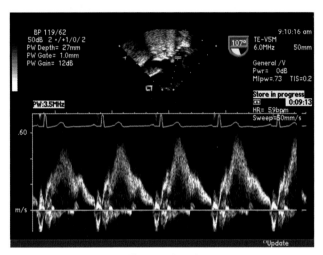

Figure 24-1

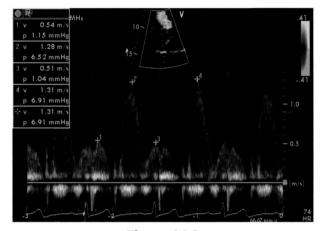

Figure 24-2

A. Repeat left atrial ablation procedure
B. Amiodarone antiarrhythmic
C. CT scan of the chest
D. Coronary angiography

QUESTION 1. On the basis of the pulsed wave Doppler of the right upper pulmonary vein (Fig. 24-1), the left atrial pressure is likely:

A. High
B. Normal

QUESTION 2. The patient returns 3 months after ablation. The palpitations have resolved; however, she has persistent fatigue and now exertional shortness of breath and occasionally chest pain. She undergoes transthoracic echocardiogram (**Videos 24-6 to 24-8** and Fig. 24-2). On the basis of the findings, appropriate next step should include:

QUESTION 3. The patient undergoes transesophageal echocardiography (**Videos 24-9 to 24-14** and Figs. 24-3 and 24-4). Doppler findings are consistent with:

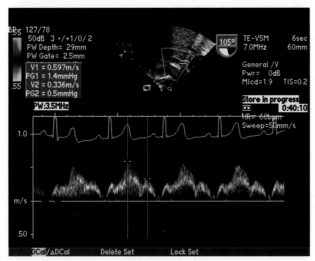

Figure 24-3

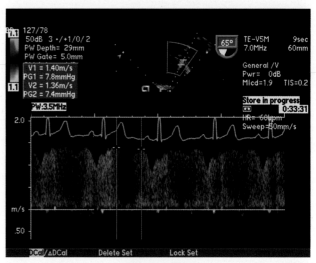

Figure 24-4

A. Severe mitral valve regurgitation
B. Severe elevation in left atrial pressure in the absence of severe mitral regurgitation
C. Pulmonary vein stenosis
D. Normal Doppler findings
E. Coronary to left atrial fistula

ANSWER 1: B. Transesophageal echocardiography shows normal left ventricular systolic function (**Video 24-1**), a normal left atrial appendage without thrombus (**Videos 24-2 and 24-3**), and normal left (**Video 24-4**) and right (**Video 24-5**) pulmonary veins. Normal pulmonary venous flow comprises two forward (positive) waves (one systolic [which may have two components] and one diastolic) and one retrograde (negative) wave with atrial contractility. The normal pattern is for the systolic wave to be greater than the diastolic wave. In the setting of high left atrial pressure, there is diminition of the systolic flow velocity with an elevation in the diastolic-filling wave.

ANSWER 2: C. In patients who have undergone left atrial ablation procedures, one complication to consider is pulmonary vein stenosis, which may occur in 1% to 3% of cases. The average onset of symptoms is within 2 to 6 months after the ablation procedure. Typical symptoms of pulmonary vein stenosis include dyspnea, cough, chest pain, and fatigue.

Here transthoracic echocardiography demonstrates a normal left atrial size. Pulse-wave interrogation of the right upper pulmonary vein demonstrates higher than expected forward flow velocities. The remaining pulmonary veins can be difficult to visualize with a transthoracic examination.

Pulmonary vein stenosis should be considered in every patient with new pulmonary symptoms after a left atrial ablation procedure. Although TEE may be diagnostic, the recommended studies to assess the pulmonary veins are CT or MRI.

ANSWER 3: C. As suggested by the surface echocardiogram and confirmed on the TEE, the flow velocities coming through the right upper pulmonary vein (Fig. 24-4) are higher than expected with early systolic velocity of 1.5 m per second and a mean gradient of 9 mm Hg. This is strongly suggestive of pulmonary vein stenosis. In contrast, interrogation of the left upper pulmonary vein (Fig. 24-3) illustrates a normal profile with early systolic velocity of 0.6 m per second.

In addition to CT scanning of the pulmonary veins, quantitative radionuclide ventilation perfusion scanning of the lungs is helpful. Percutaneous balloon dilation and stenting provides immediate symptom relief, although recurrence and the need of repeat intervention is common.[1]

Reference

1. Packer DL, Keelan P, Munger TM, et al. Clinical presentation, investigation, and management of pulmonary vein stenosis complicating ablation for atrial fibrillation. *Circulation.* 2005;111:546–554.

CASE 25

Heart Failure

A 60-year-old man presents with heart failure. Echocardiography images and Doppler tracings were obtained.

QUESTION 1. On the basis of the 2D echocardiography clips (**Videos 25-1 to 25-3**), which of the following is the most likely etiology for patient's heart failure?

A. Systolic heart failure
B. Diastolic heart failure
C. Valvular heart disease
D. Rhythm related heart failure

QUESTION 2. On the basis of Figures 25-1 to 25-6 (mitral inflow and pulmonary vein Doppler tracings), which of the following statements is correct?

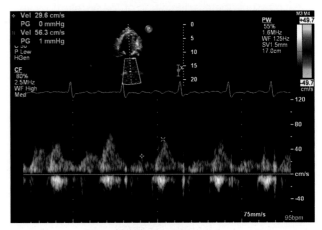

Figure 25-2

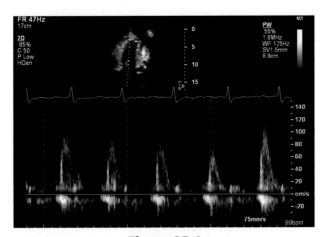

Figure 25-1

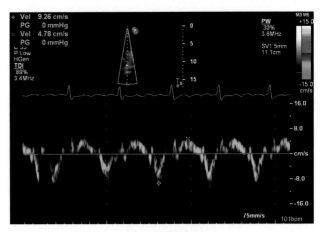

Figure 25-3

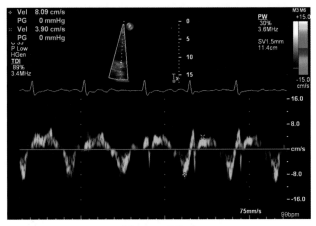

Figure 25-4

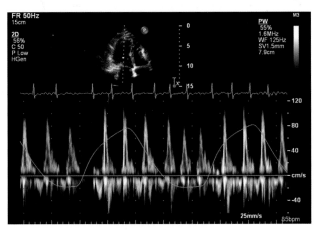

Figure 25-5

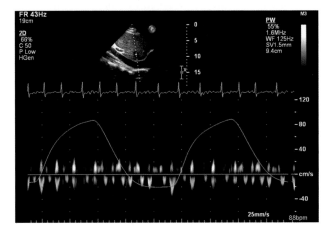

Figure 25-6

A. Left ventricular (LV) filling pressure is definitely elevated

B. Diastolic filling pressure cannot estimated because of atrial fibrillation

C. Mitral inflow deceleration time (DT) is still prognostic even in atrial fibrillation

D. E/e' does not work at all in atrial fibrillation for the estimation of filling pressure

QUESTION 3. The M-mode of LV (Fig. 25-7) indicates which of the following?

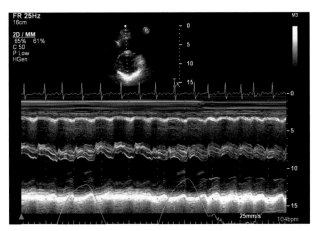

Figure 25-7

A. Atrial fibrillation

B. Translation

C. Interventricular dependence

D. Conduction delay

QUESTION 4. What would you expect to see in hepatic vein if the patient has constrictive pericarditis (Figs. 25-8 to 25-10)?

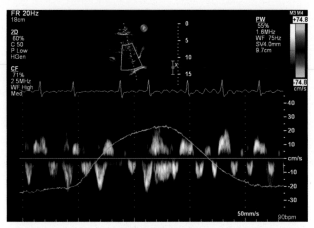

Figure 25-8

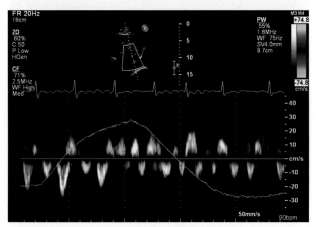

Figure 25-9

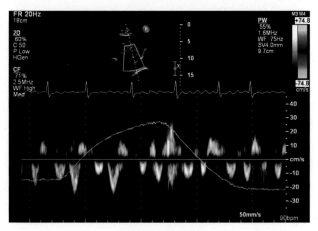

Figure 25-10

A. Diastolic flow reversals with expiration
B. Diastolic flow reversals with inspiration
C. Systolic flow reversals with expiration
D. Diastolic flow reversals with inspiration

QUESTION 5. Which of the following statements is usually correct regarding mitral annulus velocity in patients with constriction?

A. Medial, but not lateral, mitral annulus early diastolic velocity is reduced (<7 cm per second)
B. Both medial and lateral mitral annulus early diastolic velocities are reduced
C. Both medial and lateral annulus early diastolic velocities are increased, but lateral velocity is still higher
D. Medial annulus early diastolic velocity is increased and is higher than that of lateral mitral annulus velocity

QUESTION 6. Which of the following physical examination findings is characteristic for constrictive pericarditis?

A. Pulsus alternans
B. Rapid "y" descent of jugular venous pressure
C. Austin Flint murmur
D. Reduced second heart sound

ANSWER 1: B. This patient's left ventricular ejection fraction is normal, but the left atrium is enlarged suggesting diastolic dysfunction or increased filling pressure. There is no evidence for valvular heart disease. The underlying rhythm is atrial fibrillation that can also cause heart failure, but we cannot be certain without excluding other etiologies.

ANSWER 2: C. Mitral inflow shows only E velocity because of atrial fibrillation. It is difficult to assess diastolic function in patients with atrial fibrillation, but it can be done using DT of mitral inflow and E/e' as in sinus rhythm. DT <130 milliseconds in patients with atrial fibrillation has a poor prognosis. Pulmonary vein has smaller systolic forward velocity compared with diastolic forward flow velocity as shown in patients with atrial fibrillation. Such pattern usually indicates increased filling pressure when the rhythm is sinus, but not in atrial fibrillation.

There is variation in mitral E velocities that may be related to atrial fibrillation with different cycle length and/or to another mechanism such as respiratory variation in ventricular filling seen in patients with constrictive pericarditis.

ANSWER 3: C. The M-mode echocardiogram is shown with simultaneous respirometer recording. Ventricular septum moves to LV with inspiration (upstroke of the respirometer at the bottom) and to right ventricle (RV) with expiration, which is characteristic for the ventricular interdependence seen in constrictive pericarditis.

ANSWER 4: A. A specific finding in constrictive pericarditis is diastolic flow reversals with expiration in the hepatic vein. As the patient expires, there is a drop in intrathoraic pressure that leads to a relative increase in left sided filling compared with right. The intravetricular septum shifts toward the right that limits RV filling. Tricuspid inflow decreases and hepatic vein diastolic forward flow decreases with prominent diastolic flow reversals seen in expiration.

See *The Echo Manual, 3rd Edition,* **section on constrictive pericarditis on page 294 and Figure 17-23 on page 301.**

ANSWER 5: D. In patients with myocardial disease, mitral annulus early diastolic velocity (e') is almost always reduced, as e' represents the status of myocardial relaxation that is reduced in all patients with myocardial diseases. However, the lateral mitral annulus is still higher than that of medial mitral annulus. In constriction, owing to the tethering of the mitral annulus with constrictive pericardial layer, the lateral annulus velocity is usually (but not always) lower than that of the medial. Medial annulus motion is preserved or exaggerated in constriction.

ANSWER 6: B. Pulsus alternans is characteristic for patients with severe LV systolic dysfunction. Austin Flint murmur is for patients with aortic regurgitation. Reduced second heart sound is expected in patients with severe aortic stenosis. "y" descent is rapid in constriction since atrial pressure is elevated and falls very rapidly after opening of the atrio-ventricular valve.

CASE 26

Hematuria with Large Renal Mass

A 70-year-old man presents with hematuria and after a comprehensive evaluation is found to have a large renal mass, suspicious for renal cell carcinoma. He has no cardiopulmonary symptoms. On a preanesthetic evaluation, he is found to have a harsh ejection systolic murmur and is referred for transthoracic echocardiography (**Videos 26-1 to 26-5** and **Figs. 26-1 and 26-2**).

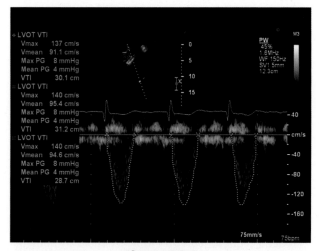

Figure 26-1

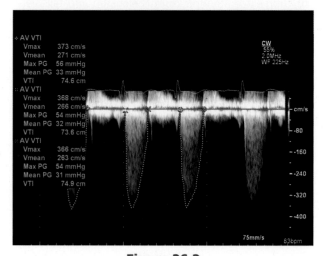

Figure 26-2

QUESTION 1. What is the calculated aortic valve (AV) area (left ventricular outflow tract [LVOT] diameter is 20 mm)?

A. 0.95 cm^2

B. 1.3 cm^2

C. 1.65 cm^2

D. 2.0 cm^2

QUESTION 2. For the same valve area, what would you expect LVOT TVI to be if AV velocity decreases to 2.5 m per second and TVI to 50 cm because of LV dysfunction?

A. 10 cm

B. 15 cm

C. 20 cm

D. 25 cm

QUESTION 3. How often the maximal velocity from the AV is obtained from nonapical transducer location?

A. 10%

B. 20%

C. 30%

D. 40%

QUESTION 4. Which of the following conditions will make the application of continuity equation most difficult in patients with aortic stenosis?

A. Aortic regurgitation
B. Mitral regurgitation
C. Low cardiac output
D. LVOT obstruction

QUESTION 5. What is the most likely etiology for the unexpected finding seen on **Videos 26-6 to 26-9** and Figure 26-3 and further evaluated on transesophageal echocardiography (**Videos 26-10 to 26-13** and Fig. 26-4)?

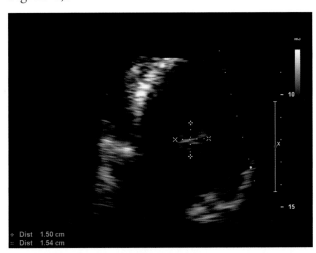

Figure 26-3

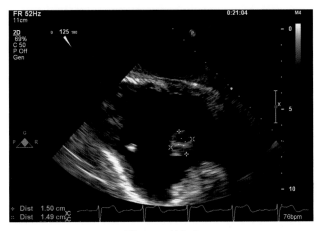

Figure 26-4

A. Metastatic renal cell carcinoma
B. Myxoma
C. Papillary fibroelastoma
D. Thrombus

QUESTION 6. The patient underwent successful nephrectomy and 6 weeks of anticoagulation. Repeat imaging was unchanged (**Video 26-14**). The patient is referred for surgical resection. Should the AV also be replaced (**Videos 26-15 and 26-16**)?

A. Yes
B. No

QUESTION 7. What is the mean reduction in AV area per year in patients with aortic stenosis?

A. 0.05 cm^2
B. 0.10 cm^2
C. 0.15 cm^2
D. 0.20 cm^2

QUESTION 8. Which coronary artery is identified by the arrow (Fig. 26-5)?

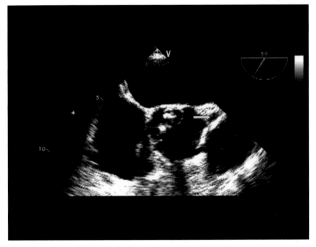

Figure 26-5

A. Left main coronary artery
B. Right coronary artery

ANSWER 1: B.

AV area = [(LVOT TVI) × (LVOT area)]/Ao TVI
= [(LVOT TVI) × (0.785 (LVOT D)^2]/Ao TVI
= [(30) × (3.14)]/75
= 94/75
= 1.3 cm^2

ANSWER 2: C. For the same valve area, LVOT TVI/AV TVI ratio should be same with the same LVOT diameter. The ratio was 30/75 initially. If AV TVI decreases by a third (from 75 to 50 cm), LVOT TVI is expected to decrease by a third (from 30 to 20 cm).

ANSWER 3: B. It is mandatory that all transducer positions are used for interrogation of AV velocity. Otherwise, the peak velocity and gradient will be missed in 20% of patients.

ANSWER 4: D. It is difficult to measure an accurate LVOT velocity when there is LVOT dynamic obstruction. In this situation, stroke volume can be calculated from the right ventricular outflow tract, or using the bi-plane Simpson's calculation of LV volumes.

See *The Echo Manual, 3rd Edition*, Doppler Echocardiography (in aortic stenosis) on pages 190 and 191.

ANSWER 5: C. Echocardiography demonstrates a large mobile mass associated with the anterior leaflet of the tricuspid valve. Tumors associated with cardiac valves are rare. By far, the most common pathology is a papillary fibroelastoma accounting for 85% to 90% of valvular tumors. The remainder is usually either myxomas or fibromas. Metastatic involvement of heart valves is rare. Renal cell carcinoma classically involves the heart through direct intravascular tumor extension through the inferior vena cava into the right atrium. Potentially, a tumor embolus or thrombus has become attached to the tricuspid apparatus, although this is less likely.

ANSWER 6: A. Patients undergoing elective cardiac surgery who have concomitant moderate or greater degrees of aortic stenosis should be considered for elective replacement of the AV.

ANSWER 7: B. On average, peak aortic valve velocity increases by 0.3 m/sec per year and aortic valve area decreases by 0.1 cm^2

ANSWER 8: A. In this view, we see a heavily calcified AV. Below the valve (between 7 and 5 o'clock) is the right ventricular outflow tract, which associates with the right coronary cusp. To the left (between 7 and 10 o'clock) is the right atrium with the tricuspid valve mass coming in and out of plane. At 10 o'clock is the intra-atrial septum, which associates with the noncoronary cusp. Above and to the upper right of the valve is the left atrium, and seen at 2 o'clock is the left main coronary artery.

Pathology of the resected tricuspid valve lesion confirmed it to be a papillary fibroelastoma. The tricuspid valve was repaired and the AV replaced. The patient did well postoperatively.

See *The Echo Manual, 3rd Edition*, discussion of papillary fibroelastomas on pages 311 to 315.

CASE 27

Transthoracic Echocardiography on a Sonography Student

A 25-year-old asymptomatic sonography student undergoes a transthoracic echocardiogram while training (**Videos 27-1 to 27-6** and Fig. 27-1).

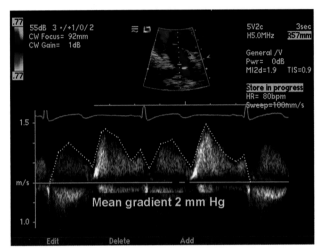

Figure 27-1

QUESTION 1. What is the finding found on transthoracic echocardiography (identified by the green arrow on **Video 27-7**)?

A. Artifact
B. Mitral valve stenosis
C. Cor triatriatum
D. Papillary fibroelastoma
E. Left atrial thrombus

QUESTION 2. Complications of this defect may include all of the following *except*:

A. Development of mitral valve regurgitation
B. Progressive pulmonary hypertension
C. Atrial fibrillation
D. Thromboembolic disease
E. Decreased vascular markings on chest radiography

QUESTION 3. What is the most likely explanation for this finding (**Video 27-8**, yellow arrow)?

A. Normal anatomy
B. Persistent left superior vena cava
C. Venous hypertension secondary to severe tricuspid valve regurgitation
D. Hiatal hernia

QUESTION 4. What is the left ventricular diastolic function (Figs. 27-2 and 27-3)?

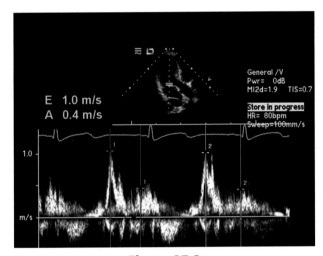

Figure 27-2

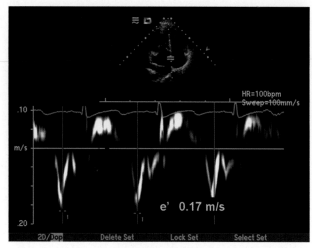

Figure 27-3

A. Normal
B. Mild (Grade 1) dysfunction
C. Moderate (Grade 2) dysfunction
D. Severe (Grade 3) dysfunction

ANSWER 1: C. Cor triatriatum is a rare congenital abnormality and is often a hemodynamically insignificant finding. There is a discrete membrane that divides the left atrium into upper and lower chambers. The membrane is attached medially to the atrial septum at the inferior margin of the fossa ovalis membrane and laterally to the junction of the left upper pulmonary vein and the left atrial appendage.

ANSWER 2: E. Occasionally, the membrane causes significant obstruction to flow, and a patient presents early with progressive left heart failure and/or pulmonary hypertension. Other complications may include mitral valve dysfunction induced by a postobstructive turbulent jet. Typically, color flow mapping (as in this case) demonstrates only mild increases in velocities, suggesting minimal obstruction. This lesion, however, is usually resected early in life, as it may lead to atrial dilation and symptomatic atrial arrhythmia. The most distinctive radiographic finding that is present in almost all patients with hemodynamically significant cor triatriatum is increased pulmonary vascular markings because of pulmonary venous hypertension.[1-3]

ANSWER 3: A. The arrow indicates the descending thoracic aorta that is normally placed. This should not be confused with a dilated coronary sinus (not present in this case), which would be found in the atrioventricular groove inside the pericardium. Common causes of a dilated coronary sinus may include a persistent left superior vena cava or elevated right atrial pressure.

ANSWER 4: A. Normal diastolic filling pattern. There is a normal mitral inflow pattern with E = 1.0 m per second, A = 0.4 m per second. It is, however, difficult to tell whether this recording is truly normal or represents pseudonormal filling. The tissue Doppler recording of the medial mitral annulus is very normal, with an e' velocity of 0.17 m per second (to be expected in an asymptomatic 25-year-old subject) and an E/e' ratio <8. This clarifies that indeed the diastolic function in this case is normal. Of note, the sample volume position (Fig. 27-2) was not optimal because the left ventricular outflow tract is seen. Mitral inflow recording is best taken from an apical four-chamber view.

References

1. O'Murchu B, Seward JB. Images in cardiovascular medicine. Adult congenital heart disease. Obstructive and nonobstructive cor triatriatum. *Circulation.* 1995;92:3574.

2. Buchholz S, Jenni R. Doppler echocardiographic findings in 2 identical variants of a rare cardiac anomaly, "subtotal" cor triatriatum: a critical review of the literature. *J Am Soc Echocardiogr.* 2001;14:846–849.

3. van Son JA, Danielson GK, Schaff HV, et al. Cor triatriatum: diagnosis, operative approach, and late results. *Mayo Clin Proc.* 1993;68:854–859.

CASE 28

Class III Exertional Shortness of Breath without Angina

A 73-year-old woman is referred to the echocardiographic laboratory for the evaluation of class III exertional shortness of breath without angina. Her medical history is significant for hyperlipidemia and systemic hypertension for which she takes simvastatin 20 mg orally, hydrochlorothiazide 12.5 mg orally, and amlodipine 5 mg orally. On examination, her blood pressure is 148/80 mm Hg, and she has trace pedal edema. The remainder of the cardiovascular examination is normal. Her 12-lead ECG demonstrates sinus rhythm with lateral ST segment depression.

She is referred for a treadmill stress echocardiogram to assess for ischemia.

She exercises for 4 minutes on a standard Bruce treadmill protocol (5 METS) and stops secondary to dyspnea. Her stress ECG is nondiagnostic secondary to resting ST-T changes. Her heart rate increases from 77 to 120 beats per minute, and her systemic blood pressure from 148/80 to 176/85 mm Hg. Please see Videos 28-1 and 28-2 for the rest and stress images (Please note that the apical 4 chamber images are displayed in the Mayo Clinic format with the left ventricle on the left).

QUESTION 1. In patients referred for exercise echocardiography for the suspicion of coronary artery disease, those with dyspnea have an equivalent or higher risk of coronary artery disease than those with typical angina.

A. True
B. False

QUESTION 2. 2D echocardiographic findings (see **Videos 28-1 and 28-2**) are suggestive of:

A. Ischemia in the left anterior descending artery territory
B. Ischemia in the setting of the right coronary artery
C. No evidence of ischemia

QUESTION 3. Before exercise, the measured left atrial volume index was 34 cc per m². Please see the following figures for the mitral inflow (Fig. 28-1), the medial mitral annulus tissue Doppler (Fig. 28-2), and the peak tricuspid regurgitant velocity (Fig. 28-3).

On the basis of the available echocardiographic data, an elevation in left ventricular filling pressures is the likely cause of the patient's dyspnea.

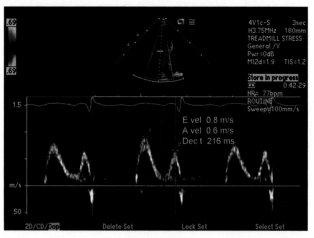

Figure 28-1

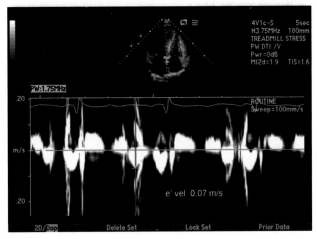

Figure 28-2

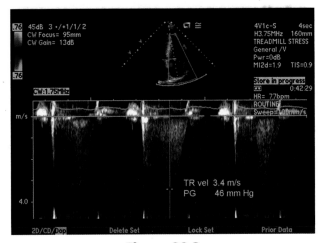

Figure 28-3

A. True
B. False
C. Unclear

QUESTION 4. Which of the following factors would not support a diagnosis of pseudonormalized diastolic dysfunction?

A. Mid-diastolic flow on the mitral inflow pattern
B. A reversal of the E/A ratio after sitting/ standing up
C. The mitral A duration exceeding the pulmonary A wave duration
D. A decrease in the rate of flow propagation on color M-mode imaging of mitral inflow

---

QUESTION 5. Immediately after the postexercise regional wall motion assessment, the mitral inflow (Fig. 28-4), the medial mitral annulus tissue Doppler (Fig. 28-5), the peak tricuspid regurgitant velocity (Fig. 28-6), and the summary of hemodynamics (Fig. 28-7) were obtained again.

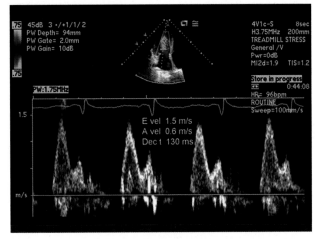

Figure 28-4

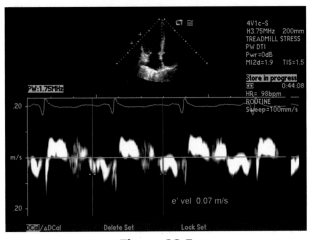

Figure 28-5

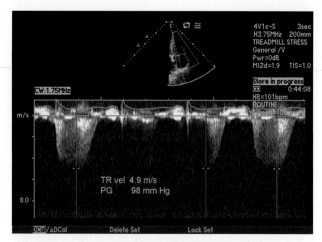

Figure 28-6

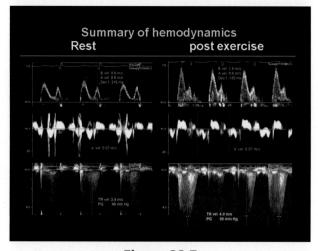

Figure 28-7

On the basis of the available echocardiographic data, an elevation in left ventricular filling pressures is the likely cause of the patient's dyspnea.

A. True
B. False
C. Unclear

ANSWER 1: A. True. Patients with dyspnea referred for exercise echocardiography for the evaluation of coronary artery disease have a high likelihood of ischemia and a high incidence of cardiac events during follow-up. Bergeron and colleagues found rates of myocardial ischemia at exercise echocardiography of 42% in patients with dyspnea compared with 19% with chest pain. Over 3 years of follow up, rates of cardiac death (5.2% vs. 0.9%, $P < .0001$) and nonfatal myocardial infarction (4.7% vs. 2.0%, $P < .0001$) were higher in dyspneic patients compared with those with chest pain.[1]

ANSWER 2: C. Poststress images demonstrate a normal left ventricular response to exercise with a left ventricular ejection fraction increasing from 65% to 70%, a decline in end-diastolic volume, and a normal increase in myocardial thickening in all segments.

ANSWER 3: C. In patients with normal left ventricular size and systolic function, a mitral inflow pattern where the early peak velocity (E) is greater than the late peak velocity (A) with an E/A ratio between 1 and 1.5 and a deceleration time between 160 and 220 millisecond may reflect either normal diastolic function or pseudonormalized, Grade 2 diastolic dysfunction. The best way to distinguish a pseudonormalized pattern from a normal one is to demonstrate impaired myocardial relaxation by e′ <7 cm per second and increased filling pressure by E/e′ >15, although e′ is borderline at 7 cm per second and the E/e′ of 11 falls in the indeterminate gray zone. Of note, the left atrium while enlarged is only mildly so. Although the picture is not entirely normal, there are insufficient data to classify the diastolic dysfunction as moderately abnormal and therefore a likely explanation of the patient's shortness of breath.

ANSWER 4: C. In addition to a decreased e′ and an E/e′ ratio >15, the following factors help distinguish a pseudonormal from a true normal pattern:

1. Mid-diastolic flow because of marked impairment of myocardial relaxation.

2. A decrease in preload, by having the patient sit, perform the Valsalva maneuver, or take sublingual nitroglycerin, may be able to unmask the underlying impaired relaxation of the left ventricle (LV), causing the E/A ratio to decrease by 0.5 or more and reversal of the E/A ratio. In normal people, both the E and A velocities decrease more proportionally with a decrease in filling.

3. A pseudonormal pattern is demonstrated by showing a shortening of mitral A duration in the absence of a short PR interval or by demonstrating prolonged pulmonary vein 'a' duration exceeding mitral A duration.

4. Color M-mode of mitral inflow can determine the rate of flow propagation in the LV. With worsening diastolic function, myocardial relaxation is always impaired and flow propagation is slow, even when left atrial pressure and mitral E velocity are increased.

See *The Echo Manual, 3rd Edition,* **pages 134 to 135 and Figure 8-8 on page 125.**

ANSWER 5: A. In this case, repeat measure of data immediately after exercise demonstrated a clear change from preexercise findings. The normal findings after exercise are a modest increase in mitral inflow velocities associated with a modest increase in early myocardial relaxation (e′). These are related to increased flow into the LV seen with the increased cardiac output of exercise and an increased rate of relaxation seen in the normal myocardium. This proportional rise in E and e′ results in a similar or sometimes lower E/e′ ratio. Assessment of E/e′ during or immediately after exercise has also been demonstrated to correlate with an elevation in left ventricular filling pressures. Here the mitral inflow pattern becomes "restrictive" with an E/A ratio of 2.5 and a deceleration time of 130 milliseconds. The e′ does not change, so the E/e′ ratio increases from 11 to 21. There is also evidence of increasing pulmonary hypertension with an estimated right ventricular systolic pressure more than 100 mm Hg, a finding that increases the specificity for the left-sided echo Doppler data. The hemodynamics of preserved ejection fraction heart failure was confirmed at cardiac catheterization (Fig. 28-8).[2-6]

See *The Echo Manual, 3rd Edition,* **discussion of estimation of filling pressures at rest and with exercise on page 138, and Tables 8-4 and 8-5 on page 139.**

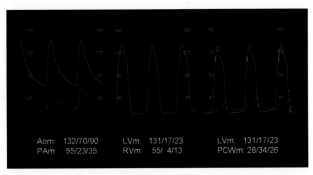

Figure 28-8

References

1. Bergeron S, Ommen SR, Bailey KR, et al. Exercise echocardiographic findings and outcome of patients referred for evaluation of dyspnea. *J Am Coll Cardiol.* 2004;43:2242–2246.

2. Ha JW, Lulic F, Bailey K, et al. Effects of treadmill exercise on mitral inflow and annular velocities in healthy adults. *Am J Cardiol.* 2003;91:114–115.

3. Ha JW, Oh JK, Pellikka PA, et al. Diastolic stress echocardiography: a novel noninvasive diagnostic test for diastolic dysfunction using supine bicycle exercise Doppler echocardiography. *J Am Soc Echocardiogr.* 2005;18:63–68.

4. Burgess MI, Jenkins C, Sharman JE, et al. Diastolic stress echocardiography: hemodynamic validation and clinical significance of estimation of ventricular filling pressure with exercise. *J Am Coll Cardiol.* 2006;47:1891–1900.

5. Talreja DR, Nishimura RA, Oh JK. Estimation of left ventricular filling pressure with exercise by Doppler echocardiography in patients with normal systolic function: a simultaneous echocardiographic-cardiac catheterization study. *J Am Soc Echocardiogr.* 2007;20:477–479.

6. Holland DJ, Prasad SB, Marwick TH. Prognostic implications of left ventricular filling pressure with exercise. *Circ Cardiovasc Imaging.* 2010;3(2):149–156.

CASE 29

Acute Pleuritic Chest Pain and Lightheadedness

*A*65-year-old man presents with acute pleuritic chest pain and lightheadedness. His systolic blood pressure varies between 90 and 100 mm Hg. He undergoes a CT scan of the chest with contrast (Figs. 29-1 and 29-2). On the basis of the findings, he undergoes transthoracic echocardiography (**Videos 29-1 to 29-8** and Figs. 29-3 to 29-5).

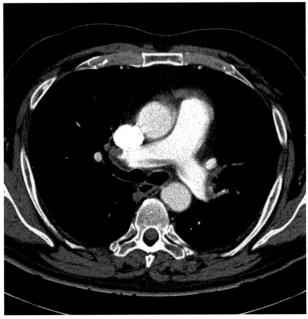

Figure 29-1

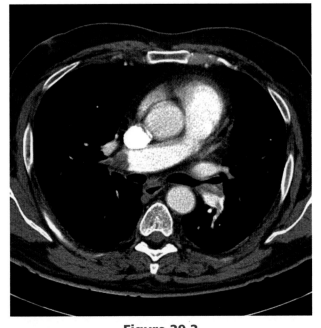

Figure 29-2

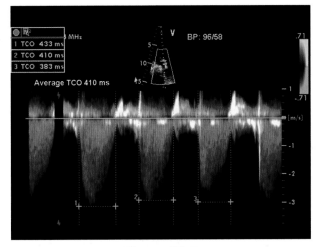

Figure 29-3

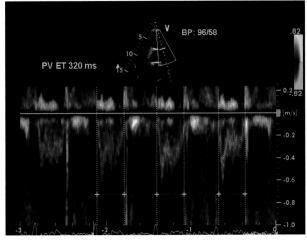

Figure 29-4

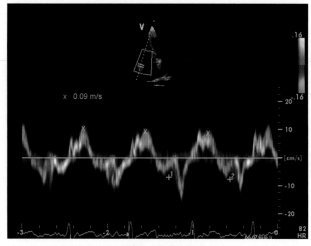

Figure 29-5

QUESTION 1. The RIMP (Tei index) is:

A. 0.22

B. 0.28

C. 0.34

D. 0.56

QUESTION 2. Which of the following is true with regard to right ventricular (RV) function?

A. The RIMP (Tei index) likely underestimates the severity of the RV dysfunction because of the acute high afterload

B. The RIMP (Tei index) likely underestimates the severity of the RV dysfunction because of the acute high preload

C. The RIMP (Tei index) and lateral tricuspid annulus tissue Doppler systolic velocity are concordant

D. The lateral tricuspid tissue Doppler systolic velocity likely overestimates the RV dysfunction

---

QUESTION 3. What do the right atrial mobile masses represent?

A. Renal tumor

B. Venous cast

C. Thrombi in situ

D. Atrial myxoma

QUESTION 4. With regard to the use of echocardiography in a patient with suspected or confirmed pulmonary embolism, which of the following statements is true?

A. Transthoracic echocardiography cannot stratify the risk of shock and death in patients presenting with pulmonary embolism who are normotensive

B. Transthoracic echocardiography will demonstrate the evidence of proximal pulmonary arterial thrombus or thrombus-in-transit in 20% to 25% of patients presenting with pulmonary embolism

C. Routine transthoracic echocardiography performed 6 weeks after acute pulmonary embolus should be considered to identify patients at risk for chronic thromboembolic pulmonary hypertension

D. Peak tricuspid regurgitant systolic velocity correlates with the severity of the pulmonary embolism

---

QUESTION 5. With regard to the use of thrombolytic therapy in a patient with confirmed pulmonary embolism, which of the following statements is true?

A. Fibrinolytic therapy is indicated in all patients with acute pulmonary embolism

B. Fibrinolytic therapy is indicated in patients with evidence of shock in the setting of acute pulmonary embolism

C. Fibrinolytic therapy is contraindicated in patients with acute pulmonary embolism and evidence of thrombus-in-transit on echocardiography

ANSWER 1: B. The myocardial performance index of the RV is a global estimate of RV systolic and diastolic function and is defined as the ratio of isovolumic time (nonejection work) divided by the ejection time (ejection work) (Fig. 29-6).

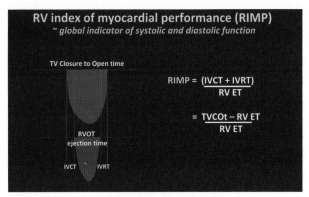

Figure 29-6

Reprinted from Tei C, Dujardin KS, Hodge DO, et al. Doppler echocardiographic index for assessment of global right ventricular function. *J Am Soc Echocardiogr* 1996:9;838-847, with permission from Elsevier.

It is calculated as the (tricuspid valve closure to opening time) − (RV ejection time)/(RV ejection time), with an upper reference limit being 0.40.

Here RIMP = (410 − 320)/320 = 0.28

ANSWER 2: B. The RIMP (Tei index), feasible in most patients, is reproducible, relatively independent of afterload and heart rates and avoids the geometric assumptions of some other global measures of RV function. However, it has been demonstrated to be unreliable when the right atrial pressure is high particularly in the acute setting. This leads to a more rapid equalization of right atrial and RV pressures, shortening the isovolumic relaxation time and resulting in an inappropriately small RIMP. The lateral tricuspid systolic velocity by pulsed tissue Doppler is a reproducible measure of basal longitudinal systolic function with a level <10 to 12 cm per second indicating abnormal contractility.[1,2]

ANSWER 3: B. Seen in the right atrium is thrombi-in-transit. These thrombi are highly mobile and have the appearance of a snake or popcorn. The mobile mass comes from en bloc embolization of venous thrombi cast.

ANSWER 4: C. Although there has been an assortment of criteria used that is a large body of data that demonstrates echocardiography identifies patients at increased risk for shock and death in the setting of acute pulmonary embolism and is particularly helpful in patients who are normotensive. Prospectively performed echocardiography studies in 209 consecutive patients who had acute pulmonary embolism demonstrated that 31% of normotensive patients did have RV dysfunction (RV dilatation, paradoxical septal motion, or tricuspid regurgitation velocity >2.8 m per second) and 10% of them developed shock and 5% died in hospital.[3]

Occasionally, thrombi-in-transit are detected in the chambers on the right side of the heart. In the international cooperative pulmonary embolism registry, this finding was observed in 42 (4%) of 1,135 patients with pulmonary embolism who had echocardiography studies. These thrombi are highly mobile and have the appearance of popcorn or a snake. The mobile mass comes from en bloc embolization of venous thrombi cast. The yield of visualizing proximal pulmonary arterial thrombus, although occasionally seen on transthoracic, is higher with transesophageal echocardiography.

Chronic thromboembolic pulmonary hypertension is a syndrome of pulmonary hypertension and right heart failure that occurs after one or more episodes of pulmonary emboli fail to resorb and triggers a chronic distal pulmonary vascular remodeling process. Although more than half of patients presenting with chronic thromboembolic disease were not previously aware of pulmonary emboli, screening echocardiography approximately 6 weeks after a clinical event of pulmonary embolic event will identify those patients who are at high risk for persistent pulmonary hypertension. In the acute setting, the RV is unable to generate a RV systolic pressure much higher than 50 to 60 mm Hg. Hence, markers of severity in acute pulmonary embolism include degree of RV dilation or dysfunction, markers of elevated right atrial pressure, and indicators of poor left ventricular filling. However, estimates of pulmonary artery pressure, although often mostly abnormal overall, reflect disease severity less well.[3–6]

ANSWER 5: B. Fibrinolysis, in addition to systemic anticoagulation with heparin-based therapy, is indicated in patients with *massive* pulmonary embolism (i.e., associated with shock) or *submassive* (i.e., clinical evidence of adverse prognosis, for example, severe RV dysfunction on echocardiography, new hemodynamic instability, or major myocardial necrosis). Fibrinolysis is not recommended for patients with pulmonary embolus that is of low risk. In patients with a large burden of thrombus-in-transit like in this case, consideration should be given to therapy in addition to heparin-based anticoagulation alone—specifically thrombolytic therapy or percutaneous or surgical embolectomy. Decisions should be based on patient characteristics including bleeding risk and expert availability. Our patient proceeded with successful emergent surgical embolectomy and did well.

References

1. Tei C, Dujardin KS, Hodge DO, et al. Doppler echocardiographic index for assessment of global right ventricular function. *J Am Soc Echocardiogr.* 1996:9;838–847.

2. Rudski LG, Lai WW, Afilalo J, et al. Guidelines for the echocardiographic assessment of the right heart in adults: a report from the American Society of Echocardiography: endorsed by the European Association of Echocardiography, a registered branch of the European Society of Cardiology, and the Canadian Society of Echocardiography. *J Am Soc Echocardiogr.* 2010:23;685–713.

3. Grifoni S, Olivotto I, Cecchini P, et al. Short-term clinical outcome of patients with acute pulmonary embolism, normal blood pressure, and echocardiographic right ventricular dysfunction. *Circulation.* 2000;101:2817–2822.

4. Jaff MR, McMurtry MS, Archer SL, et al. Management of massive and submassive pulmonary embolism, iliofemoral deep vein thrombosis and chronic thromboembolic pulmonary hypertension. *Circulation.* 2011;123:1788–1830.

5. Sanchez O, Trinquart L, Colombet I, et al. Prognostic value of right ventricular dysfunction in patients with haemodynamically stable pulmonary embolism: a systematic review. *Eur Heart J.* 2008;29:1569–1577.

6. Pengo V, Lensing AW, Prins MH, et al. Incidence of chronic thromboembolic pulmonary hypertension after pulmonary embolism. *N Engl J Med.* 2004;350:2257–2264.

Acute Severe Retrosternal Chest Discomfort

*A*n 80-year-old woman presents 24 hours after an episode of acute severe retrosternal chest discomfort. She no longer has chest pain; however, she feels weak. Her blood pressure is 90/60 mm Hg. Her ECG is shown in Figure 30-1. She undergoes an emergent transthoracic echocardiogram (see **Videos 30-1 to 30-8** and Figs. 30-2 to 30-4).

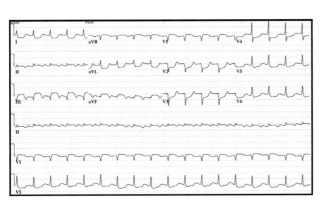

Figure 30-1

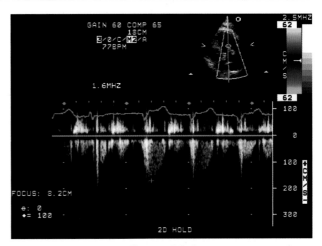

Figure 30-3

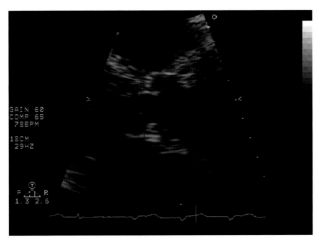

Figure 30-2

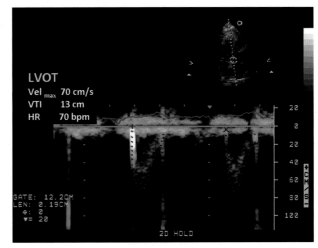

Figure 30-4

QUESTION 1. The calculated cardiac index is (body surface area = 1.6 cm^2):

A. 1.8
B. 2.2
C. 2.5
D. 2.9

QUESTION 2. On the basis of the echocardiographic findings, the appropriate management steps include:

A. Heparin intravenous anticoagulation and CT chest scan
B. Intravenous fluid and inotrope administration
C. Urgent surgical consultation
D. Intravenous diuresis and intra-aortic balloon pump
E. Intravenous nitroglycerin and intra-aortic balloon pump

QUESTION 3. The expected tricuspid annular systolic plane excursion (TAPSE) in this case would be:

A. 4 mm
B. 14 mm
C. 24 mm
D. 34 mm

QUESTION 4. The next day the patient became progressively more short of breath with low oxygen saturations. Oxygen saturations remained 85% despite high-flow supplemental oxygen. An emergent echocardiogram is ordered. Which of the following components of the echocardiogram is most likely to be diagnostic?

A. 2D and color Doppler assessment of the mitral valve
B. 2D and color Doppler assessment of the interventricular septum
C. 2D assessment of the pericardium
D. 2D regional wall motion assessment of the left ventricle
E. Agitated saline contrast study

QUESTION 5. On reviewing **Video 30-9**, the likely pathology is:

A. Normal echo contrast study
B. Evidence of an intracardiac left-right shunt
C. Evidence of an intracardiac right-left shunt
D. Evidence of an intrapulmonary shunt

ANSWER 1: A. Stroke volume (SV) is calculated from the left ventricular outflow tract (LVOT) as a product of the LVOT area ([LVOT diameter/2]² × 3.14) and the LVOT time velocity integral.

Here SV = 3.14 × (2/2 cm)² × 13 cm = 41 ml at a heart rate of 70 beats per minute = cardiac output of 2.9 L per minute and a cardiac index of 1.8 L/min/m²

See *The Echo Manual, 3rd Edition*, Figure 4-16 on pages 71 and 72.

ANSWER 2: B. There is evidence of right ventricular enlargement and dysfunction in the setting of inferior wall hypokinesis. These findings are consistent with infarction in the distribution of the right coronary artery. Hypotension is mediated through poor right-sided cardiac output and decreased left ventricular filling. Management should involve avoidance of agents that drop left ventricular preload further (e.g., diuretics and nitroglycerin); instead, the use of intravenous fluids and inotropes is indicated. Heparin and chest CT would be the appropriate line of management if an acute pulmonary embolus was the consideration, which is not the case here.

ANSWER 3: A. An easy to obtain measure that reflects right ventricular longitudinal systolic function is the absolute distance of excursion of the lateral tricuspid annulus toward the apex during systole. A normal value is being ≥20 mm. A reduction in TAPSE (<15 mm) has been shown to strongly associate with a high risk of adverse events following acute myocardial infarction.[1]

ANSWER 4: E. Echocardiography is a key test in the evaluation of a new complication following myocardial infarction. The presence of hypoxemia that persists despite oxygen supplementation is highly suggestive of shunt physiology. An agitated saline study to assess for right-left shunt is needed.

ANSWER 5: C. On agitated saline administration and filling of the right atrium, there is almost immediate presence of contrast bubbles in the left-sided chambers, initially the left atrium and the left ventricle. This is diagnostic of a right to left shunt at the atrial level. The degree of shunting and hence peripheral hypoxemia is exacerbated by the high right atrial pressures seen in the setting of acute right ventricular infarction that open up a patent foramen ovale. This condition was difficult to manage before the application of a percutaneous closure devise.

Reference

1. Antoni ML, Scherptong RW, Atary JZ, et al. Prognostic value of right ventricular function in patients after acute myocardial infarction treated with primary percutaneous coronary intervention. *Circ Cardiovasc Imaging.* 2010;3:264–271.

CASE 31

Lightheadedness and Severe Fatigue

*M*r. VD is a 46-year-old man with a history of diabetes mellitus and hypertension who presents to the emergency department after the onset of lightheadedness and severe fatigue. Three days before, he had spent the day in bed with a bad case of indigestion. On examination, he has a systolic blood pressure of 75 mm Hg and an audible systolic murmur. He undergoes a bedside transthoracic echocardiogram (see **Video 31-1, Fig. 31-1**).

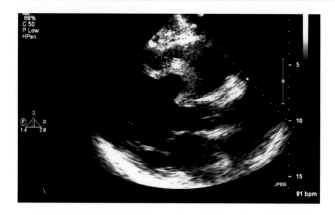

Figure 31-1

QUESTION 1. Which of the following mechanisms likely underlies the findings?

A. Anterolateral papillary muscle rupture

B. Postmyocardial infarction rupture of the ventricular septum

C. Left ventricular (LV) outflow tract obstruction

D. Free wall rupture

QUESTION 2. Diagnostic findings on invasive catheterization include:

A. Oxygen saturation samples

B. Pulmonary capillary wedge tracing

C. LV end-diastolic pressure change following a premature ventricular contraction

D. Thermodilution cardiac output measurements

QUESTION 3. The findings on coronary angiography are likely:

A. Occluded left circumflex coronary artery

B. Occluded left anterior descending coronary artery (LAD)

C. Occluded right coronary artery

D. High-grade obstructive three-vessel coronary disease

QUESTION 4. The right ventricular (RV) systolic pressure is:

A. 50 mm Hg

B. 25 mm Hg

C. 25 mm Hg plus right atrial pressure

D. 60 mm Hg

QUESTION 5. The appropriate management is:

A. Intra-aortic balloon pump and surgical consultation

B. Intra-aortic balloon pump and percutaneous coronary intervention

C. Percutaneous coronary intervention and percutaneous defect closure

ANSWER 1: B. Ventricular septal rupture occurs in 1% to 3% of patients after myocardial infarction, and it occurs during the early phase of acute infarction (within the first week). As in free wall rupture, ventricular septal rupture is more common in elderly women who have not had a previous myocardial infarction. The typical clinical presentation is a new systolic murmur, with abrupt and progressive hemodynamic deterioration.

The differential diagnosis of a new systolic murmur in patients with acute myocardial infarction includes infarct-related ventricular septal rupture, papillary muscle dysfunction or rupture, pericardial rub, acute LV outflow tract obstruction, and free wall rupture. After physical examination, echocardiography is the next logical noninvasive diagnostic procedure for all patients with a new murmur, especially for those who are hemodynamically unstable. Infarct-related ventricular septal defect is diagnosed by the demonstration of a disrupted ventricular septum with a left-to-right shunt, as in this case. It is interesting that the patient's main symptom was fatigue and light-headedness, but no shortness of breath which is a predominant symptom of severe acute mitral regurgitation due to papillary muscle rupture. Another important condition to keep in mind for patients with a new systolic murmur after acute myocardial infarction is acute LVOT obstruction.

The defect is located in the region of thinned myocardium with dyskinetic motion. Here echocardiography demonstrates a mildly enlarged LV with depressed systolic function, and LV ejection fraction is 30% to 35%. There is anterior and apical akinesis. The LV anteroseptum is dyskinetic, and there is a serpiginous defect through the basal portion with left-to-right shunting.

See *The Echo Manual, 3rd Edition,* page 162.

ANSWER 2: A. Oxygen saturation samples. The characteristic findings at right heart catheterization of a patient with an acute ventricular septal defect are of an oxygen saturation "setup" with a pulmonary arterial oxygen saturation 10% greater than the oxygen saturation in the right atrium.

See *The Echo Manual, 3rd Edition,* Table 10-2 on page 162.

ANSWER 3: B. An increased risk of ventricular septal rupture is seen in patients with high-grade single-vessel coronary disease (especially the left anterior descending

artery). The prevalence is higher in the setting of first myocardial infarction. Septal rupture may occur in the setting of acute infarction with a large wrap around left anterior descending artery or an acute infarction involving the right coronary artery. When the rupture is in the inferoseptum, the myocardial infarction usually involves the RV, which portends a poor prognosis. An inferoseptal ventricular septal rupture can be a serpiginous septal tear, and an antero-apical septal ventricular septal rupture may evolve into an LV free wall rupture. Seen here the extensive wall motion abnormalities involving the septum, anterior wall, and apex point toward the LAD as being the infarct-related artery.

See *The Echo Manual, 3rd Edition,* page 162.

ANSWER 4: A. The peak velocity from the continuous wave Doppler interrogation across the ventricular septal defect corresponds to the peak gradient between the LV and RV. Seen here the continuous wave Doppler tracing indicates a continuous shunt through the ventricular septal defect except during early diastole. The peak systolic flow velocity is 2.5 m per second (Fig. 31-2), corresponding to a 25 mm Hg pressure gradient between the LV and the RV. Systolic blood pressure was 75 mm Hg, hence RV systolic pressure = 50 mm Hg.

See *The Echo Manual, 3rd Edition,* page 162 and Figure 10-11 on page 164.

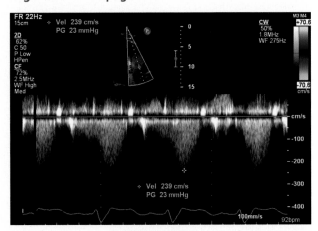

Figure 31-2

ANSWER 5: B. Intra-aortic balloon pump and surgical consultation. The current recommended approach to an infarct-related ventricular septal rupture is afterload reduction, intra-aortic balloon pump counterpulsation, and urgent surgical intervention.[1]

Reference

1. Reeder GS. Identification and treatment of complications of myocardial infarction. *Mayo Clin Proc.* 1995;70:880–884.

CASE 32

Retrosternal Chest Pain

A 65-year-old woman presents to the emergency department after 1 hour of retrosternal chest pain. She is observed for 6 hours, and serial ECG and troponin T measurements are normal. Her exercise capacity is limited secondary to severe arthritis in her knee. She is referred for dobutamine stress echocardiography (see **Videos 32-1 to 32-4**) (Please note that the apical 4 chamber view is in the Mayo Clinic format with the left ventricle displayed on the left).

QUESTION 1. Stress echocardiography demonstrates evidence of:

- A. Normal study
- B. Anterior ischemia
- C. Anterior infarction and inferior ischemia
- D. Inferior and lateral ischemia
- E. Lateral infarction

QUESTION 2. Which of the following findings at dobutamine stress echocardiography is suggestive of myocardial ischemia?

- A. Normal resting wall motion, an initial hyperdynamic response with low-dose dobutamine followed by a decline in function at higher doses
- B. A dobutamine-induced deterioration in normal wall motion without a change at low-dose dobutamine
- C. A hypokinetic apex at rest that becomes akinetic at higher doses of dobutamine
- D. A hypotensive response to peak doses of dobutamine
- E. A, B, and C

QUESTION 3. Decreasing the mechanical index to optimize contrast images can be accomplished by:

- A. Increasing the ultrasound frequency
- B. Lowering the ultrasound frequency
- C. Decreasing the output power of the transducer
- D. Decreasing the gain settings of the transducer
- E. A and C
- F. B and D

QUESTION 4. Appropriate indications for dobutamine stress echocardiography might include all of the following except?

- A. Preoperative cardiac risk assessment in a 55-year-old diabetic man being considered for aortobifemoral bypass for symptomatic peripheral arterial disease
- B. A 70-year-old woman complaining of atypical angina that occurs with brisk activity with 1.5 mm of downsloping lateral ST depression on her resting ECG
- C. A 68-year-old man with typical angina occurring after climbing three flights of stairs
- D. A 58-year-old woman with an exertional chest pain syndrome who had a negative stress ECG test, stopping at a peak heart rate of 110 beats per minute because of limiting knee pain
- E. A and D

ANSWER 1: D. Regional contractility was normal at rest; however, with incremental dobutamine infusion, the patient developed inferior and lateral hypokinesis with left ventricular dilation and a reduction in ejection fraction from 65% to 50% at peak stress. Findings that are highly suggestive of left circumflex +/− right coronary artery disease. Coronary angiography demonstrated 90% left circumflex (Fig. 32-1) and 70% right coronary artery (Fig. 32-2) stenoses.

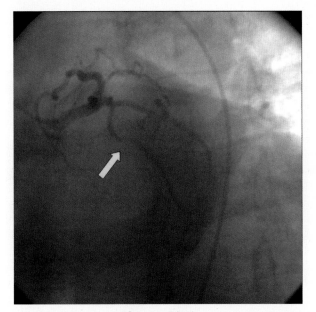

Figure 32-1

ANSWER 2: E. The typical finding of ischemia during a dobutamine stress echocardiogram is the development of new/worsening wall motion abnormalities with dobutamine infusion. These segments may or may not initially display hypercontractility at lower doses of dobutamine. A hypotensive response to dobutamine is typically related to the vasodilatory effects of peripheral β-receptor stimulation in the setting of a small hyperdynamic left ventricle and does not necessarily represent the presence of coronary artery disease. Hypotension may also occur in the setting of severe dynamic outflow tract obstruction induced by dobutamine. Patients with chronically ischemic myocardial segments may demonstrate myocardial hibernation. This is characterized by a biphasic myocardial response to dobutamine infusion with an improvement in resting wall motion abnormalities at low doses of dobutamine with a subsequent decline in myocardial contractility at higher doses.

ANSWER 3: E. Mechanical index is proportional to the peak power and inversely proportional to the square root of the frequency.

ANSWER 4: E. Dobutamine stress echocardiography is appropriate in patients who have valid indications for stress echocardiography but are unable to exercise. Patient A likely has a limited exercise capacity, is at more than mild clinical risk of ischemic heart disease, and will undergo a high-risk nonemergent surgical procedure. Patient B requires imaging because her stress ECG will be nondiagnostic, but an exercise stress should be considered. Patient C has exertional symptoms and a high pretest probability for coronary artery disease. Patient D has an equivocal stress ECG test because of noncardiac limitation and is appropriate to undergo a pharmacologic stress test to evaluate her chest pain syndrome.[1]

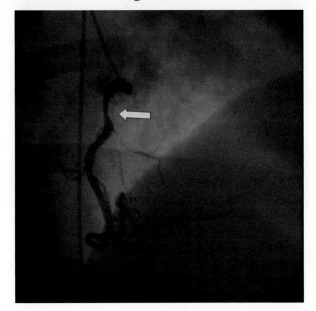

Figure 32-2

References

1. Douglas PS, Khandheria B, Stainback RF, et al. ACCF/ASE/ACEP/AHA/ASNC/SCAI/SCCT/SCMR 2008 appropriateness criteria for stress echocardiography. *J Am Coll Cardiol.* 2008;18:1127–1147.

CASE 33

Dyspnea and Chest Tightness

A 72-year-old woman with dyspnea and chest tightness on mild to moderate exertion presents for evaluation. She has had two recent hospitalizations for acute respiratory failure. Her medical history is significant for systemic hypertension, cardiomyopathy, atrial fibrillation, and defibrillator placement.

QUESTION 1. On the basis of the 12-lead ECG (Fig. 33-1), what is the likely type of cardiomyopathy?

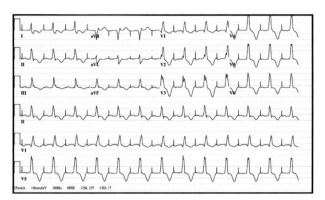

Figure 33-1

A. Septal hypertrophic cardiomyopathy
B. Apical variant of hypertrophic cardiomyopathy
C. Ischemic cardiomyopathy
D. Right ventricular dysplasia

QUESTION 2. On the basis of the transthoracic echocardiographic images (**Videos 33-1 to 33-5** and Figs. 33-2 to 33-6), the findings are consistent with:

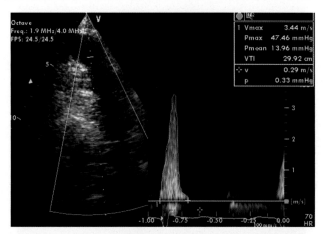

Figure 33-2

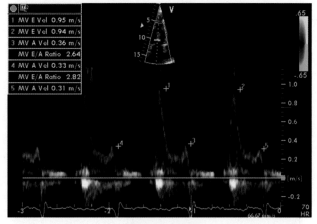

Figure 33-3

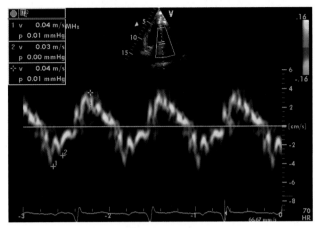

Figure 33-4

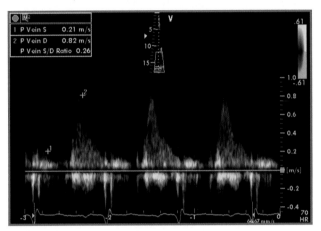

Figure 33-5

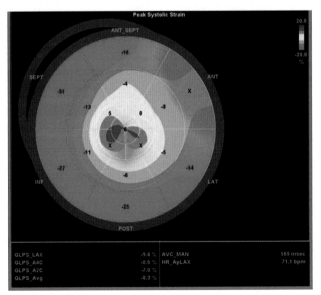

Figure 33-6

A. Normal left ventricular regional wall contractility
B. Apical infarct with aneurysmal formation
C. Apical hypertrophic cardiomyopathy
D. Contained apical rupture

QUESTION 3. Diastolic function is:

A. Normal
B. Mildly abnormal
C. Moderately abnormal
D. Severely abnormal

QUESTION 4. Given these findings, a limited exercise capacity, and significant symptoms, which of the following is a likely beneficial management option?

A. Left ventricular assist device
B. Alcohol ablation
C. Surgical myectomy
D. None of the choices

QUESTION 5. The patient underwent successful treatment and left ventriculography 2 weeks later (**Video 33-6**).

After 3 months, the patient represents with acute left ventricular failure. She undergoes repeat echocardiography (**Videos 33-7 to 33-9** and Figs. 33-7 to 33-9). The likely mechanism for the patient's acute pulmonary edema is:

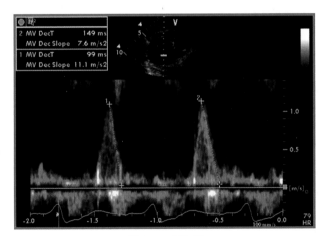

Figure 33-7

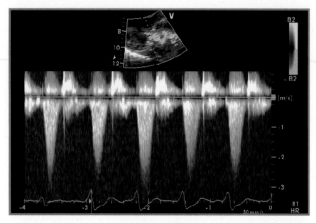

Figure 33-8

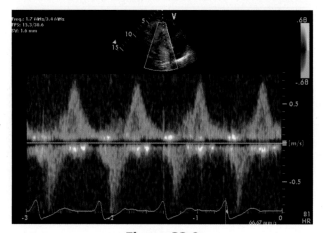

Figure 33-9

A. Severe mitral valve regurgitation
B. Apical ballooning syndrome
C. Acute anterior wall myocardial infarction
D. Severe diastolic dysfunction

QUESTION 6. The patient is referred back to the operating room for mitral valve replacement. On the basis of the intraoperative study (**Videos 33-10 to 33-13**), the next step should be:

A. Cancel the case
B. Obtain a confirmatory contrast left ventriculogram
C. Intravenous dobutamine
D. Intravenous phenylephrine

ANSWER 1: A. The ECG demonstrates deep symmetrical precordial T-waves typical for the pattern seen with apical hypertrophic cardiomyopathy.

ANSWER 2: C. 2D images demonstrate severe hypertrophy of the mid and apical two-thirds of the left ventricle with systolic obliteration at this level and near diastolic obliteration of the neck into the apical pouch.

ANSWER 3: D. The functional ventricular chamber is essentially the basal one-third that results in restrictive filling typified by the mitral inflow pattern with a high early (E) velocity that is much greater than a diminutive A velocity, diastolic predominant pulmonary vein flow, and a markedly reduced early diastolic medial annulus tissue velocity (e′).

ANSWER 4: C. In patients with symptomatic apical hypertrophic cardiomyopathy refractory to medical management, a surgical apical (and here midventricular) myectomy has been performed with a reasonable success. There is no role for alcohol ablation in the apical variant of hypertrophic cardiomyopathy.[1]

ANSWER 5: A. Repeat transthoracic echocardiography demonstrates mitral valve leaflet tethering with resultant severe mitral valve regurgitation.

ANSWER 6: D. Transesophageal images demonstrate that there appears to be only mild mitral valve regurgitation (Fig. 33-10). This striking difference compared with the transthoracic echocardiogram is likely because of differences in the loading conditions brought about by anesthesia. Infusion of phenylephrine that increased the systolic blood pressure from 90 mm Hg to 150 mm Hg resulted in the unmasking of severe mitral valve regurgitation (Fig. 33-11) associated with a rise in the mean pulmonary artery pressure from 25 to

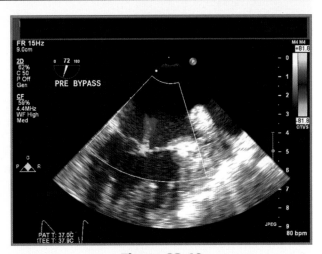

Figure 33-10

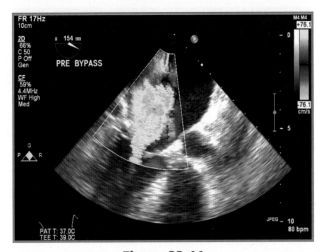

Figure 33-11

50 mm Hg. The patient underwent successful mitral valve replacement and did very well.

Differences in loading conditions with anesthesia may lead to underestimation of mitral valve regurgitation by reduction in preload that leads to a decrease in mitral annulus diameter and improved leaflet coaptation and/or a reduction in afterload that decreases the pressure gradient across the mitral valve.[2,3]

References

1. Schaff HV, Brown ML, Dearani JA, et al. Apical myectomy: a new surgical technique for management of severely symptomatic patients with apical hypertrophic cardiomyopathy. *J Thorac Cardiovasc Surg.* 2010;139:634–640.

2. Grewal KS, Malkowski MJ, Piracha AR, et al. Effect of general anesthesia on the severity of mitral regurgitation by transesophageal echocardiography. *Am J Cardiol.* 2000;85:199–203.

3. Mihalatos DG, Gopal AS, Kates R, et al. Intraoperative assessment of mitral regurgitation: role of phenylephrine challenge. *J Am Soc Echocardiogr.* 2006;19:1158–1164.

CASE 34

Exertional Dyspnea

A 36-year-old woman presents with 4 days of exertional dyspnea. She is 6 days after delivery of a healthy baby boy at 41 weeks of gestation. This was her first pregnancy and was uncomplicated. She has no medical history. On examination, her heart rate is 130 beats per minute. There is evidence of neck vein distension and peripheral edema. Her body surface area is 1.8 and her body mass index 27 (**Videos 34-1 to 34-5** and Figs. 34-1 to 34-6).

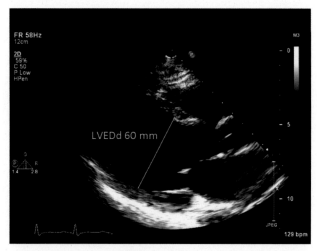

Figure 34-1

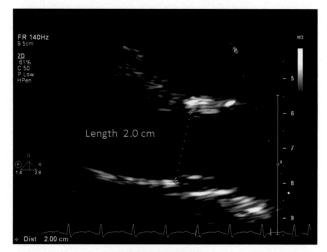

Figure 34-3

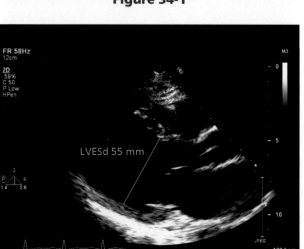

Figure 34-2

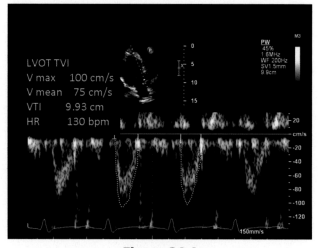

Figure 34-4

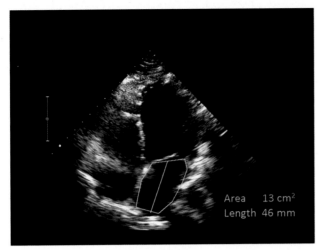

Area   13 cm²
Length 46 mm

Figure 34-5

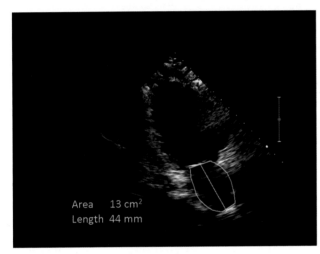

Area   13 cm²
Length 44 mm

Figure 34-6

QUESTION 1. What is the calculated left ventricular ejection fraction (LVEF)?

   A. 11%
   B. 16%
   C. 21%
   D. 26%
   E. 31%

QUESTION 2. The Doppler-derived left ventricular cardiac index is:

   A. 1.9 L/min/m²
   B. 2.2 L/min/m²
   C. 2.6 L/min/m²
   D. 3.5 L/min/m²
   E. 4.0 L/min/m²

QUESTION 3. The calculated left atrial (LA) volume index by the biplane area length method is:

   A. 18 mL/m²
   B. 21 mL/m²
   C. 24 mL/m²
   D. 28 mL/m²
   E. 32 mL/m²

QUESTION 4. The likely etiology for the clinical and echocardiographic findings is:

   A. Chronic idiopathic dilated cardiomyopathy exacerbated by the postpartum state
   B. Amniotic fluid embolus
   C. Peripartum cardiomyopathy
   D. Spontaneous coronary artery dissection

QUESTION 5. Appropriate steps in this patient's management might include all of the following *except:*

   A. Angiotensin-converting enzyme (ACE) inhibition
   B. Counseling to avoid lactation
   C. ß-Adrenoceptor antagonism
   D. Bromocriptine
   E. Immunosuppression

QUESTION 6. The patient returns 9 months later after medical therapy. On the basis of repeat transthoracic echocardiography (**Video 34-6** and Fig. 34-7), recommendations include:

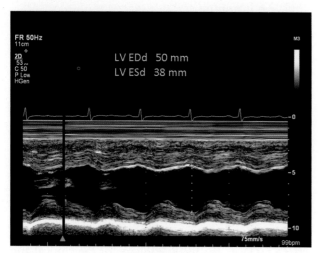

Figure 34-7

A. Further pregnancies are contraindicated
B. ACE inhibition may be stopped, but further pregnancies should be avoided
C. ACE inhibition may be stopped, and it is likely safe to consider a future pregnancy

ANSWER 1: B. As recommended by the American Society of Echocardiography, the long- and short-axis dimensions can be obtained directly from the ESd and EDd, measured at the level of the mitral tips as the smallest and largest diameters, respectively. If there are no regional wall motion abnormalities, the left ventricular dimensions measured from the level of the papillary muscles can be used to calculate the LVEF as follows:

$$\text{Uncorrected LVEF (uLVEF)} = [(EDd)^2 - (ESd)^2] / (EDd)^2] \times 100$$
$$\text{Corrected LVEF} = uLVEF + [(100 - uLVEF) \times \text{correction factor}\%]$$

The correction factor is 15% if apical function is normal, 5% if apical function is hypokinetic, or 0% if apical function is severely hypokinetic or akinetic.

Here,

$$uLVEF = [(60)^2 - (55)^2] / (60)^2] \times 100 = 16\%$$
$$\text{Corrected LVEF} = 16 + [(100 - 16) \times 0\%] = 16\%$$

ANSWER 2: B. Stroke volume (SV) is calculated as the product of the cross-sectional area of the left ventricular outflow tract (LVOT) and the time velocity integral (TVI) of a pulse-wave sample from the LVOT.

$$\begin{aligned} SV \text{ (ml)} &= [(D/2)^2 \times \pi] \times [\text{LVOT TVI}] \\ &= [(2/2)^2 \times \pi] \times [10] \\ &= 3.14 \times 10 \\ &= 31 \text{ ml} \end{aligned}$$

Cardiac output is the product of SV and heart rate $= 31 \times 130 = 4{,}030$ ml per minute

Cardiac index = cardiac output/body surface area
$$= 4/1.8 = 2.2 \text{ L/min/m}^2$$

See *The Echo Manual, 3rd Edition*, **Figure 4-16 on page 71.**

ANSWER 3: A. The biplane area–length method requires measuring LA area from two orthogonal apical views (apical four chamber and apical two chamber) and LA length. The average of the two lengths is used.

LA volume = $(0.85 \times \text{area}_1 \times \text{area}_2)$/Average length
LA volume = $(0.85 \times 13 \times 13)/4.5^*$

*It is important to use consistent units: cm² for area and cm for length.

LA volume = 32 cc
When indexed to body surface area = 18 cc per m²

ANSWER 4: C. The echocardiogram demonstrates mild to moderate left ventricular dilatation, severe global reduction in left ventricular contractility with depressed ejection fraction and SV. The LA size is normal. The most likely etiology is peripartum cardiomyopathy that can present anytime between the last trimester of pregnancy and 6 months postpartum, most commonly becoming clinically apparent in the first month after delivery. It is more common in patients older than 30 years and/or who are African American. A chronic cardiomyopathy is less likely in the setting of an entirely normal LA size, and if it were to have given rise to clinical heart failure, would more likely have done so either in the second to third trimester or immediately postpartum. An amniotic fluid embolus is a rare complication occurring in the immediate postpartum period, and although left ventricular dysfunction may occur, the primary insult is seen with the right ventricle (dilation and dysfunction). A spontaneous coronary artery dissection would be expected to have an associated clinical chest pain syndrome and left ventricular regional dysfunction.

ANSWER 5: E. Standard medical therapy for systolic heart failure including ACE inhibition and ß-blockade is critical. It is important to recognize that ACE inhibitors are contraindicated if the diagnosis is made prior to delivery as they are highly teratogenic. Recent studies have identified a potentially pathophysiologic role by a defective antioxidant defense mechanism triggering pathogenic prolactin fragments, and hence, suppression prolactin production with bromocriptine is indicated (warfarin anticoagulation also needed). For the same reasons, counseling against lactation is reasonable. Immunosuppression is only indicated in the setting of cases of biopsy-proven giant cell myocarditis or other acute inflammatory cardiomyopathies but not idiopathic peripartum cardiomyopathy.[1]

ANSWER 6: A. Repeat echocardiography demonstrates that the left ventricular size has normalized and the LVEF has improved, though remaining depressed, with a calculated LVEF 41%. In this setting, the patient needs to remain on heart failure therapy, and future pregnancy should be avoided because it would come with a high risk to the mother.

Reference

1. Sliwa K, Blauwet L, Tibazarwa K, et al. Evaluation of bromocriptine in the treatment of acute severe peripartum cardiomyopathy: a proof-of-concept pilot study. *Circulation*. 2010;121:1465–73.

CASE 35

Severe Angina

A 53-year-old woman presents to the emergency department for the evaluation of severe angina (**Videos 35-1 and 35-2**).

QUESTION 1. Which of the following scenarios may explain the patient's echo findings?

- A. Subarachnoid hemorrhage
- B. Pheochromocytoma
- C. Recent emotional stress
- D. Coronary artery atherosclerosis
- E. All of the scenarios

QUESTION 2. Appropriate treatment strategies for the patient's hypotension might include all of the following *except*:

- A. Intravenous dopamine
- B. Intravenous metoprolol
- C. Intravenous phenylephrine
- D. Intravenous fluids

QUESTION 3. If the systemic blood pressure is 80/50 mm Hg, the peak left ventricular pressure is approximately:

- A. 60 mm Hg
- B. 80 mm Hg
- C. 110 mm Hg
- D. 130 mm Hg

QUESTION 4. Which of the following statements is correct?

- A. This condition occurs more frequently in young women with stress
- B. LV function does not recover fully in most of patients
- C. Myocardial contrast echo shows a large perfusion defect
- D. This condition can occur repeatedly

ANSWER 1: E. Transthoracic echocardiography demonstrates hyperdynamic basal left ventricular contractility with akinesis of the mid and distal left ventricle. Although these findings may occur in the setting of severe coronary artery diease, the appearance is consistent with that which occurs in the setting of an acute myocardial infarction with normal coronary arteries.

See *The Echo Manual, 3rd Edition*, page 167.

ANSWER 2: A. Echocardiography demonstrates a dynamic left ventricular outflow tract obstruction secondary to the hyperdynamic basal contractility that occurs in approximately 15% of stress-induced cardiomyopathy. There is systolic anterior motion of the anterior mitral valve leaflet with posterior-directed mitral valve regurgitation. Appropriate management in this setting includes intravenous fluids, β-blockers, peripheral vasoconstrictors, and the avoidance of inotropic agents.[1]

ANSWER 3: D. The peak left ventricular systolic pressure will be the sum of the systemic systolic blood pressure (80 mm Hg) and the left ventricular outflow tract pressure gradient $(4 \times [3.5]^2) = 129$ mm Hg.

ANSWER 4: D. Stress induced cardiomyopathy is a phenomenon that most commonly affects post-menopausal women. Patients typically present with a chest pain syndrome and ECG abnormalities (frequently ST segment elevation) but are found to have normal coronary arteries at angiography (and echo contrast perfusion). Left ventricular function is depressed but recovers in the majority to normal within days to a few weeks. While most patients do well, up to 10% have have a recurrence.[1,2]

Reference

1. Bybee KA, Kara T, Prasad A, et al. Systemic review: transient left ventricular apical ballooning: a syndrome that mimics ST-segment elevation myocardial infarction. *Ann Intern Med.* 2004:141(11):858–865.

2. Madhavan M, Rihal CS, Lerman A, Prasad A. Acute heart failure in apical ballooning syndrome (TakoTsubo/stress cardiomyopathy): clinical correlates and Mayo Clinic risk score. J Am Coll Cardiol 2011;57(12):1400-01.

Exertional Fatigue, Dyspnea, and Two-Pillow Orthopnea

A 30-year-old man presents with exertional fatigue, dyspnea, and two-pillow orthopnea. He is referred for transthoracic echocardiography (**Video 36-1**).

QUESTION 1. Potential underlying etiologies for the findings include all of the following *except*:

    A. Idiopathic

    B. Iron overload

    C. HIV infection

    D. Scleroderma

    E. Myocarditis

QUESTION 2. The Doppler-derived cardiac output (see Figs. 36-1 and 36-2) is:

    A. 2.9 L per minute

    B. 3.5 L per minute

    C. 4.2 L per minute

    D. 6.5 L per minute

    E. 7.4 L per minute

QUESTION 3. An appropriate next step may include:

    A. Iron studies

    B. Endomyocardial biopsy

    C. Coronary angiography

    D. Systemic anticoagulation

    E. All of the choices

QUESTION 4. Endomyocardial biopsy (**Video 36-2**) is associated with a risk of ventricular thrombus.

    A. True

    B. False

QUESTION 5. With regard to testing for hemochromatosis, which of the following is true?

    A. A serum ferritin level >300 ng per ml is diagnostic for hemochromatosis

    B. A negative endomyocardial biopsy excludes the diagnosis

    C. Shortened relaxation times of cardiac MRI signals is highly sensitive for the diagnosis

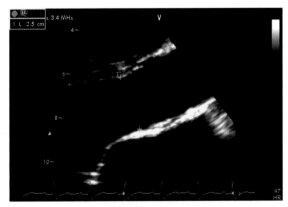

Figure 36-1

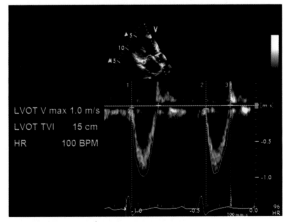

Figure 36-2

ANSWER 1: D. An unexpected finding of dilated cardiomyopathy in a young person should raise the suspicion for genetic idiopathic dilated cardiomyopathy or a secondary cause such as hemochromatosis (iron overload), HIV infection, and postviral myocarditis. Scleroderma may lead to a serositis, valve dysfunction, and/or pulmonary arterial hypertension. Marked global left ventricular systolic dysfunction is not a feature typically seen in patients with sarcoidosis.[1]

ANSWER 2: E. The cardiac output can be calculated as $= (\pi r^2)(LVOT\ TVI)(HR)$

$$= 0.785(D)^2 (LVOT\ TVI)(HR)$$
$$= 0.785 \times (2.5)^2 \times (15) \times (100)$$
$$= 7.4\ L\ per\ minute$$

See *The Echo Manual, 3rd Edition*, stroke volume on page 116.

ANSWER 3: E. All of the choices. In patients who present with heart failure in the setting of unexplained left ventricular global hypokinesis, one should consider potential primary etiologies. This should include coronary artery disease, hemochromatosis, and other primary etiologies of dilated cardiomyopathy. Furthermore, owing to the presence of mobile masses, highly suspicious for thrombus, the patients should also be anticoagulated.

ANSWER 4: A. True. Despite therapeutic anticoagulation with unfractionated heparin, the day after endomyocardial biopsy repeat transthoracic echocardiography (**Video 36-3**) demonstrates more mobility to the thrombus in the left ventricular apex and new mobile thrombus attached to the ventricular septal surface of the right ventricle at the site of endomyocardial biopsy.

ANSWER 5: C. Although a serum ferritin level >300 ng per ml (>200 ng per ml in women) is the suggested cutoff for screening in patients; it must be recognized that serum ferritin is an acute phase reactant and may increase with stress. Endomyocardial biopsy is the traditional gold standard for the diagnosis of cardiac hemochromatosis; however, the iron deposition in the heart is not uniform and may be missed on biopsy. In iron-loaded tissue, the paramagnetic effect of iron shortens the relaxation time of tissue signals. Cardiac magnetic resonance relaxation times correlate not only with the presence or absence of iron overload but also with the risk of clinical decompensation in patients with cardiac hemochromatosis.[2]

With medical therapy (lisinopril, carvedilol, warfarin, and chelation therapy), the patient gradually improved left ventricular contractility (see **Video 36-4**).

References

1. Varess G, Bruce CJ, Andreen K, et al. Acute thrombus formation as a complication of right ventricular biopsy. *J Am Soc Echocardiogr*. 2010;23:1039–1044.

2. Gujjs P, Rosing DR, Tripodi DJ, et al. Iron overload cardiomyopathy. *J Am Coll Cardiol*. 2010;56:1–12.

Three-Month History of Progressive Exertional Shortness of Breath

*A*60-year-old man presents with a 3-month history of progressive exertional shortness of breath. He is referred for transthoracic echocardiogram (**Videos 37-1 to 37-11** and Figs. 37-1 to 37-3).

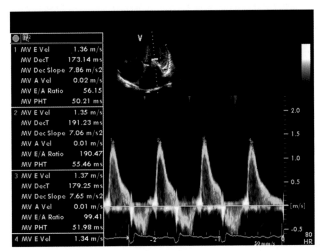

Figure 37-1

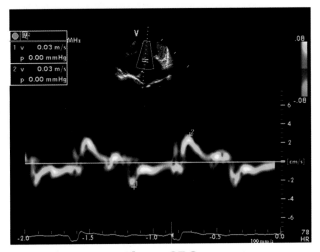

Figure 37-3

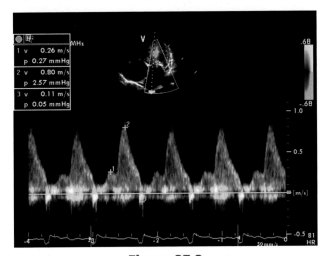

Figure 37-2

QUESTION 1. The left ventricular filling pressures are:

   A. Normal
   B. Mildly elevated
   C. Moderately elevated
   D. Severely elevated

QUESTION 2. Which of the following blood tests is most likely to aid in the diagnosis in this patient?

   A. Immunoassay for serum free light chains
   B. Iron studies
   C. Serum brain natriuretic peptide level
   D. Serum angiotensin converting enzyme level
   E. Serum protein electrophoresis

QUESTION 3. Which of the following systolic longitudinal strain patterns would be most consistent with the 2D findings and diagnosis?

A. Figure 37-4A
B. Figure 37-4B
C. Figure 37-4C
D. Figure 37-4D

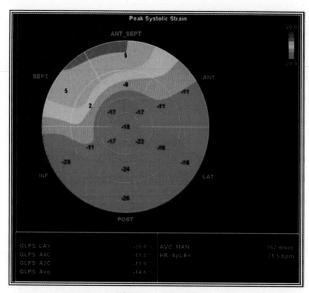

Figure 37-4C

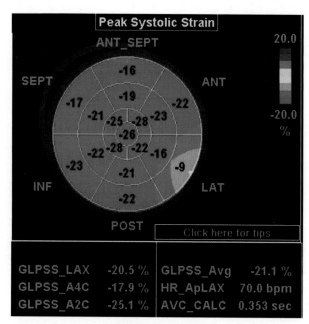

Figure 37-4A

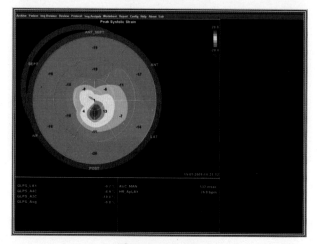

Figure 37-4D

QUESTION 4. Factor or factors that are helpful in determining the appropriate treatment strategies and prognosis in this disorder include:

A. Cardiac troponin T
B. N terminal pro-brain natriuretic peptide (NT-pro BNP)
C. Serum uric acid
D. Serum free light chains
E. All of the choices

QUESTION 5. What is the likely incidence of intracardiac thrombus in this patient?

A. 0% to 10%
B. 11% to 25%
C. 26% to 40%
D. >40%

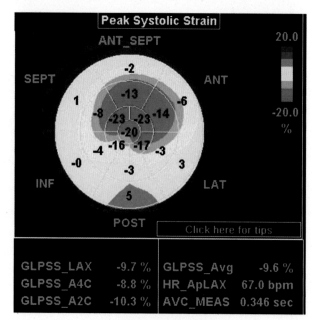

Figure 37-4B

ANSWER 1: D. Mitral inflow peak early (E) velocity is high at 1.4 m per second with a marked reduction in early diastolic medial tissue velocity (e') at 3 cm per second. An E/e' ratio >40 is compatible with a marked elevation in left ventricle filling pressure analogous to grade 3 diastolic dysfunction seen in patients with sinus rhythm.

ANSWER 2: A. The 2D findings of increased thickness of all ventricular and atrial walls, all four heart valve leaflets, and a pericardial effusion are very suspicious for a systemic infiltrative disorder such as amyloidosis. Serum immunoglobulins will almost certainly be abnormal with an abnormal increase in serum free light chains characterizing a clonal excess of circulating plasma cells. Although serum and urine protein electrophoresis are often abnormal, they lack sensitivity and if negative do not exclude the diagnosis. Serum iron studies (abnormal in hemochromatosis—which can be associated with a dilated cardiomyopathy) and serum angiotensin converting enzyme level (often elevated in sarcoidosis) would both be expected to be normal. The degree of elevation in brain natriuretic peptide levels provides prognostic information in systemic amyloidosis; however, it is nonspecific and would not help in characterizing the cardiomyopathy. Evidence of amyloid deposition in tissue will also be required to confirm the presence of amyloidosis. Common sites of biopsy with high yields (often obviating the need for cardiac biopsy) include abdominal fat pad, rectum, and bone marrow.

See *The Echo Manual, 3rd Edition,* pages 274 to 276.

ANSWER 3: B. The typical strain pattern seen with AL amyloidosis is a marked reduction in global left ventricular longitudinal systolic strain with preservation of apical function (B). The global average of −10% is markedly reduced. For comparison, Figure 37-4A demonstrates a normal left ventricular strain pattern (normal more negative than −18%). Figure 37-4C with overall normal pattern apart from a focal marked reduction in strain in the septum and Figure 37-4D with marked reduction in apical strain would be the typical patterns of regional dysfunction seen with hypertrophic cardiomyopathy of the septal (C) or apical (D) variants. Systolic longitudinal strain by speckle tracking provides a sensitive, reproducible assessment of left ventricular systolic function identifying global and regional abnormality patterns that are helpful in evaluating patients with suspected cardiomyopathies.[1,2]

ANSWER 4: E. The presence and degree of cardiac involvement dominates prognosis in patients with systemic amyloidosis. Various markers are very helpful in assessing both prognosis as well as suitability for tolerating stem cell transplantation. These include serum uric acid and serum free light chains. A simple prognostic model is based on three variables: a serum uric acid >8 mg per dl, an NT-pro-BNP >332 ng per L, and a cardiac troponin T >0.035 μg per L.[1-4]

ANSWER 5: D. There are a host of factors that suggest this patient is at a particularly high risk of intracardiac thrombosis. The study by Feng et al.[5] evaluated the characteristics associated with intracardiac thrombosis seen in patients with amyloidosis. Factors that were associated with intracardiac thrombosis included AL amyloidosis, atrial fibrillation, and worse diastolic function. Patients with restrictive filling pattern (grade 3 or 4 diastolic dysfunction) were 17-fold more likely to have intracardiac thrombosis compared with those with a nonrestrictive filling pattern (grade 1 or 2) even in the setting of sinus rhythm. Intracardiac thrombus is present in ventricles as well as in atria. TEE should be considered in patients with cardiac amyloidosis and a restrictive diastolic filling pattern.

References

1. Bellavia D, Pellikka PA, Al-Zahrani GB, et al. Independent predictors of survival in primary systemic (Al) amyloidosis, including cardiac biomarkers and left ventricular strain imaging: an observational cohort study. *J Am Soc Echocardiogr.* 2010;23:643–652.

2. Dispenzieri A, Gertz MA, Kyle RA, et al. Prognostication of survival using cardiac troponins and *N*-terminal pro-brain natriuretic peptide in patients with primary systemic amyloidosis undergoing peripheral blood stem cell transplantation. *Blood.* 2004;104:1881–1887.

3. Dispenzieri A, Lacy MQ, Katzmann JA, et al. Absolute values of immunoglobulin free light chains are prognostic in patients with primary systemic amyloidosis undergoing peripheral blood stem cell transplantation. *Blood.* 2006;107:3378–3383.

4. Gertz M, Lacy M, Dispenzieri A, et al. Troponin T level as an exclusion criterion for stem cell transplantation in light-chain amyloidosis. *Leuk Lymphoma.* 2008;49:36–41.

5. Feng D, Syed IS, Martinez M, et al. Intracardiac thrombosis and anticoagulation therapy in cardiac amyloidosis. *Circulation.* 2009;119:2490–2497.

CASE 38

Progressive Exertional Dyspnea

*M*r. SA is an 81-year-old man who presents with a 6-month history of progressive exertional dyspnea, now functional class III. He denies angina or orthopnea. He has modest peripheral edema controlled by a low-dose loop diuretic. He has long-standing systemic hypertension and chronic kidney disease with a baseline creatinine of 2 mg per dl. On examination, his blood pressure was 110/50 mm Hg and pulse rate 80 beats per minute and regular. His central venous pressure was elevated to 15 cm. Carotid pulses are of normal intensity. His chest is clear. He had a 3/6 pansystolic murmur at the lower left sternal border and an audible third heart sound. He was referred for transthoracic echocardiography (see **Video 38-1**).

QUESTION 1. Diastolic function (see **Video 38-1** and Figs. 38-1 through 38-3) is:

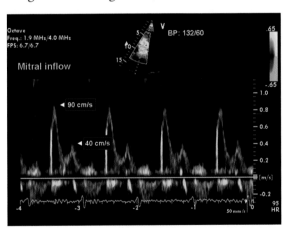

Figure 38-1

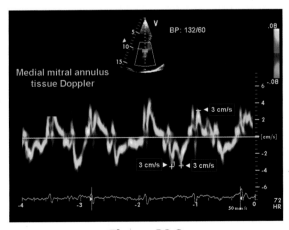

Figure 38-2

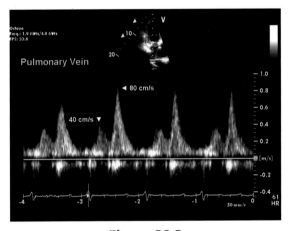

Figure 38-3

A. Normal

B. Mildly abnormal (delayed relaxation)

C. Moderate to severely abnormal with restrictive filling

QUESTION 2. Doppler profile across the patent foramen ovale (see **Video 38-1** and Fig. 38-4) suggests:

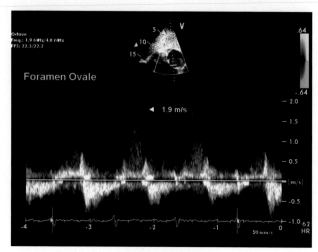

Figure 38-4

A. Severe right–left shunt
B. Left atrial hypertension
C. Severe tricuspid valve regurgitation
D. Severe mitral valve regurgitation

QUESTION 3. The likely diagnosis (see **Video 38-1**) is:

A. Eosinophilic heart disease
B. Cardiac amyloidosis
C. Idiopathic (primary) pulmonary hypertension
D. Hypertrophic obstructive cardiomyopathy
E. Dilated cardiomyopathy

QUESTION 4. Which of the following statements regarding senile cardiac amyloidosis compared with primary (AL) amyloidosis is *false*?

A. Patients with senile cardiac amyloidosis tend to be older
B. Patients with senile cardiac amyloidosis almost always are male
C. Left ventricular (LV) wall thicknesses tend to be less in senile amyloidosis
D. Survival in senile amyloidosis may be up to five times greater

ANSWER 1: C. Diastolic function is moderate to severely abnormal. Mitral inflow pattern demonstrates restrictive filling pattern with E>>A and a short deceleration time, although it can be normal by itself especially in a young individual who can have a short DT as well. However, the main difference between normal and pseudonormal mitral inflow is that pseudonormal inflow is a result of delayed myocardial relaxation that decreases E velocity and prolongs deceleration time (DT), and elevated filling pressure that increases E velocity and shortens DT. Peak early diastolic velocity (e′) on tissue Doppler of medial mitral annulus indicates the status of myocardial relaxation and is reduced (e′ = 3 cm per second) resulting in a ratio of E/e′ of 30, consistent with a severe elevation in LV filling pressures. E/e′ >15 usually indicates elevated diastolic LV filling pressure. Pulmonary vein Doppler profile of diastolic predominant forward flow is also consistent with an elevation in left atrial pressure, although similar pulmonary vein Doppler velocity pattern can be seen in a young healthy individual. It should also be noted that pulmonary vein atrial flow reversal velocity is not prominent as expected in a patient with increased filling pressure. It is related to prolonged PR interval on the electrocardiogram so that the onset of atrial contraction takes place before the diastolic forward flow is completed. Pulmonary vein atrial flow reversal pattern of prolonged flow duration and increased velocity is specific, but not sensitive for detecting increased left ventricular end diastolic pressure.

See *The Echo Manual, 3rd Edition,* page 120.

ANSWER 2: B. Doppler profile across the patent foramen ovale suggests left atrial hypertension. Doppler profile across patent foramen ovale demonstrates flow from the left to right atrium, implying an LA pressure higher than right atrial pressure. On the basis of the modified Bernoulli equation ($P = 4v^2$), the pressure gradient between these chambers equals $4(1.9)^2$, that is, 14 mm Hg. Subcostal imaging demonstrating significant enlargement of the inferior vena cava signifies that right atrial pressure is high (10 to 15 mm Hg). Therefore, left atrial pressure at the end of systole is in the range of 24 to 29 mm Hg.

See *The Echo Manual, 3rd Edition,* Figure 4-14 on page 69.

ANSWER 3: B. The likely diagnosis is cardiac amyloidosis. Two-dimensional imaging demonstrates increased left and right ventricular wall thickness, thickened valve leaflets, and a pericardial effusion. The constellation of findings coupled with the severe diastolic function abnormalities points toward a diagnosis of cardiac amyloidosis. Although many disorders may give rise to an increase in LV wall thickness, involvement of all heart chambers, the valves, and pericardium is characteristic of an infiltrative disorder. Cardiac amyloidosis caused by the deposition of amyloid fibrils predominantly in the myocardial interstitium gives rise to an increase in LV wall thickness and profound relaxation abnormalities but preservation in LV chamber size and ejection fraction until late in the disease. ECG abnormalities are common and classically demonstrate low voltage with a pseudoinfarct pattern (see Fig. 38-5).

In this patient, endomyocardial biopsy confirmed the presence of the senile–cardiac restricted subtype (transthyretin positive) on amyloidosis (positive sulfated alcian blue staining).

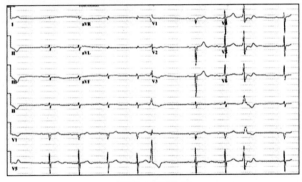

Figure 38-5

See *The Echo Manual, 3rd Edition,* amyloidosis on pages 274 to 279.

ANSWER 4: C. Patients with senile cardiac amyloidosis tend to be male, be older, and have a greater degree of LV wall thickening than do patients with primary (AL) cardiac amyloidosis. Survival estimates are much longer with senile amyloidosis despite the older ages of the patients.[1,2]

References

1. Kyle RA, Spittell PC, Gertz MA, et al. The premortem recognition of systemic senile amyloidosis with cardiac involvement. *Am J Med.* 1996;101:395–400.

2. Ng B, Connors LH, Davidoff R, et al. Senile systemic amyloidosis presenting with heart failure: a comparison with light chain-associated amyloidosis. *Arch Intern Med.* 2005;165:1425–1429.

CASE 39

Loud Systolic Murmur

A 30-year-old woman presents for the evaluation of a loud systolic murmur heard on a preemployment medical examination. She has no symptoms. Her heart rate is 70 beats per minute and her blood pressure 128/64 mm Hg.

QUESTION 1. On the basis of the lesion (**Videos 39-1 to 39-3**, Fig. 39-1, **Videos 39-4 to 39-6**, and Figs. 39-2 and 39-3), what lesion is present?

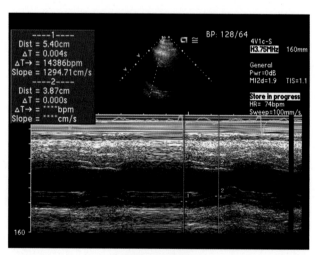

Figure 39-1

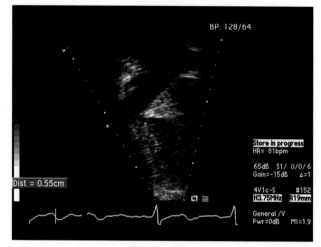

Figure 39-2

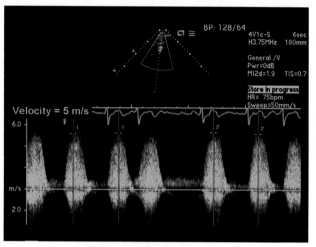

Figure 39-3

A. Membranous ventricular septal defect
B. Muscular ventricular septal defect
C. Inlet ventricular septal defect
D. Primum atrial septal defect

QUESTION 2. What is the calculated right ventricular systolic pressure (RVSP)?

A. 100 mm Hg plus right atrial pressure
B. 28 mm Hg
C. 28 mm Hg plus right atrial pressure
D. 100 mm Hg

QUESTION 3. The most common form of ventricular septal defect in young children is:

A. Membranous ventricular septal defect
B. Muscular ventricular septal defect
C. Inlet ventricular septal defect
D. Supracristal ventricular septal defect

QUESTION 4. In the parasternal short-axis view (Fig. 39-4), a membranous septal defect will typically be located in which of the following locations (illustrated in the figure as A, B or C)?

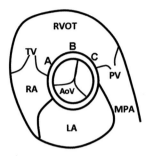

Figure 39-4

AoV, aortic valve; LA, left atrium; RA, right atrium; TV, tricuspid valve; RVOT, right ventricular outflow tract; PV, pulmonary valve; MPA, main pulmonary artery.

A. Location A
B. Location B
C. Location C

QUESTION 5. Complications of ventricular septal defect include:

A. Pulmonary hypertension
B. Aortic valve regurgitation
C. Right ventricular outflow tract obstruction
D. All of the choices

ANSWER 1: B. Best seen in the apical four-chamber view, there is a small muscular ventricular septal defect measuring approximately 4 mm in width. The left and right ventricles are of normal size.

ANSWER 2: B. The peak velocity across the ventricular septal defect is high (5 m per second) consistent with a restrictive defect and a normal RVSP. There is a low-velocity left–right diastolic gradient indicating that right ventricular diastolic pressures are also low. The peak velocity from the continuous wave Doppler interrogation across the ventricular septal defect corresponds to the peak gradient between the left and right ventricles. The peak systolic flow velocity of 5 m per second corresponds to a 100 mm Hg pressure gradient between the left ventricle and the right ventricle. Given the systolic blood pressure is 128 mm Hg, then the RVSP = 28 mm Hg.

See *The Echo Manual, 3rd Edition,* page 162 and Figure 10-1 on page 164.

ANSWER 3: B. The most common form of ventricular septal defect in children is the muscular type. These defects typically are small and surrounded entirely by cardiac muscle. Usually, they are located in the distal two-thirds of the left ventricular septum. They frequently close during the course of childhood such that by adulthood the most common form of ventricular septal defect is the membranous type.

ANSWER 4: A. Membranous ventricular septal defects are located at the base of the heart, at the junction of the muscular, AV atrio-ventricular, and outlet portions of the septum. The membranous septum is the thinnest portion of the normal septum, and ventricular septal defects in this location are immediately adjacent to the aortic and tricuspid valves, which can easily be appreciated in the short-axis view. The proximity of membranous defects to the tricuspid and aortic valves leaves the adjacent leaflets somewhat unsupported. Consequently, the patients require prolonged surveillance for the development of progressive regurgitation, even if the defect is small.

See *The Echo Manual, 3rd Edition,* Figure 20-13 on page 343.

ANSWER 5: D. Right ventricular outflow tract obstruction occurs secondary to muscular infundibular obstruction. A supracristal ventricular septal defect leads to a lack of support of the right coronary cusp resulting in aortic valve regurgitation. A large ventricular septal defect will lead to a large degree of shunting through the pulmonary vasculature, the development of severe pulmonary hypertension, and a reversal of the shunt.

CASE 40

Exertional Shortness of Breath with No Medical History

A 26-year-old woman comes for the evaluation of exertional shortness of breath. She has no medical history of note. She is referred for transthoracic echocardiogram (**Videos 40-1 to 40-11** and Figs. 40-1 to 40-10).

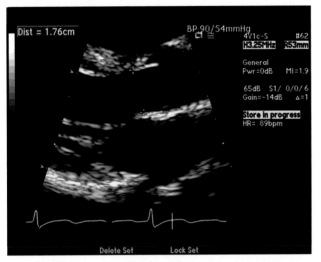

Figure 40-1

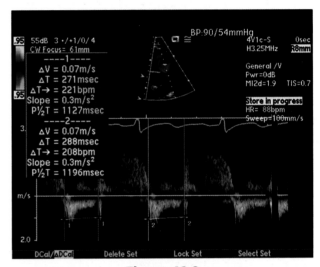

Figure 40-3

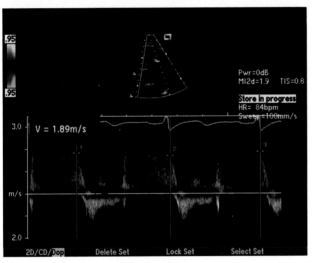

Figure 40-2

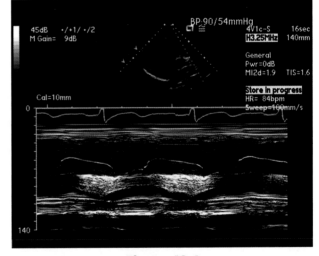

Figure 40-4

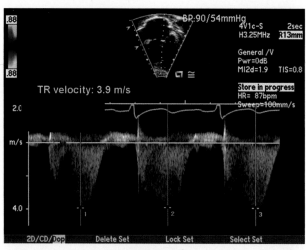

Figure 40-5

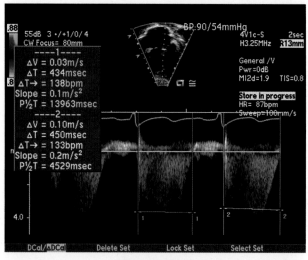

Figure 40-6

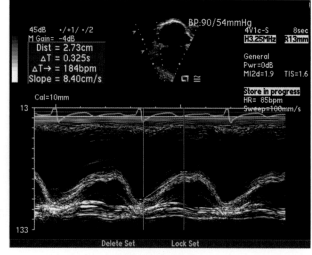

Figure 40-7

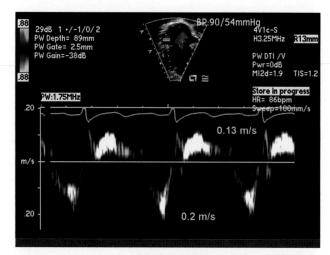

Figure 40-8

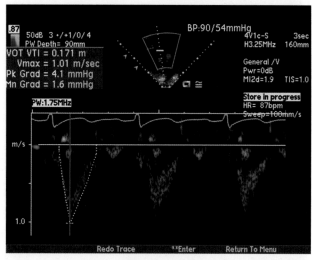

Figure 40-9

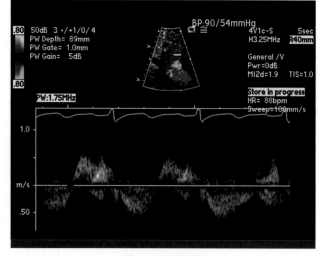

Figure 40-10

QUESTION 1. What are the estimated pulmonary artery pressures?

   A. 21/9 mm Hg
   B. 21/13 mm Hg
   C. 36/18 mm Hg
   D. 60/15 mm Hg
   E. 65/20 mm Hg

QUESTION 2. What is the Doppler-derived cardiac output?

   A. 4 L per minute
   B. 5 L per minute
   C. 6 L per minute
   D. 7 L per minute

QUESTION 3. The right ventricular index of myocardial performance (RIMP) (Tei index) is:

   A. 0.40
   B. 0.45
   C. 0.50
   D. 0.55
   E. 0.60

QUESTION 4. Measures of right ventricular longitudinal systolic function are:

   A. Normal
   B. Mild to moderately reduced
   C. Severely reduced

QUESTION 5. What are the structure and cause of blood flow indicated with the arrow in **Videos 40-12 and 40-13**?

   A. Coronary sinus
   B. Left inferior pulmonary vein
   C. Left circumflex coronary artery to left atrial fistula
   D. Artifact

QUESTION 6. The M-mode tracing (Fig. 40-4) through the pulmonary valve is associated with which finding?

   A. Pulmonary valve stenosis
   B. Pulmonary valve regurgitation
   C. Pulmonary hypertension
   D. Bicuspid pulmonary valve
   E. Normal finding

QUESTION 7. What is the cause for right ventricular enlargement?

   A. Primum atrial septal defect
   B. Sinus venosus atrial septal defect
   C. Secundum atrial septal defect
   D. Intact atrial septum and primary severe tricuspid valve regurgitation

QUESTION 8. After transesophageal echocardiography (**Video 40-14** and Fig. 40-11), the appropriate next step includes:

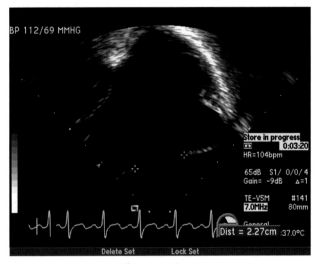

Figure 40-11

   A. Surgical repair or replacement of the tricuspid valve
   B. Percutaneous closure of the atrial septal defect
   C. Surgical closure of the atrial septal defect
   D. Hemodynamic catheterization

ANSWER 1: E. Pulmonary artery systolic pressure is estimated as four times the peak (tricuspid regurgitant velocity)^2 plus an estimate of right atrial pressure. Pulmonary artery diastolic pressure is estimated as four times the (end pulmonary regurgitant velocity)^2 plus an estimate of right atrial pressure. Here the inferior vena cava is of normal size and collapses normally with respiration, and hence, the right atrial pressure is normal (5 mm Hg). Here pulmonary artery systolic pressure is estimated as 4(3.9)^2 plus 5 = 65 mm Hg and 4(1.9)^2 plus 5 = 20 mm Hg.

ANSWER 2: B. Stroke volume (SV) is calculated as the product of the cross-sectional area of the left ventricular outflow tract (LVOT) and the time velocity integral (TVI) of a pulse-wave sample from the LVOT.

$$
\begin{aligned}
\text{SV (ml)} &= [(D/1.8)^2 \times \pi] \times [\text{LVOT TVI}] \\
&= (2/1.8)^2 \times \pi] \times [17] \\
&= 3.88 \times 17 \\
&= 66 \text{ ml}
\end{aligned}
$$

Cardiac output is the product of SV and heart rate $= 66 \times 87 = 5.7$ L per minute

See *The Echo Manual, 3rd Edition*, Figure 4-16 on page 71.

ANSWER 3: E. The RIMP is a relatively load-independent parameter of global function that is a ratio of the sum of the isovolumic relaxation and contraction times to the right ventricular ejection time. It can be easily calculated by the following equation:

RIMP = [Tricuspid valve closure to opening time] − [right ventricular ejection time]/[Right ventricular ejection time]
= 445 − 280/280 = 0.60

ANSWER 4: A. Unlike the left ventricle, the predominant orientation of myocardial fibers in the right ventricle runs in the longitudinal plane with a much greater proportion of right ventricular contraction determined by the base moving up toward the apex rather than radial contractility. This study has two measures of longitudinal motion of the tricuspid annulus as measures of right ventricular longitudinal systolic motion. The first is a measure of the distance of annular excursion during systole, the tricuspid annular plane systolic excursion. A normal value in a young patient should be >20 to 22 mm (here 27 mm). Alternatively, one can measure the peak systolic tissue velocity of the tricuspid lateral annulus (S'), here

13 cm per second is also normal. The American Society of Echocardiography recommends at least one of these two measures is performed to assess right ventricular systolic function.

ANSWER 5: B. Echocardiography demonstrates normal anatomy of the left inferior pulmonary vein draining into the left atrium with normal laminar flow.

ANSWER 6: C. An M-mode recordings from the pulmonary valve shows the characteristic appearance of pulmonary hypertension with a "W" shape with mid-systolic interruption of valve opening producing the notching and "W" shape. This is because of pressures waves reflected back to the proximal pulmonary artery in the setting of high pulmonary vascular resistance.

See *The Echo Manual, 3rd Edition*, Figure 9-8B on page 148.

ANSWER 7: C. Atrial septal defects comprise approximately 10% of congenital heart disease. The most common form is the secundum defect accounting for 60% to 75% of atrial septal defects. Large atrial septal defects result in a large left-to-right shunt that causes right heart volume overload and chamber enlargement as in this case. Secundum atrial septal defects are typically found in the central portion of the septum, surrounding the foramen ovale, and are frequently oblong or elliptical.

See *The Echo Manual, 3rd Edition*, atrial septal defect discussion on pages 334 to 335.

ANSWER 8: D. Closure of an atrial septal defect (whether percutaneously or surgically) is indicated in the setting of right-sided chamber enlargement regardless of the presence of symptoms. Given the associated severe tricuspid valve regurgitation, consideration would be given to surgical closure with concomitant tricuspid valve repair rather than percutaneous closure alone, despite the adequate rim surrounding the defect. However, the presence of significant pulmonary hypertension would warrant hemodynamic catheterization to discern the magnitude of fixed intrinsic pulmonary arterial hypertension rather than that simply because of increased transpulmonary flow. Indeed, at cardiac catheterization, the patient had significant pulmonary hypertension and marked increase in pulmonary vascular resistance and was recommended to receive pulmonary vascular targeted therapy rather than ASD closure.

Progressive Fatigue and Marked Lower Extremity Edema

A 45-year-old man presents to the emergency department for the evaluation of progressive fatigue and marked lower extremity edema. His medical history is significant for right innominate vein stenosis secondary to a clotted dialysis catheter. He has undergone uncomplicated percutaneous revascularization for 2 years before. He continues to dialyze three times a week through a left forearm fistula. He has diabetes mellitus.

On examination, his heart rate is 70 beats per minute and his blood pressure 170/70 mm Hg. His central venous pressure is elevated. He has a 2/6 pansystolic murmur that increases on inspiration. He has pitting edema of the lower extremities to midthigh.

QUESTION 1. What is the most likely explanation for the abnormal finding seen on parasternal long-axis imaging (**Videos 41-1 to 41-3** and Fig. 41-1)?

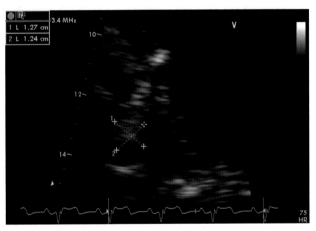

Figure 41-1

A. Metastatic carcinoma to pericardium
B. Pericardial fat
C. Myxoma

QUESTION 2. The findings demonstrated at the level of the tricuspid valve (**Videos 41-4 to 41-6**) likely represent:

A. Thrombus
B. Myxoma
C. Tricuspid prosthesis
D. Foreign material

QUESTION 3. On the basis of the hepatic vein Doppler (Fig. 41-2), which of the following is *false*?

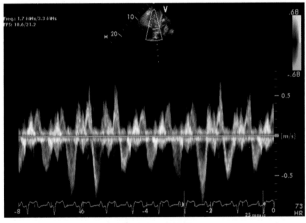

Figure 41-2

A. Systolic flow reversals secondary to tricuspid valve regurgitation tend to peak later in systole
B. Forward flow decreases during expiration
C. An increase in systolic flow reversals with expiration suggests the presence of constrictive hemodynamics
D. The sum of the peak systolic forward flow velocity and the peak velocity of atrial reversal is associated with the right atrial pressure

ANSWER 1: B. Fat may accumulate around the epicardial surface of the heart or between the pericardial layers. In the setting of a pericardial effusion, fat may appear as an irregular, hyperechoic mass mobile in the pericardial space or on the epicardial surface and may be mistaken as a metastatic tumor. Lipomatous tissue is easily distinguished by CT as hypodense appearing tissue with attenuation of between −20 to 50 Hounsfield units and on MRI, where its tissue will display high signal intensity on T_1- and T_2-weighted imaging and signal dropout on fat-saturation imaging.[1,2]

ANSWER 2: D. Echocardiography demonstrates two large tubular structures crossing the tricuspid valve causing significant valvular regurgitation and probably interfering with the filling of the right ventricle. They have a diameter of 1 cm each, have the appearance of metallic stents, and represent the migration of the previously placed venous vascular stents. They were successfully removed percutaneously with a snare (Fig. 41-3).

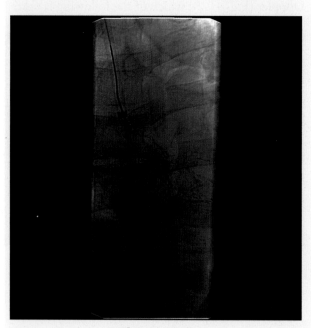

Figure 41-3

ANSWER 3: D. See Figure 41-4. Although there is no simultaneous respirometer recording, forward flow (below the baseline) increases with inspiration (INSP) and decreases with expiration (EXP). Throughout the respiratory cycle, there is diastolic predominant forward flow (DFW). Systolic flow is predominantly reversal flow (SR) indicative of elevated right atrial pressure and illustrating a signal that peaks in later systole, in keeping with systolic flow reversals seen with significant tricuspid valve regurgitation. Here systolic flow reversals tend to fall in expiration. A marked decrease in diastolic forward flow and an increase in diastolic flow reversals observed with expiration (not seen here, see case 16) are highly suggestive of constrictive hemodynamics.[3]

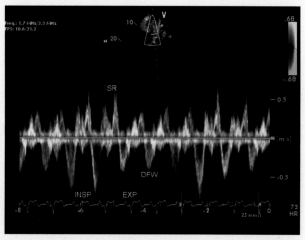

Figure 41-4

See *The Echo Manual, 3rd Edition*, discussion of echo findings in constrictive pericarditis on pages 294 to 299.

References

1. Ahn YK, Park JC, Park WS, et al. A case of prominent epicardial fat mimicking a tumor on echocardiography. *J Korean Med Sci.* 1999;14:571–574.

2. Pressman G, Verma N. Pericardial fat masquerading as tumor. *Echocardiography.* 2010;27:E18–E20.

3. Ommen SR, Nishimura RA, Hurrell DG, et al. Assessment of right atrial pressure with 2-dimensional and Doppler echocardiography: a simultaneous catheterization and echocardiographic study. *Mayo Clin Proc.* 2000;75:24–29.

CASE 42

Progressive Exertional Dyspnea, Atypical Chest Discomfort, Abdominal and Lower Extremity Swelling

*M*s. HA is a 38-year-old woman with a medical history of bipolar affective disorder, migraines, asthma, and gastroesophageal reflux disease. She presents with a 1-year history of progressive exertional dyspnea, atypical chest discomfort, abdominal and lower extremity swelling. On examination, her blood pressure is 130/60 mm Hg and heart rate 98 beats per minute. Her apical impulse is displaced laterally, and she has systolic and diastolic murmurs. There is evidence of ascites and significant lower extremity edema. She is referred for transthoracic echocardiography (see **Video 42-1**).

QUESTION 1. Echo two-dimensional and Doppler findings are consistent with:

A. Mild aortic valve regurgitation

B. Mild–moderate aortic valve regurgitation

C. Moderate–severe aortic valve regurgitation

QUESTION 2. In addition to aortic valve regurgitation, what other cardiovascular pathology can cause diastolic flow reversal in the descending aorta?

A. Coarctation of the aorta

B. Patent ductus arteriosus (PDA)

C. Aortic dissection

D. Supravalvular aortic stenosis

QUESTION 3. Which of the following chronic medical therapies is likely responsible for the patient's findings?

A. Omeprazole for gastroesophageal reflux disease

B. Montelukast for asthma

C. Lithium for bipolar affective disorder

D. Ergotamine for migraine headaches

QUESTION 4. Which of the following settings could also likely explain the echocardiographic findings?

A. Primary bronchial carcinoid

B. Hepatic carcinoid metastases with patent foramen ovale

C. Primary ovarian carcinoid

QUESTION 5. Which of the following is correct with regard to the "reverse-dagger" shape of the tricuspid regurgitation (TR) velocity (Fig. 42-1)?

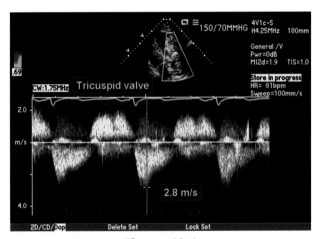

Figure 42-1

A. The shape is because of high right atrial pressure

B. The shape is characteristic for all TR velocities

C. The shape is because of rapid rise of right atrial pressure

D. The shape is because of pulmonary hypertension

ANSWER 1: C. There is moderate–severe aortic valve regurgitation.

See *The Echo Manual, 3rd Edition*, pages 207 to 210 and Appendix 20 on page 413.

In assessment of aortic valve regurgitation, the width of the regurgitant jet at its origin relative to the dimension of the left ventricular outflow tract (LVOT) is a good predictor of the angiographic severity of aortic regurgitation. Other Doppler features that should be used in determining the severity of regurgitation include pressure halftime of the continuous wave Doppler signal of the regurgitant jet, diastolic reversal flow in the descending aorta, and the deceleration time of the mitral flow E velocity. Vena contracta is the smallest neck of the flow region at the level of the aortic valve, immediately below the flow convergence region. This is smaller than the width of the jet of aortic regurgitation in the LVOT. The vena contracta is usually measured from the parasternal long-axis view, and a vena contracta width larger than 6 mm is specific for severe aortic regurgitation.

In severe aortic regurgitation, systemic diastolic pressure decreases quickly, so that the aortic regurgitation signal (corresponding to the pressure difference between the aorta and the left ventricle) has a shortened deceleration time and thus shortened pressure halftime. A pressure halftime between 200 and 500 milliseconds would be compatible with moderate aortic valve regurgitation. Diastolic retrograde flow can be demonstrated in the descending thoracic aorta and even in the abdominal aorta. Holodiastolic reversal of flow is also compatible with severe aortic valve regurgitation.

ANSWER 2: B. Patent ductus arteriosus (PDA). Persistent patency of the ductus arteriosus is an arterial communication between the upper descending aorta and the pulmonary artery and usually arises from the upper descending aorta and connects to the distal main pulmonary artery, near the origin of the left pulmonary artery. This results in a diastolic run off of aortic pressure and may be associated with diastolic flow reversals seen in the proximal descending thoracic aorta (see Case 19, Fig. 19-3). Most persistent PDAs are small but are associated with a somewhat increased risk for infective endarteritis (relative to the normal heart), even when the volume load is insignificant. In the absence of other cardiac abnormalities, closure of the PDA decreases the risk of endarteritis to that of the general population, and therefore, closure by surgery or catheter device is generally recommended for any PDA that has an audible murmur. A large PDA can lead to pulmonary hypertension and left atrial and left ventricular volume overload.

ANSWER 3: D. Ergotamine for migraine headaches. Omeprazole is not noted for cardiac toxicity. Montelukast, like all leukotriene inhibitors, has been linked with triggering or unmasking Churg–Strauss syndrome in patients with severe asthma. Characterized by asthma, peripheral and tissue hypereosinophilia, and small vessel vasculitis, Churg–Strauss syndrome can affect the heart in up to 25% of cases. Cardiac manifestations include endomyocardial thickening and thrombus formation, left ventricular dysfunction, and pericardial inflammation. Lithium is most notable for causing cardiac rhythm abnormalities including sinus node dysfunction and bradycardia. The ergot derivatives ergotamine and methysergide were previously used widely for the prophylaxis and treatment of migraines but are used less frequently because of available alternatives with better adverse risk profiles. Their notable cardiac toxicity is the induction of valvular abnormalities similar to those seen with carcinoid syndrome.

Other agents linked with similar valvular findings include the appetite suppressant combination of fenfluramine and dexfenfluramine ("Fen-Phen") and the dopamine agonists, pergolide and cabergoline, used for the treatment of Parkinson disease. The link between these agents and disease states appears to be stimulation of the serotonin 2B receptors that in turn stimulates fibroblast proliferation and valvular thickening. In severe cases, valve leaflets become retracted and progressive immobile with significant valvular regurgitation.

ANSWER 4: B. Hepatic carcinoid metastases with patent foramen ovale. Because the substances that are secreted by a carcinoid tumor are inactivated by the lung, it is predominantly the right side of the heart that is involved. However, the left-sided cardiac valves are involved in 5% to 7% of cases. This is most likely because of the presence of a patent foramen ovale that allows the tumor substances to pass from the right atrium to the left atrium or because of pulmonary metastasis. Although bronchial carcinoid if it is secretory may give rise to left-sided valve involvement, these tumors typically do not secrete. The notable fact about carcinoid involvement of the testes or ovaries is that they are distinct from other abdominal tumor sites because they may give rise to right-sided cardiac involvement even in the absence of hepatic disease. This is because of exceptional venous supply of the gonads that bypass the liver.

ANSWER 5: C. The shape is because of a rapid rise of right atrial pressure. Typically, the shape of the tricuspid regurgitant jet is a symmetrical parabolic curve. However, in the setting of torrential tricuspid valve regurgitation, the large volume of blood reentering the right atrium during systole causes a rapid rise in right atrial pressure that equilibrates with the right ventricular pressure and terminates the regurgitant waveform to be more triangular.

Monomorphic Ventricular Tachycardia after Cardiac Arrest

A 9-year-old girl suffers a cardiac arrest at school. She is appropriately resuscitated by her teacher with an automated external defibrillator. She has a further run of monomorphic ventricular tachycardia in hospital and undergoes implantation of a defibrillator. She is referred for further evaluation (**Video 43-1**).

QUESTION 1. The likely etiology of her dysrhythmia is:

   A. Long QT interval syndrome
   B. Cardiac fibroma
   C. Cardiac rhabdomyosarcoma
   D. Metastatic carcinoma
   E. Myxoma

QUESTION 2. The most appropriate management of further dysrhythmia is:

   A. Antiarrhythmic therapy
   B. Tumor resection
   C. Cardiac transplantation
   D. Chemotherapy

ANSWER 1: B. Transthoracic echocardiography demonstrates a large, discrete, homogenous mass present in the lateral wall of the left ventricle. The appearance in light of the history is most suggestive of a cardiac fibroma.

Cardiac fibromas are benign neoplasms arising from myocardial fibroblasts. Arising most commonly in the left ventricle (typically the free wall), they are the second most common tumor in the pediatric population; however, they are rarely also seen in adults. The manifestations of the tumor vary depending on their size and location. Typical presentations include malignant ventricular dysrhythmia and heart failure.

Cardiac fibromas are typically echocardiographically well circumscribed and contain calcification in up to 50% of cases.

See *The Echo Manual, 3rd Edition*, page 311.

ANSWER 2: B. Cardiac fibromas are benign tumors, for which there is no role for chemotherapy. Surgical resection is indicated whenever the tumor is associated with significant clinical manifestations. Typically, fibromas can be "peeled away from the underlying myocardium after hypothermic cardiopulmonary arrest and cardioplegic myocardial protection." Although a few patients may require cardiac transplantation for very extensive tumors, most fibromas may be resected without complication. The long-term outcome after resection, as in this patient (Fig. 43-1), is generally excellent.[1,2]

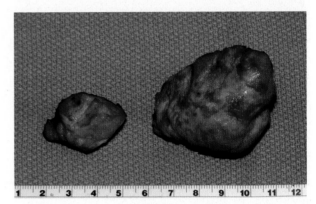

Figure 43-1. Resected cardiac fibroma.

References

1. ElBardissi AW, Dearani JA, Daly RC, et al. Analysis of benign ventricular tumors: long-term outcome after resection. *J Thorac Cardiovasc Surg.* 2008;135:1061–1068.

2. ElBardissi AW, Dearani JA, Daly RC, et al. Survival after resection of primary cardiac tumors: a 48-year experience. *Circulation.* 2008;118(14)(suppl):S7–S15.

CASE 44

Exertional Chest Pain

A 77-year-old man with a history of hyperlipidemia is referred for exercise echocardiogram for the assessment of new onset exertional chest pain.

His resting ECG demonstrates non specific ST-T changes.

Prior to stress, his rest echocardiogram demonstrates normal left ventricular size with an ejection fraction of 60%. He has grade 1 diastolic dysfunction, a left atrial volume index of 30 cc per m², and normal cardiac valves. Images were suboptimal, and echo contrast was given for left ventricular opacification.

QUESTION 1. What was the intervention that likely improved the image with regard to the use of echo contrast for left ventricular opacification (see **Video 44-1**):

A. More contrast was given
B. The mechanical index was decreased
C. The dose of contrast was decreased

QUESTION 2. Which of the following statements concerning mechanical index is *false*?

A. Mechanical index is a measure of acoustic power
B. Mechanical index is proportional to the acoustic pressure
C. Mechanical index is proportional to the square root of the ultrasound frequency
D. Mechanical index greater than 0.7 is likely to destroy microbubbles

QUESTION 3. The patient exercised on a standard Bruce treadmill protocol for 6 minutes (98% of predicted), developing chest pain. The stress ECG was nondiagnostic secondary to resting ST-T segment change. Exercise stress echocardiography demonstrates

evidence of (see **Videos 44-2 and 44-3**. Orientation in both clips is as follows: top left, apical 4 chamber in the Mayo format with left ventricle displayed on the left; top right, apical 3 chamber; bottom left, apical short axis; bottom right, apical 2 chamber):

A. Anterior infarction
B. Lateral wall ischemia
C. Anterior ischemia
D. Inferior infarction
E. No evidence of ischemia

QUESTION 4. The following is/are true with respect to findings suggesting evidence of severe ischemia on exercise stress echocardiography:

A. The development of multiple wall motion abnormalities with stress
B. Dilation of the left ventricular cavity and/or a reduction in left ventricular ejection fraction are more common in exercise rather than dobutamine stress
C. Hypotension is more specific for severe coronary disease with exercise rather than dobutamine stress
D. All of the choices

ANSWER 1: B. The first part of the clip demonstrates absence of contrast in the distal two-thirds of the left ventricle. Although this may be related to the insufficient contrast, the first step is to ensure that the myocardial index is low. Indeed here the MI was reduced from 0.6 to 0.25 resulting in the avoidance of bubble destruction without the need for further contrast administration. If excessive contrast is present in the left ventricle, there will be attenuation effects and relative drop-out of contrast seen in the distal part of the image. Here a relative reduction in the concentration of contrast will aid in allowing uniform opacification.

See *The Echo Manual, 3rd Edition*, page 101.

ANSWER 2: C. The ultrasound acoustic power is expressed as the mechanical index, which is proportional to the acoustic pressure and inversely proportional to the square root of the ultrasound frequency. A mechanical index higher than 0.7 is likely to destroy the microbubbles:

$$\text{Mechanical index} = \frac{\text{Acoustic pressure}}{\sqrt{fo}}$$

See *The Echo Manual, 3rd Edition*, gas-filled microbubbles discussion on pages 100 to 101.

ANSWER 3: C. At rest, left ventricular wall motion is normal. Following exercise stress there is hypokinesis/severe hypokinesis of the anterior wall (base to apex), septum (mid and apex), and apical lateral and inferior segments, suggesting ischemia in the territory of the proximal left anterior descending coronary artery. Subsequent coronary angiography demonstrated high-grade stenotic lesions in the left anterior descending coronary artery and a diagonal artery (see Fig. 44-1).

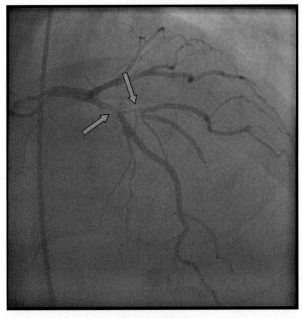

Figure 44-1

See *The Echo Manual, 3rd Edition*, pages 176 to 180.

ANSWER 4: D. In addition to the development of multiple regional wall motion abnormalities, other factors that are specific for the presence of severe coronary artery disease include left ventricular dilation, and a decline in left ventricular systolic function (both findings less commonly seen with dobutamine stress, despite a high burden of coronary disease). Hypotension with exercise is also a specific finding for severe disease unlike with dobutamine where hypotension may also be related to systemic vasodilation from β-2 stimulation or dynamic outflow tract obstruction.

See *The Echo Manual, 3rd Edition*, Table 11-4 on page 179.

CASE 45

Dyspnea and Presyncope

A 74-year-old woman presents with dyspnea and presyncope. On examination, her blood pressure is 120/80 mm Hg and her heart rate 80 beats per minute. Her apex beat is non-displaced. There is a 3/6 harsh systolic murmur with a single second heart sound. She is referred for transthoracic echocardiogram (**Videos 45-1 and 45-2** and Figs. 45-1 through 45-3).

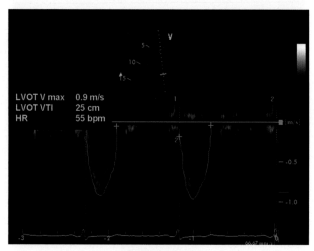

Figure 45-1

LVOT V max   0.9 m/s
LVOT VTI   25 cm
HR   55 bpm

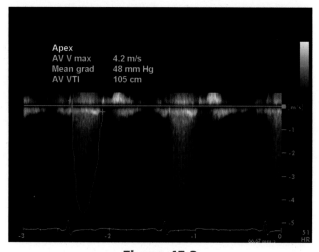

Figure 45-3

Apex
AV V max   4.2 m/s
Mean grad   48 mm Hg
AV VTI   105 cm

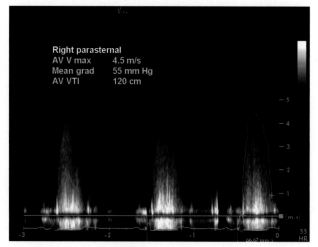

Figure 45-2

Right parasternal
AV V max   4.5 m/s
Mean grad   55 mm Hg
AV VTI   120 cm

QUESTION 1. What is the calculated cardiac output, given a left ventricular outflow tract diameter of 20 mm (Fig. 45-1)?

- A. 3.9 L per minute
- B. 4.3 L per minute
- C. 5.5 L per minute
- D. 6.2 L per minute

QUESTION 2. How often is the peak velocity of aortic stenosis obtained from a nonapical window?

- A. Rarely
- B. 5%
- C. 10%
- D. 20%
- E. 30%

QUESTION 3. What is the calculated aortic valve area (**Videos 45-1 and 45-2** and Figs. 45-1 and 45-3)?

    A. 0.65 cm^2

    B. 0.7 cm^2

    C. 0.75 cm^2

    D. 0.8 cm^2

    E. 0.85 cm^2

QUESTION 4. Coronary angiography demonstrated three-vessel coronary disease, and the patient underwent aortic valve replacement with a tissue bioprosthesis and a left internal mammary graft to left anterior descending coronary artery and saphenous vein grafts from the aorta to the distal right and obtuse marginal arteries. The procedure was uncomplicated.

On postoperative day 6, the patient acutely becomes nauseated, complains of abdominal pain, and passes out. She had no palpable blood pressure. She requires 2 minutes of chest compressions and received vasopressin, and her systolic blood pressure improved to 80 mm Hg.

A 12-lead ECG was obtained (see Fig. 45-4). The next appropriate step includes:

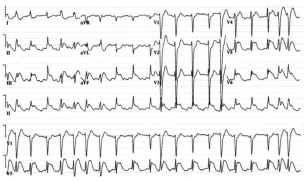

Figure 45-4

    A. Surgical reexploration of coronary grafts

    B. Coronary angiography

    C. CT scan of cardiac function, arteries, and grafts

    D. Intravenous thrombolytic therapy

QUESTION 5. Following this test or intervention, a transthoracic echocardiogram was performed (see **Videos 45-3 through 45-7**). An appropriate next step involves:

    A. Diuresis and ongoing inotropic support

    B. A transesophageal echocardiogram to better assess chamber size and function

    C. CT scan to evaluate pulmonary arteries for pulmonary embolus

ANSWER 1: B. The cardiac output can be calculated as = (πr^2)(LVOT TVI)(HR)

$$= 0.785 \ (D^2)(\text{LVOT TVI})(\text{HR})$$
$$= 0.785(2^2)(25)(55)$$
$$= 4.3 \text{ L per minute}$$

See *The Echo Manual, 3rd Edition*, pages 69 to 71 and Figure 4-16 on page 71.

ANSWER 2: D. Here two continuous wave Doppler signals are shown, one from the apex and one from the right parasternal area. In a comprehensive examination of a patient with aortic stenosis, it is critical to perform a Doppler evaluation from all available transducer windows. Approximately 20% of the time, the peak signal will be obtained from a window other than the apex.

See *The Echo Manual, 3rd Edition*, Doppler echocardiography (in aortic stenosis) on pages 190 and 191.

ANSWER 3: A.

Aortic valve area = [(LVOT TVI) × (LVOT area)]/Ao TVI

$$= [(\text{LVOT TVI}) \times 0.785$$
$$(\text{LVOT D})^2]/\text{Ao TVI}$$
$$= [(25) \times (3.14)]/120$$
$$= 78.5/120$$
$$= 0.65 \text{ cm}^2$$

ANSWER 4: B. ECG demonstrates acute injury pattern in the inferior and anterolateral leads. The patient remains in shock. Angiography allows for simultaneous assessment of native and graft patency and the potential for placement of an intra-aortic balloon pump and if required percutaneous coronary and or graft intervention. Thrombolytic therapy would be contraindicated in the immediate postoperative period.

Coronary angiography demonstrates unchanged severe native vessel coronary disease with patent grafts. An intra-aortic balloon pump is placed. The patient receives intravenous fluid resuscitation and dopamine. The right atrial pressure is 19 mm Hg, pulmonary capillary wedge pressure is 23 mm Hg, and cardiac output is 1.5 L per minute.

ANSWER 5: B. Transthoracic images are suboptimal; however, there is an impression of external clot in the pericardial space. Although this could be assessed by a CT scan, a transesophageal echocardiogram can be performed rapidly at the bedside in the intensive care unit. A transesophageal echocardiogram demonstrates significant pericardial fluid and solid material (presumed clot) in the pericardial space (**Videos 45-8 through 45-11**). The patient went to the operating room where the mediastinal and pericardial clot was evacuating leading to an immediate improvement in hemodynamics.

This case illustrates characteristics of tamponade that may occur in the early postoperative state. Typically, transthoracic imaging is difficult and classic findings of tamponade, and/or fluid collections are seen in only approximately two-thirds of patients. Transesophageal echocardiography is required in the remainder to adequately visualize the fluid. Effusions occurring early after surgery are often small and frequently localized. Surgical exploration is preferred over percutaneous pericardiocentesis.[1]

Reference

1. Price S, Prout J, Jaggar SI, et al. "Tamponade" following cardiac surgery: terminology and echocardiography may both mislead. *Eur J Cardiothoracic Surg.* 2004;26:1156–1160.

CASE 46

Severe Ischemic Cardiomyopathy and Functional Class IV Left Heart Failure

A76-year-old man with known severe ischemic cardiomyopathy and functional class IV left heart failure is referred for echocardiography (see **Videos 46-1 through 46-4** and Figs. 46-1 through 46-5).

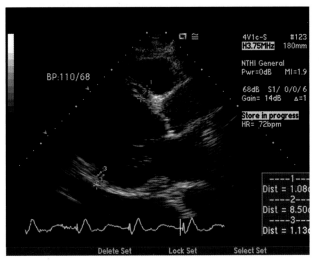

Figure 46-1

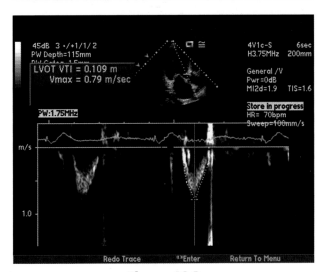

Figure 46-3

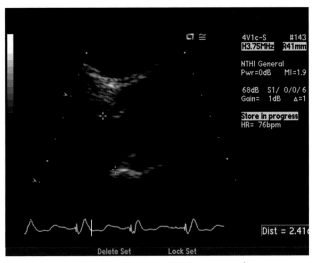

Figure 46-2

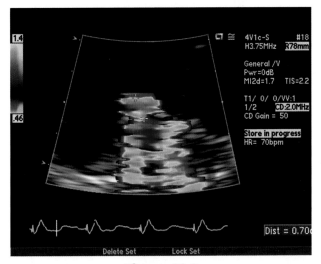

Figure 46-4

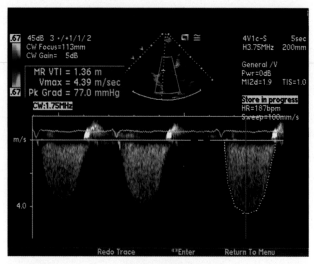

Figure 46-5

and 46-7). The status of aortic valve opening (see **Video 46-5**) is influenced by:

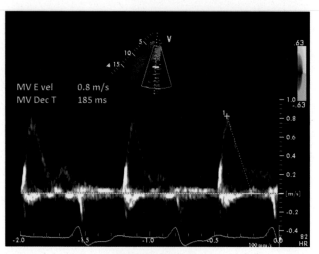

Figure 46-7

QUESTION 1. The Doppler-derived left ventricular (LV) cardiac output is:

    A. 3.0 L per minute   C. 4 L per minute
    B. 3.5 L per minute   D. 4.5 L per minute

QUESTION 2. The calculated mitral effective regurgitant orifice (ERO) area by the proximal isovelocity surface area method is:

    A. 0.28 cm^2 C. 0.38 cm^2
    B. 0.32 cm^2 D. 0.46 cm^2

QUESTION 3. The patient is referred for implantation of a continuous flow LV assist device (LVAD, Heart Mate II) as destination therapy for his heart failure. He is referred for followup echocardiography (see **Videos 46-6 through 46-9** and Figs. 46-6

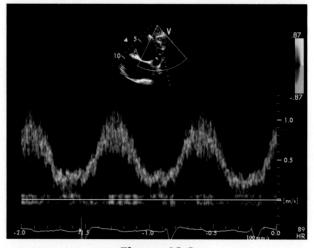

Figure 46-6

    A. LVAD function
    B. LV contractility
    C. LV end-diastolic pressure
    D. All of the choices

QUESTION 4. The patient's LV filling pressures are likely:

    A. Normal
    B. High
    C. Unable to assess based on available data

QUESTION 5. The inflow cannula systolic velocity profile (see Fig. 46-6) is:

    A. Too low, the velocity should be >2 m per second
    B. Normal
    C. Too high, the velocity should be <1 m per second

QUESTION 6. In patients with LV assist devices, the limitation to cardiac output is by the:

    A. LV
    B. Right ventricle
    C. LVAD
    D. There is no limitation to output

ANSWER 1: B. Stroke volume (SV) is calculated as the product of the cross-sectional area of the LV outflow tract and the velocity time integral of a pulse wave sample from the LVOT.

$$SV \ (ml) = [(D/2)^2 \times \pi] \times [LVOT \ TVI]$$
$$= [(2.4/2)^2 \times \pi] \times [11]$$
$$= 4.52 \times 11$$
$$= 50 \ ml$$

Cardiac output is the product of SV and heart rate = 50 × 70 = 3500 ml per minute.

ANSWER 2: B. $0.32 \ cm^2$

The regurgitant flow can be calculated as follows:

Flow rate $= (r)^2 \times 6.28 \times$ aliasing velocity
$= (0.70 \ cm)^2 \times 6.28 \times 46 \ cm$
per second
$= 142 \ cc$ per second

ERO = Flow rate/Peak MR velocity
ERO = 142 cc per second/439 cm per second
$= 0.32 \ cm^2$

ANSWER 3: D. The aortic valve opening status is a complex phenomenon that is affected by many factors and reflects the pressure/function relationship of the LV to the LV assist device. The aortic valve will open if the degree of LV flow supersedes LVAD flow. Factors that lead to an increase in LV flow include high LV end diastolic pressure or an increase in LV contractility. Factors that lead to a fall in LVAD flow may include obstruction to the inflow cannula, the pump, or the outflow cannula, or a reduction in the rate of the pump.

ANSWER 4: A. A critical function of the LVAD is unloading of the LV. Echocardiography is critical in the noninvasive assessment of loading status. Markers of high left atrial (LA) pressure include an intra-atrial septum that bows toward the right (particular in the setting of a dilated, noncollapsing inferior vena cava), a restrictive mitral inflow filling pattern with a short deceleration time. Here the intra-atrial septum is shifted toward the right (see **Video 46-7**), and the vena cava is small and collapses normally (see **Video 46-8**), indicating the LA pressure is less than the right atrial (RA) pressure and that the RA pressure is not high. The mitral inflow deceleration time is also not shortened.

ANSWER 5: B. In assessing the patient with an LV assist device, imaging of the inflow cannula is critical. The inflow cannula must be sitting centrally in the LV apex directed toward the mitral valve (best evaluated in the four- and two-chamber views). There should be laminar color flow without any turbulence. At the entrance to the inflow cannula, pulse wave Doppler should demonstrate modal pulsatile flow between 1 and 2 m per second. If it is low, it is because the patient is volume depleted or there is a problem with the inflow cannula. If it is high, there is typically some obstruction to the inflow cannula.

ANSWER 6: B. In patients with an LV assist device, the limiting factor in cardiac output is the right ventricle. If the LVAD output exceeds the flow into the LV (determined by the right ventricular output), a life-threatening "suck-down event" occurs with physical collapse of the LV manifested by immediate drop in perfusion, acute ventricular dysrhythmia, and right ventricular dilatation (see **Video 46-9**).

Progressive Exertional Dyspnea, Weight Gain, and Peripheral Edema

*A*65-year-old woman presents with a 6-year history of progressive exertional dyspnea, weight gain, and peripheral edema. Her history is notable for a mitral valve surgical commissurotomy 20 years before.

QUESTION 1. On the basis of her transthoracic images (**Videos 47-1 to 47-14** and Figs. 47-1 to 47-11), the calculated tricuspid effective regurgitant orifice (ERO) area by the proximal isovelocity surface area (PISA) method is:

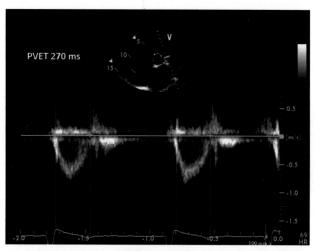

Figure 47-3

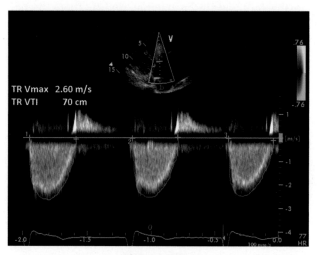

Figure 47-1

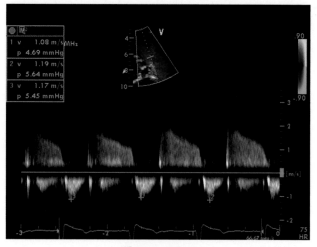

Figure 47-4

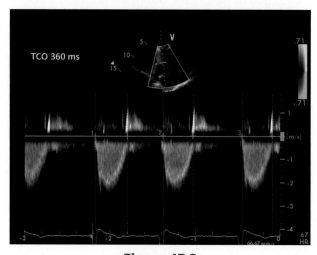

Figure 47-2

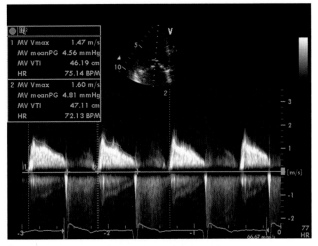

Figure 47-5

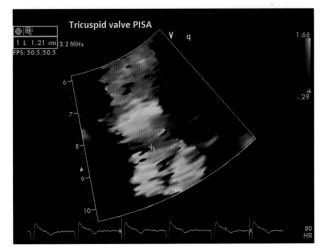

Figure 47-8

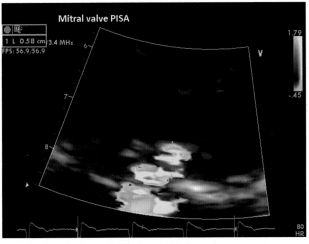

Figure 47-6

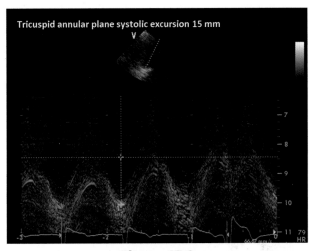

Figure 47-9

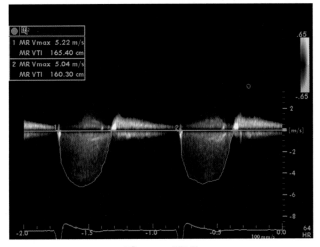

Figure 47-7

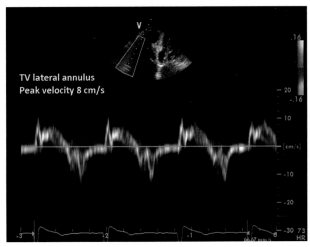

Figure 47-10

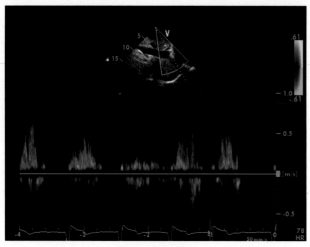

Figure 47-11

A. 0.65 cm²
B. 0.80 cm²
C. 0.95 cm²
D. 1.2 cm²

QUESTION 2. Which of the following findings is consistent here with the presence of severe tricuspid valve regurgitation?

A. Incomplete tricuspid valve leaflet coaptation
B. Coronary sinus dilatation
C. Systolic flow reversals in the hepatic veins
D. A PISA radius >0.9 cm²
E. All of the choices

QUESTION 3. Which of the following is the potential cause of an enlarged coronary sinus?

A. Anomalous drainage of the left pulmonary veins
B. Persistent left superior vena cava
C. Severe pulmonary arterial hypertension
D. A and B
E. A, B, and C

QUESTION 4. Calculate the right ventricular (Tei) index of myocardial performance (RIMP).

A. 0.25
B. 0.33
C. 0.60
D. 0.72

QUESTION 5. With regard to the following parameters of right ventricular function:

A. The RIMP, TAPSE, and Lateral S' are consistent with normal right ventricular systolic function
B. The TASPSE and Lateral S' are falsely low because of the preload
C. The RIMP is falsely low because of the preload
D. The RIMP, TAPSE, and Lateral S' are consistent with reduced right ventricular systolic function

(TAPSE, tricuspid annular plane systolic excursion; Lateral S', tricuspid annulus lateral peak systolic tissue velocity).

QUESTION 6. Appropriate management steps following coronary angiography include:

A. Percutaneous mitral valve balloon valvuloplasty
B. Mitral valve repair and tricuspid valve replacement
C. Mitral valve replacement and tricuspid valve repair
D. Mitral and tricuspid valve replacements

ANSWER 1: D. 1.2 cm^2

The regurgitant flow can be calculated as follows:

Flow rate = $(r)^2$ × 6.28 × aliasing velocity
× angle correction factor*
= $(1.2$ cm$)^2$ × 6.28 × 29 cm
per second × 220/180
= 321 cc per second

*Unlike the mitral valve where the leaflets are flat, the tricuspid valve leaflets are funnel shaped. This needs to be accounted for when calculating PISA. The assumption of a hemispheric shape of the flow convergence needs to be corrected for by measuring the angle of the leaflets. Typically, the angle of the tricuspid leaflets is 220° rather than the 180° of the mitral valve. Without this adjustment, the additional area of flow convergence would not be accounted for if the angle of the leaflets were not measured, which would lead to an underestimate of the regurgitation severity.

ERO = Flow rate/Peak tricuspid regurgitation velocity
ERO = 321 cc per second/260 cm per second = 1.2 cm^2

ANSWER 2: E. All of the choices. Incomplete tricuspid valve leaflet coaptation, coronary sinus dilatation, systolic flow reversals in the hepatic veins and a PISA radius >0.9 cm^2 when present in the setting of tricuspid valve regurgitation are all suggestive that the regurgitation is severe.

See *The Echo Manual, 3rd Edition*, discussion of echo findings in severe tricuspid valve regurgitation on pages 119 to 220, and Appendix 21 on page 414.

ANSWER 3: E. All of the choices. Although not specific for tricuspid valve regurgitation, a dilated coronary sinus is commonly a sign of longstanding right atrial hypertension (frequently a feature of severe tricuspid valve regurgitation).

See *The Echo Manual, 3rd Edition*, explanation of causes of enlarged coronary sinus on page 346.

ANSWER 4: B. The RIMP incorporates both systolic and diastolic time intervals to give a global ventricular index of myocardial performance.

The index can be easily derived from the tricuspid valve opening to closing time (TCO) and the pulmonary valve ejection time (PVET) as RIMP = TCO − PVET/PVET

Here RIMP = 360 − 270/270 = 0.33

See *The Echo Manual, 3rd Edition*, pages 137 and 138.

ANSWER 5: C. Measures of the extent (TAPSE) and the peak velocity (Lateral S') of longitudinal right ventricular contraction may be easily obtained from apical long-axis four-chamber view. Here both these measures are significantly reduced reflecting a reduction in right ventricular systolic function. The RIMP, however, is normal. The likely reason for this discordance is "pseudonormalization" of the RIMP caused by a relative reduction in the isovolumic contraction time in the setting of very high right atrial and right ventricular end-diastolic pressures.

ANSWER 6: D. Transthoracic echocardiography demonstrates rheumatic aortic, mitral valve, and tricuspid valve disease. The aortic valve is no more than mildly affected and does not require intervention. The mitral valve has the classic anterior leaflet "hockey-stick" deformity with nodular leaflet calcification typically of rheumatic involvement. There is mild–moderate stenosis (mean gradient 5 mm Hg) with moderate mitral valve regurgitation (regurgitant volume 35 cc). The tricuspid valve is moderately thickened (particularly the anterior leaflet) with a dilated annulus and severe regurgitation and is the primary source of the patient's symptoms. The patient should be referred for tricuspid valve replacement. The mitral valve should be addressed at the same time and is not amenable for repair. The patient underwent successful mitral and tricuspid valve replacements and is doing well in follow-up.

CASE 48

Progressive NYHA Class II and III Exertional Dyspnea and Palpitations

A 40-year-old male patient presents for the evaluation of progressive New York Heart Association functional class II to III exertional dyspnea and palpitations. Over the past month he has developed exertional presyncope. His only medication is metoprolol succinate 100 mg two times daily. On examination, his blood pressure is 115/70 mm Hg and heart rate 50 beats per minute (bpm). He has a brisk carotid upstroke and normal central venous pressure. His left ventricular apical impulse is sustained and localized. He has a 2/6 systolic ejection murmur at the apex that does not change with Valsalva with little change from squat to stand. His 12-lead ECG is shown in Figure 48-1. He is referred for transthoracic echocardiogram (see **Video 48-1**).

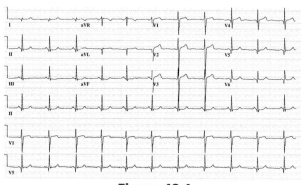

Figure 48-1

QUESTION 1. The findings in the parasternal long-axis evaluation are consistent with:

   A. Normal examination
   B. Mitral valve stenosis
   C. Hypertrophic cardiomyopathy with systolic anterior motion of the mitral valve
   D. Hypertrophic cardiomyopathy without evidence of outflow tract obstruction

QUESTION 2. The expected effect on the systolic ejection murmur with inhalation of amyl nitrite would be:

   A. Increase in murmur
   B. No change
   C. Decrease in murmur

QUESTION 3. Peak continuous wave Doppler gradients were recorded through the left ventricular outflow tract (LVOT) at rest (see Fig. 48-2), with Valsalva (see Fig. 48-3), and with amyl nitrite (see Fig. 48-4). The appropriate next step for this patient would be:

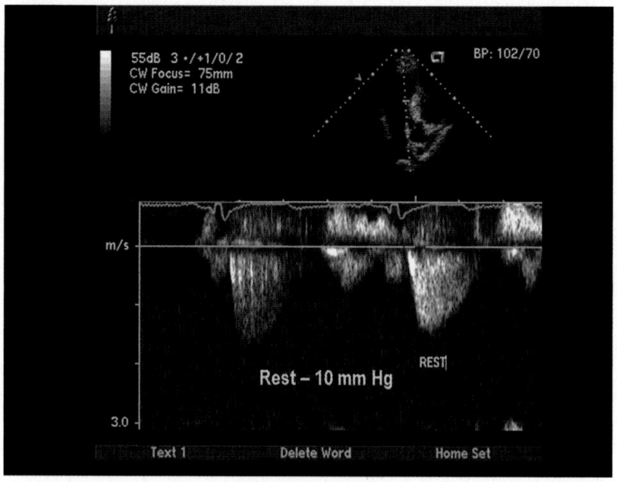

Figure 48-2

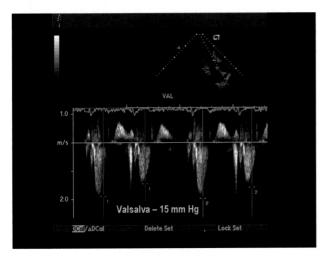

Figure 48-3

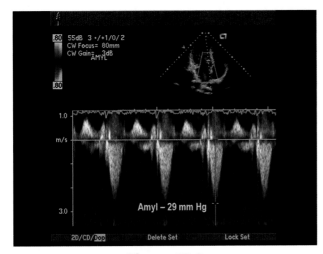

Figure 48-4

A. Refer for Doppler stress echocardiography
B. Refer for hemodynamic left and right heart catheterization
C. Refer for alcohol septal ablation
D. Refer for surgical septal myectomy

QUESTION 4. The patient is referred for a treadmill stress echocardiogram to assess functional capacity, and clinical and left ventricular hemodynamics. He exercised on a Bruce protocol for a little over 9 minutes and stopped secondary to dyspnea and lightheadedness. His preexercise heart rate was 58 bpm and blood pressure 122/70 mm Hg. His peak heart rate was 160 bpm and blood pressure 100/70 mm Hg. The regional wall motion assessment (see **Videos 48-2 and 48-3**) demonstrates:

A. No evidence of ischemia
B. Evidence of anterior ischemia
C. Evidence of inferior ischemia

QUESTION 5. On the basis of the findings from the stress echocardiogram (see **Video 48-4** and Fig. 48-5), the next step in management should include:

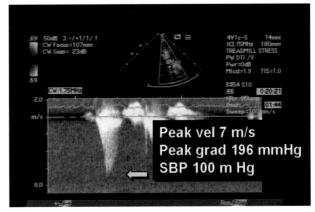

Figure 48-5

A. Refer for hemodynamic left and right heart catheterization
B. Refer for alcohol septal ablation
C. Refer for surgical septal myectomy
D. Nothing further, medical management only

QUESTION 6. The following still M-mode tracing (see Fig. 48-6) demonstrates evidence of:

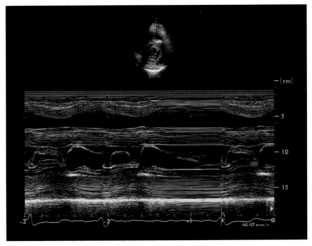

Figure 48-6

A. Systolic anterior motion of the anterior mitral valve leaflet
B. Mitral stenosis
C. Posterior leaflet mitral valve prolapse

QUESTION 7. Who is responsible for describing the echo finding in Figure 48-6 first?

A. Dr. Harvey Feigenbaum
B. Dr. Jamil Tajik
C. Dr. Pravin Shah
D. Dr. Liv Hatle

CASE 48 / 159

ANSWER 1: D. The left ventricle is of normal size with normal contractility. There is increased septal wall thickening particularly of the basal septum, suggestive of hypertrophic cardiomyopathy. There is no evidence of resting outflow tract obstruction or systolic anterior motion of the mitral valve at rest.

ANSWER 2: A. Amyl nitrite is a rapidly active vasodilator that is often used as a diagnostic tool to reveal a dynamic LVOT obstruction. Other maneuvers include a Valsalva or squat to stand.

ANSWER 3: A. In this patient with hypertrophic cardiomyopathy, it is likely that exertional symptoms of dyspnea are related to a dynamic outflow tract obstruction. If one can document a significant instantaneous gradient (50 mm Hg or greater) on maximal medical therapy, a septal reduction procedure such as alcohol septal ablation or surgical myectomy is an appropriate consideration. However, so far despite attempts with the Valsalva maneuver or inhaled amyl nitrite, no outflow tract gradient has been induced. An exercise Doppler study is the next appropriate step.

ANSWER 4: A. Echocardiographic images at rest demonstrate normal left ventricular contractility with normal poststress incremental increase in contractility with decrease in left ventricular size.

ANSWER 5: C. The exercise stress test reproduced the patient's typical symptoms of exertional dyspnea and lightheadedness associated with systemic hypotension. Doppler echocardiography was able to demonstrate that this occurred in the setting of dynamic outflow tract obstruction with a high gradient. Given that these findings occurred on high-dose ß-blockers, a referral for a septal reduction procedure is appropriate. In a young person without significant comorbidities, a surgical septal myectomy is the preferred option over alcohol septal ablation. With a similar in-hospital mortality (0.6% for myectomy and 1.6% for ablation), a lower rate of permanent pacemaker implantation for complete heart block (3.3% vs. 18.4%) and a higher success rate (required repeat procedure 0.6% in

myectomy patients vs. 5.5% in ablation patients)[1-4]. The patient here underwent successful surgical myectomy (Fig. 48-7).

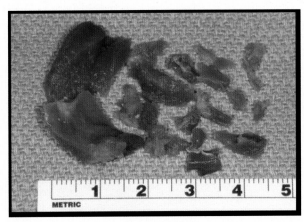

Figure 48-7

There is a Doppler signal recorded at 7 m per second (which corresponds to a peak instantaneous gradient of 196 mm Hg). It is unclear if this all represents the dynamic gradient or a signal contaminated with mitral regurgitation. However, even if this is the peak mitral regurgitant velocity, this implies that the LVOT gradient is high regardless.

Left ventricular systolic pressure equals the peak gradient across the mitral valve ($4v^2$, where v is the peak mitral regurgitant velocity) plus an estimate of left atrial pressure. In this case, $4(7)^2 + 20 = 215$ mm Hg. Alternatively (in the absence of aortic valve disease), left ventricular pressure also equals systolic blood pressure plus the intracavitary gradient. Therefore, in this case (if the Doppler signal is mitral regurgitation), the intracavitary gradient = $215 - 100 = 115$ mm Hg.

ANSWER 6: A. M-mode of hypertrophic cardiomyopathy demonstrates the evidence of systolic anterior motion of the anterior mitral valve leaflet.

See *The Echo Manual, 3rd Edition,* **Figure 2-19 on page 23.**

ANSWER 7: C. Dr. Pravin Shah first described the echo finding in Figure 48-6.

References

1. Ommen SR, Maron BJ, Olivotto I, et al. Long-term effects of surgical septal myectomy on survival in patients with obstructive hypertrophic cardiomyopathy. *J Am Coll Cardiol.* 2005;46:470–476.

2. Qin JX, Shiota T, Lever HM, et al. Outcome of patients with hypertrophic obstructive cardiomyopathy after percutaneous transluminal septal myocardial ablation and septal myectomy surgery. *J Am Coll Cardiol.* 2001;38:1994–2000.

3. Sorajja P, Valeti U, Nishimura RA, et al. Outcome of alcohol septal ablation for obstructive hypertrophic cardiomyopathy. *Circulation.* 2008;118:131–139.

4. Talreja DR, Nishimura RA, Edwards WD, et al. Alcohol septal ablation versus surgical septal myectomy: comparison of effects on atrioventricular conduction tissue. *J Am Coll Cardiol.* 2004;44:2329–2332.

5. Shah PM, Gramiak R, Kramer DH. Ultrasound localization of left ventricular outflow obstruction in hypertrophic obstructive cardiomyopathy. *Circulation.* 1969;40:3–11.

CASE 49

Progressive Exertional Fatigue and Lower Extremity Edema

A 42-year-old woman presents with progressive exertional fatigue and lower extremity edema.

QUESTION 1. On the basis of your review of the echocardiogram (**Videos 49-1 through 49-9**), the predominant pathology present is:

A. Tricuspid valve atresia

B. Ebstein anomaly

C. Right ventricular dysplasia with annular dilation and secondary tricuspid valve regurgitation

D. Carcinoid syndrome

QUESTION 2. Concerning this right heart abnormality, 25% of patients are prone to primary ventricular tachydysrhythmia.

A. True

B. False

QUESTION 3. Typical examination findings may include all of the following *except*:

A. Normal jugular venous pulsations

B. Cyanosis

C. A pan-systolic murmur that increases on inspiration

D. A narrowly split second heart sound

QUESTION 4. The likely secondary finding on this echocardiogram (**Videos 49-10 through 49-13** and Fig. 49-1, arrow) is:

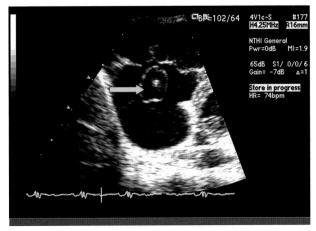

Figure 49-1

A. Papillary fibroelastoma

B. Vegetation

C. Blood cyst

D. Artifact

QUESTION 5. All of the following congenital cardiac lesions are associated with maternal rubella infection *except*:

A. Ebstein anomaly

B. Tetralogy of Fallot

C. Coarctation of the aorta

D. Patent ductus arteriosus

ANSWER 1: B. Seen here is a marked example of Ebstein anomaly[1] characterized by a morphologically and functionally abnormal tricuspid valve. The posterior and septal leaflets fail to delaminate from the ventricular wall leading to apical displacement of the tricuspid annulus (Fig. 49-2). Ebstein anomaly is defined as a displacement of septal tricuspid valve insertion 8 mm per m^2 toward the ventricular apex. This leads to atrialization of the right ventricle.

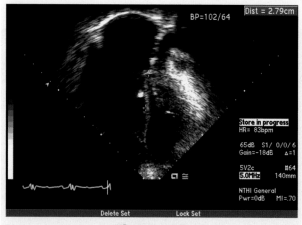

Figure 49-2

ANSWER 2: B. False. Ebstein anomaly is associated with the presence of accessory pathways and the Wolff–Parkinson–White syndrome in 20% to 25% of cases. Patients are prone to supraventricular rhythm abnormalities mediated either through the accessory pathway or through the atrial dysrhythmias caused by atrial enlargement. Unlike right ventricular dysplastic cardiomyopathies, primary ventricular dysrhythmia is uncommon, although atrial dysrhythmia, particularly if conducted down an accessory pathway, is poorly tolerated and potentially may degenerate into secondary ventricular dysrhythmias.

ANSWER 3: D. Unlike most other cases of severe tricuspid valve regurgitation, patients with Ebstein anomaly typically have normal jugular pulsations because of the compliance of the huge right atrial enlargement. Patients may be cyanotic because of right-to-left shunting through either an associated atrial septal defect or a patent foramen ovale (one or either of which is present in 50% of cases). Typical of right-sided murmurs, the murmur of tricuspid valve regurgitation will augment with the increased right-sided filling on inspiration. Patient's with Ebstein anomaly will have either a widely split S_2 (because of a delay in pulmonary valve closure) or a fixed split S_2 in the setting of an atrial septal defect.

ANSWER 4: C. The differential diagnosis for freely mobile lesions present on heart valves, or here attached to the Eustachian valve, includes tumors, vegetation, thrombus, and artifacts. Here, though, the thin-wall and central echo-free space is characteristic of a benign blood cyst. More common in children, cysts are typically found on cardiac valves and typically regress with age. They are of little clinical importance except for the potential for the echocardiographer to misdiagnose them as something more sinister leading to unnecessary invasive diagnostic or therapeutics.

ANSWER 5: A. Unlike the other defects listed, Ebstein anomaly is not associated with maternal rubella infection. Ebstein anomaly has been linked with maternal lithium use.

See *The Echo Manual, 3rd Edition,* pages 563 to 565 for discussion of Ebstein's anomaly.

Reference

1. Attenhofer Jost CH, Connolly HM, Dearani JA, et al. Ebstein's anomaly. *Circulation.* 2007;115:277–285.

CASE 50

Progressive Exertional Shortness of Breath and Lower Extremity Edema

A 52-year-old man presents with a 6-month history of progressive exertional shortness of breath and lower extremity edema. He is now New York Heart Association functional class IV. On examination, his blood pressure is 95/50 mm Hg and he has a heart rate of 100 beats per minute. He has distended neck veins and three-plus bilateral pedal edema. His chest is clear. He is referred for transthoracic echocardiography (see **Video 50-1**).

QUESTION 1. In this case, all of the following are true *except*:

A. The absence of right atrial collapse suggests against echo evidence of tamponade physiology
B. The presence of respiratory variation in mitral inflow supports echo evidence of tamponade physiology
C. Right ventricular (RV) end-diastolic pressure is likely higher than mean left atrial pressure
D. Hepatic vein dilation suggests an elevation in right atrial pressure
E. Left ventricular ejection fraction is increased (hyperdynamic)

QUESTION 2. In the calculation of estimated RV systolic pressure, the correct tricuspid velocity to take is:

A. In end inspiration
B. In end expiration
C. An average of all consecutive values

QUESTION 3. The most likely clinical finding in this patient is:

A. Audible fourth heart sound
B. Sclerodactyly and esophageal dilatation
C. Lung mass on chest x-ray
D. Acute pulmonary embolus
E. Muffled second heart sound

QUESTION 4. Which of the following is the most specific two-dimensional (2D) echocardiographic finding for cardiac tamponade?

A. RV diastolic collapse
B. Right atrial diastolic collapse
C. Abnormal ventricular septal motion
D. Dilated inferior vena cava

QUESTION 5. Left ventricular diastolic filling pressure based on mitral inflow is:

A. Normal
B. Reduced
C. Increased
D. Not able to be determined

ANSWER 1: A. This case is one of severe pulmonary and right atrial hypertension with superimposed cardiac tamponade. Here we see 2D evidence of left atrial collapse but not the more usual RV or right atrial collapse, indicating that pericardial pressure exceeds left atrial but not RV or right atrial pressure. This is a classic echocardiographic finding seen in tamponade patients with severe pulmonary hypertension in whom there is associated severe elevation in right-sided intracardiac pressures.

Although any degree of pericardial fluid present in a patient with pulmonary hypertension is associated with a worse prognosis (reflecting it as a marker of elevated right atrial pressure), the occurrence of moderate or greater degrees of pericardial fluid in the setting of pulmonary arterial hypertension is much less common. Assessment of the hemodynamic significance of pericardial effusions in the setting of pulmonary hypertension is challenging and largely relies on the findings of left-sided chamber diastolic collapse.

Doppler studies from mitral inflow and hepatic vein are characteristic for cardiac tamponade with respiratory variation of mitral inflow (A velocities are indicated by arrow) and increased diastolic hepatic vein flow with expiration.[1,2]

ANSWER 2: B. Hemodynamic measures of RV end-systolic or pulmonary artery pressures should be made in end expiration whether in the echocardiographic or catheterization laboratory because this is the point at which intrathoracic pressure is closest to atmospheric pressure. Typically with expiration, right-sided inflow tends to be lower with higher pulmonary artery pressures. With inspiration, flow into right-sided chambers increases and peak tricuspid regurgitant velocities tend to modestly decline. These hemodynamic changes with respiration can be magnified in cases where intrathoracic pressures swings are exaggerated such as obstructive lung disease.

ANSWER 3: B. A pericardial effusion may develop in the setting of severe pulmonary arterial hypertension because of right atrial hypertension and/or associated connective tissue disease. Although the presence of even small amounts of pericardial fluid in the setting of pulmonary hypertension is associated with a worse prognosis, sufficient fluid does not accumulate to have hemodynamic significance in most cases. In the smaller proportion of patients with pulmonary hypertension who develop moderate/severe amounts of fluid almost all have associated scleroderma/CREST syndrome.

ANSWER 4: A. When present, RV diastolic collapse is most specific for tamponade with higher intrapericardial pressure than RV pressure during early diastole. Other 2D findings are frequently present not only in tamponade but also in other conditions.

ANSWER 5: B. E velocity is much lower than that of A velocity. Respiratory variation of mitral inflow velocities is more pronounced than A velocity. Both the tamponade physiology and the RV dysfunction in the setting of pulmonary hypertension in this patient are limiting flow to the left heart chambers resulting in a grade 1 diastolic dysfunction pattern.

References

1. Eysmann SB, Palevsky HL, Reichek N, et al. Two-dimensional and Doppler-echocardiographic and cardiac catheterization correlates of survival in primary pulmonary hypertension. *Circulation.* 1989;80:353–360.

2. Plotnick GD, Rubin DC, Feliciano Z, et al. Pulmonary hypertension decreases the predictive accuracy of echocardiographic clues for cardiac tamponade. *Chest.* 1995;107:919.

CASE 51

Dyspnea with Modest Exertion

A 64-year-old woman without significant medical history presents with new-onset dyspnea with modest exertion. She denies angina, orthopnea, or edema. She is referred for exercise stress echocardiography.

QUESTION 1. On the basis of her resting study, what is the diastolic function (see **Video 51-1**)?

A. Normal
B. Mildly abnormal (grade 1)
C. Moderately abnormal (grade 2)
D. Severely abnormal (grade 3)

QUESTION 2. After review of the rest (on left of quads) and stress (on right side of quads) images (see **Video 51-2**), the stress echocardiogram (apical 4 chamber images are in Mayo format with left ventricle on the left) is:

A. Negative for ischemia
B. Positive for ischemia in the distribution of the left anterior descending artery
C. Positive for ischemia in the distribution of the right coronary artery
D. Positive for multivessel ischemia

QUESTION 3. The most likely etiology for this patient's dyspnea is:

A. Symptomatic coronary artery disease
B. Pulmonary arterial hypertension
C. Elevation in left ventricular filling pressures
D. Mitral stenosis
E. Pulmonary disease and/or deconditioning

QUESTION 4. Two weeks later, she presents to the emergency department after an episode of syncope. A repeat transthoracic echocardiogram is obtained (see **Video 51-3**). There is now evidence of:

A. Significant pulmonary hypertension
B. Severe tricuspid valve regurgitation
C. Tricuspid stenosis
D. Acute myocardial infarction because of occlusion of the left anterior descending artery

QUESTION 5. Appropriate steps might include all of the following *except*:

A. Coronary angiography
B. CT angiography
C. Emergency cardiac surgery
D. Thrombolytic therapy

ANSWER 1: B. The mitral inflow pattern here indicates where early diastolic filling (E) is less than late diastolic filling (A) related to delayed left ventricular relaxation. This corresponds to grade 1 or mildly abnormal diastolic function.

See *The Echo Manual, 3rd Edition*, **grading of diastolic function on pages 132 to 134.**

She exercised for 3 minutes 30 seconds on a Bruce protocol to a double product of 24,700 and stopped because of dyspnea. She had no chest pain, and her stress ECG was nondiagnostic because of resting ST changes.

ANSWER 2: A. Seen here is a normal left ventricular response to exercise with generalized increase in left ventricular myocardial contractility, a decline in left ventricular size, and an increase in left ventricular ejection fraction. No regional wall motion abnormalities are seen.

See *The Echo Manual, 3rd Edition*, **Table 11-3 on page 178.**

ANSWER 3: E. Exercise stress echocardiography has the capacity to evaluate/screen all major cardiac causes of dyspnea. Beyond the assessment of coronary artery disease, echocardiographic evaluation of left-sided valve disease, pulmonary pressures, and left-sided filling pressures (suggests by an elevation in the ratio of the peak velocity of early mitral filling (E) to that of the peak early diastolic velocity (e') on tissue Doppler of medial mitral annulus. An E'e' ratio >15 usually indicates elevated diastolic left ventricular filling pressure). In the absence of these findings, dyspnea is commonly related to pulmonary disease and/or deconditioning.

ANSWER 4: B. Echo images indicate a marked interval change, with a D-shaped left ventricle, severe right ventricular enlargement, tricuspid annular dilation, and severe tricuspid valve regurgitation that are new. Findings here suggestive of severe tricuspid regurgitation include a severely dilated annulus with poor leaflet coaptation, a dense continuous wave Doppler signal, and a dagger-shaped signal. One would expect to find systolic flow reversals in the hepatic veins.

ANSWER 5: B. The sudden interval change with evidence of severe right ventricular overload in the setting of syncope and recent new onset of dyspnea suggests a high likelihood of pulmonary emboli as the underlying etiology, a suspicion that could be confirmed by CT angiography of the chest. Options of therapy in this setting include consideration of either emergency thrombectomy or intravenous thrombolytic therapy.[1-5]

See *The Echo Manual, 3rd Edition*, **pages 149 to 151.**

References

1. Goldhaber SZ. Thrombolysis for pulmonary embolism. *N Engl J Med.* 2002;347:1131–1132.

2. Sadeghi HM, Kimura BJ, Raisinghani A, et al. Does lowering pulmonary arterial pressure eliminate severe functional tricuspid regurgitation? Insights from pulmonary thromboendarterectomy. *J Am Coll Cardiol.* 2004;44:126–132.

3. Konstantinides S, Geibel A, Heusel G, et al. Management strategies and prognosis of pulmonary embolism-3 trial investigators. Heparin plus alteplase compared with heparin alone in patients with submassive pulmonary embolism. *N Engl J Med.* 2002;347:1143–1150.

4. Tapson VF. Acute pulmonary embolism. *N Engl J Med.* 2008;358:1037.

CASE 52

Fevers, Malaise, and Fatigue

A 33-year-old woman presents with a 2-month history of fevers, malaise, and fatigue. She has a medical history of autoimmune thyroid disease on hormone replacement with a normal sensitive thyroid-stimulating hormone. Examination is normal. Twelve-lead ECG demonstrates T-wave inversion in her precordial leads (Fig. 52-1), and she is referred for echocardiogram (**Video 52-1**).

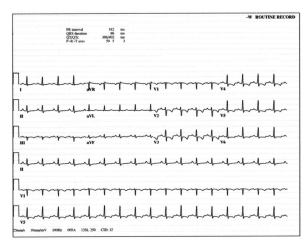

Figure 52-1

QUESTION 1. Calculate the left ventricular (LV) fractional shortening (FS) (Fig. 52-2).

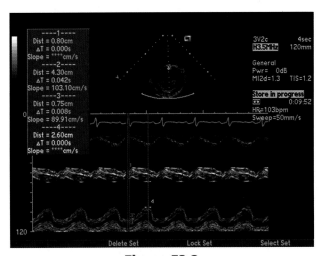

Figure 52-2

A. 33%
B. 40%
C. 60%
D. 63%

QUESTION 2. Calculate the mitral valve regurgitant volume (Figs. 52-3 and 52-4).

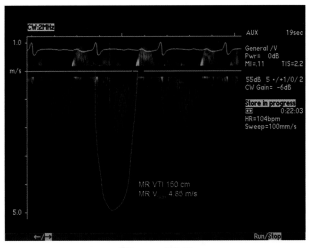

Figure 52-3

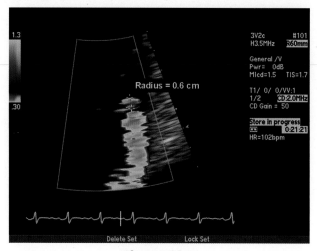

Radius = 0.6 cm

Figure 52-4

A. 15 cc
B. 21 cc
C. 29 cc
D. 40 cc
E. 45 cc

QUESTION 3. When the aliasing velocity is 30 cm per second for PISA calculation, which of the following PISA radii provides an effective regurgitant orifice (ERO) of 0.4 cm² assuming mitral regurgitation (MR) velocity of 5 m per second?

A. 0.5 cm
B. 0.75 cm
C. 1.0 cm
D. 1.5 cm

QUESTION 4. The echocardiographic findings would be most compatible with abnormalities on which of the following tests?

A. Serum protein electrophoresis
B. Serum white blood cell count
C. Urinary 5-HIAA excretion
D. Fasting transferrin saturation
E. Antinuclear antibody and anticentromere antibodies

ANSWER 1: B. 40%. FS is the percentage change in LV dimensions with each LV contraction.

$$FS = \frac{LVED - LVES}{LVED} \times 100\%,$$

where LVED is the LV end-diastolic dimension and LVES is the LV end-systolic dimension. Normal FS for men is 25% to 43% and for women is 27% to 45%.

Here LVED = 43 mm and LVES = 26 mm. Therefore, FS = (43–26)/43 × 100% = 40%.

See *The Echo Manual, 3rd Edition*, page 115.

ANSWER 2: B. 21 cc.

The regurgitant flow can be calculated as follows:

Flow = $(r)^2$ × 6.28 × aliasing velocity
= $(0.6 \text{ cm})^2$ × 6.28 × 30 cm per second
= 68 cc per second

ERO = Flow/Peak MR velocity
ERO = 68 cc per second/485 cm per second
= 0.14 cm²

Regurgitant volume = ERO × regurgitant time velocity integral
= 0.14 cm² × 150 cm
= 21 cc

See *The Echo Manual, 3rd Edition*, PISA equation on page 215.

ANSWER 3: C. When the aliasing velocity is 30 cm per second, the flow rate can be calculated as 6.28 × 30 × radius. If the flow rate is divided by the MR velocity of 500 cm per second, it gives an ERO that is 0.4 × radius. Therefore, the radius of 1 cm gives ERO of 0.4 cm².

ANSWER 4: B. The echocardiographic findings here demonstrate biventricular endocardial thickening with thrombotic-fibrotic obliteration of the ventricular apices, and myocardial contrast imaging reveals characteristic apical thrombus. These findings are characteristic of hypereosinophilic heart disease. Patients typically have markedly elevated eosinophil counts for 6 or more months.[1]

See *The Echo Manual, 3rd Edition*, hypereosinophilic syndrome and Figure 16-17 on page 284.

Reference

1. Ommen SR, Seward JB, Tajik AJ. Clinical and echocardiographic features of hypereosinophilic syndromes. *Am J Cardiol.* 2000;86:110–113.

Dyspnea and Asymmetrical Ground-glass Pulmonary Infiltrates

A 72-year-old man is referred for transthoracic echocardiogram (**Videos 53-1 to 53-16** and Figs. 53-1 to 53-10). He has been hospitalized on three occasions over the past 5 months for dyspnea and asymmetrical ground-glass pulmonary infiltrates of unclear etiology. Two months ago, he underwent an adenosine sestamibi perfusion study that was normal. His history is significant for a mitral valve bioprosthesis for mitral valve regurgitation and one vessel bypass graft 9 years ago.

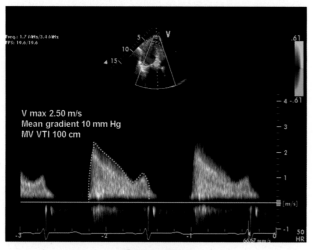

Figure 53-1

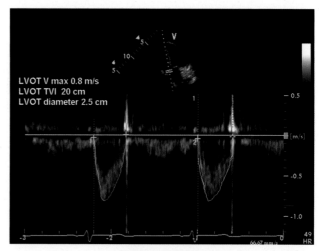

Figure 53-3

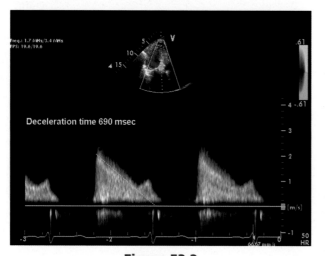

Figure 53-2

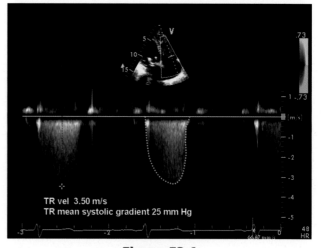

Figure 53-4

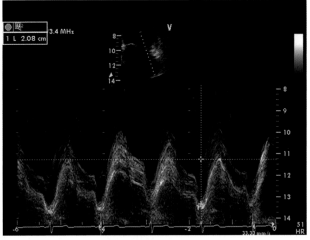

Figure 53-5

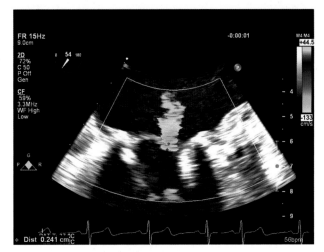

Figure 53-8

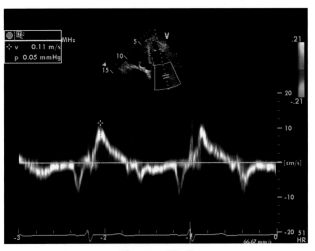

Figure 53-6

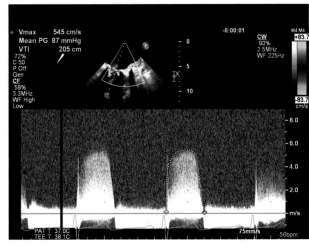

Figure 53-9

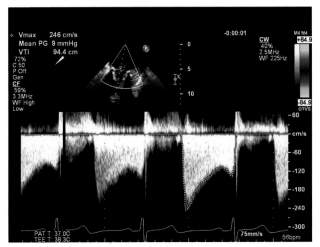

Figure 53-7

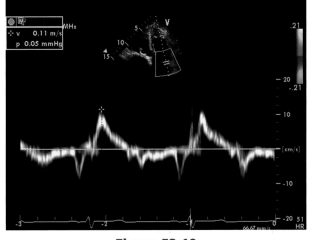

Figure 53-10

QUESTION 1. Calculate the pressure halftime of the mitral bioprosthesis.

A. 100 milliseconds
B. 150 milliseconds
C. 200 milliseconds
D. 300 milliseconds

QUESTION 2. Calculate the estimated mean pulmonary artery pressure (mPAP).

A. 25 mm Hg
B. 35 mm Hg
C. 45 mm Hg
D. 59 mm Hg
E. 69 mm Hg
F. Cannot be performed on the basis of the available data

QUESTION 3. Mitral prosthetic flow velocities are consistent with:

A. Normal mitral bioprosthetic function in the setting of high output
B. Significant prosthetic dysfunction likely related to obstruction
C. Significant prosthetic dysfunction likely related to regurgitation

QUESTION 4. Right ventricular systolic function is:

A. Normal
B. Mildly reduced
C. Markedly reduced

QUESTION 5. The next step in the assessment of this patient's dyspnea should include:

A. Hemodynamic catheterization
B. Cardiac MR scan
C. Transesophageal echocardiogram
D. Coronary angiogram

QUESTION 6. Following review of **Videos 53-17 and 53-18,** and Figures 53-11 to 53-13, the mitral valve prosthetic gradient appears related to:

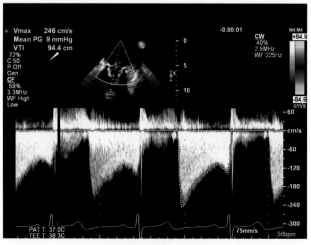

Figure 53-11

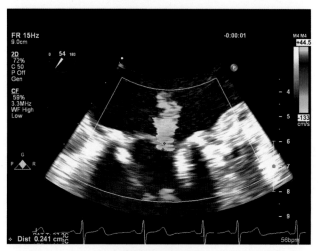

Figure 53-12

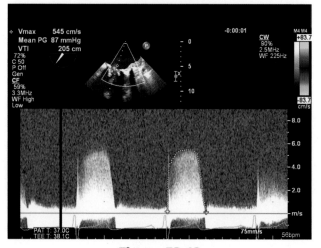

Figure 53-13

A. Normal mitral bioprosthetic function
B. Moderate–severe valvular regurgitation
C. Bioprosthetic calcific degeneration
D. Thrombotic obstruction of the bioprosthesis

QUESTION 7. In which of the following scenarios, should patients receive both warfarin and aspirin antithrombotic therapy?

A. Mitral valve bioprosthesis in the setting of left ventricular dysfunction
B. Mechanical mitral valve replacement
C. Aortic valve bioprosthesis with a history of a hypercoagulable state
D. A and B
E. All of the choices

ANSWER 1: C. The pressure halftime is calculated as 0.29 times the deceleration time that here equals to 690 × 0.29 = 200 milliseconds.

ANSWER 2: B. Assessment of mPAP is a useful measure in the assessment of patients with pulmonary arterial hypertension. Although measures of mPAP by echocardiography can be derived after integrating systolic and diastolic pulmonary artery pressure estimates or from the pulmonary valve acceleration time, derivation of mPAP from the mean gradient method appears to be the most robust and readily obtainable method. By this method, mPAP = right ventricular – right atrial mean systolic gradient to the right atrial pressure (here estimated as 10 mm Hg in the presence of a mildly dilated inferior vena cava).[1]

ANSWER 3: B. There is evidence of increased flow velocities across the mitral valve with a super evaluation in early (E) peak velocity at 2.5 m per second. Increased flow velocities may be related to flow acceleration, which is related to valve obstruction, or increased quantity of flow, which is related to valvular regurgitation or a high output state. Useful indicators for separating these mechanisms are the pressure half time and the left ventricular outflow tract (LVOT) velocities. Here the LVOT velocity profile is normal with a normal Doppler-derived cardiac output (5.4 L per minute) excluding a high output state. Although flow velocities and mean gradient may be elevated in both prosthetic obstruction and regurgitation, the pressure halftime is prolonged in the former but not in the latter. The pressure half time of 200 milliseconds here suggests an obstructive rather than regurgitant etiology.

See *The Echo Manual, 3rd Edition*, pages 229 and 230.

ANSWER 4: A. The recent American Society of Echocardiography guidelines recommend at least one measure of longitudinal systolic function be recorded to assess right ventricular systolic function in every patient. Options include the tricuspid annular plane systolic excursion (TAPSE, normal >16 to 18 mm) and the peak systolic tissue velocity of the lateral tricuspid annulus (S, normal >10 to 12 cm per second).[2]

ANSWER 5: C. As discussed in answers to Questions 2 and 3, the transthoracic echocardiogram shows evidence of mitral bioprosthesis dysfunction, more likely related to valvular obstruction and secondary pulmonary hypertension. The best test to better characterize mitral valvular function/dysfunction is a transesophageal echocardiogram.

ANSWER 6: D. Transesophageal echocardiogram demonstrates predominantly laminated thrombus involving a large surface area of the left atrial wall extending from the left-sided pulmonary veins down to the valvular sewing ring and extending up to partially obstruct flow through the prosthesis (appreciated on **Video 53-18**). The patient was commenced on systemic anticoagulation, was proceeded with left atriotomy and resection of the laminated thrombus, and underwent mitral valve replacement.

ANSWER 7: E. All of the choices. Aspirin is recommended for all patients with prosthetic heart valves. In patients with bioprosthesis and no risk factors (atrial fibrillation, hypercoagulable state, left ventricular dysfunction, previous thromboembolism), aspirin alone is sufficient. All patients with mechanical valves and patients with a bioprosthesis and risk factor should also receive warfarin anticoagulation[3].

References

1. Aduen JF, Castello R, Daniels JT, et al. Accuracy and precision of three echocardiographic methods for estimating mean pulmonary artery pressure. *Chest*. 2011;139:347–352.

2. Rudski LG, Lai WW, Afilalo J, et al. Guidelines for the echocardiographic assessment of the right heart in adults: a report from the American Society of Echocardiography endorsed by the European Association of Echocardiography, a registered branch of the European Society of Cardiology, and the Canadian Society of Echocardiography. *J Am Soc Echocardiogr*. 2010;23:685–713.

3. Bonow RO, Carabello BA, Chatterjee K, et al. 2008 focused update incorporated into the ACC/AHA 2006 guidelines for the management of patients with valvular heart disease: a report of the American College of Cardiology/American Heart Association Task Force on Practice Guidelines (Writing Committee to Revise the 1998 Guidelines for the Management of Patients with Valvular Heart Disease): endorsed by the Society of Cardiovascular Anesthesiologists, Society for Cardiovascular Angiography and Interventions, and Society of Thoracic Surgeons. *Circulation*. 2008;118:e523–e661.

CASE 54

Congenital Aortic Valve Stenosis Status Post Replacement

*A*30-year-old woman presents with a medical history significant for congenital aortic valve stenosis status postreplacement at age 5 and re-replacement with a 21-mm Medtronic Hall prosthesis at age 20. Her medications include warfarin 2 mg daily. She rarely undergoes INR monitoring.

She describes mild breathlessness while walking (functional class II). On examination, her blood pressure is 140/80 mm Hg and her heart rate 75 beats per minute. Her central venous pressure is normal. She has 3/6 late-peaking systolic murmur at the base that radiates to the carotids bilaterally and is heard throughout precordium. There are no added sounds or evidence of volume overload. Her INR is 1.2.

She is referred for transthoracic echocardiography (**Videos 54-1 through 54-5** and Figs. 54-1 through 54-3).

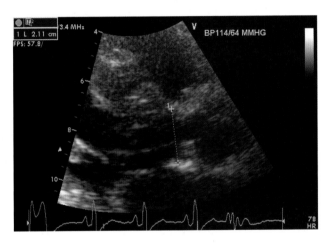

Figure 54-1

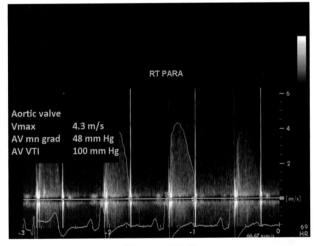

Figure 54-3

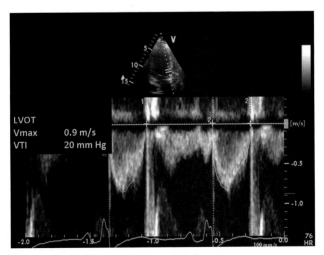

Figure 54-2

QUESTION 1. What is the calculated prosthetic function orifice area?

    A. 0.69 cm²

    B. 0.79 cm²

    C. 0.89 cm²

    D. 0.99 cm²

QUESTION 2. The next appropriate step in the management of this patient, in addition to intravenous heparin, is:

    A. Surgical consultation

    B. Continuation of intravenous heparin until INR is therapeutic

    C. A retrograde hemodynamic left heart catheterization to assess the prosthetic aortic valve area

    D. Transesophageal echocardiography

    E. Intravenous thrombolytic therapy

QUESTION 3. On the basis of your review of these additional images (**Videos 54-6 through 54-10**) in the context of the overall case, the likely pathology is:

    A. Thrombus

    B. Pannus

    C. Normal function

    D. Infective endocarditis

QUESTION 4. The patient had normal leaflet excursion on fluoroscopy and favored conservative management. The patient returned 2 months later now asymptomatic and a prosthetic mean aortic valve gradient of 25 mm Hg. She was advised to follow up in 3 months.

She returns 4 years later, acutely unwell. She describes a 2-week history of fever, severe exertional dyspnea, orthopnea, and lower extremity edema. On examination, she is pale, diaphoretic, and tachycardic and has a systemic blood pressure of 105/65 mm Hg. She has systolic and diastolic precordial murmurs.

She undergoes repeat transthoracic echocardiogram (**Videos 54-15 through 54-20**). Potential explanations for the aortic valve findings include:

    A. Aortic dissection

    B. Thrombosis

    C. Infective endocarditis

    D. Pseudoaneurysm rupture

QUESTION 5. Which of the following describes the mitral valve pathology (**Videos 54-11 through 54-14**)?

    A. Anteriorly directed mitral valve regurgitation secondary to leaflet prolapse

    B. Posteriorly directed mitral valve regurgitation secondary to leaflet prolapse

    C. Functional anteriorly directed mitral valve regurgitation

    D. Functional posteriorly directed mitral valve regurgitation

QUESTION 6. Which of the following is not a clinical scenario in which the flow marked with the arrow (Fig. 54-4) may be seen?

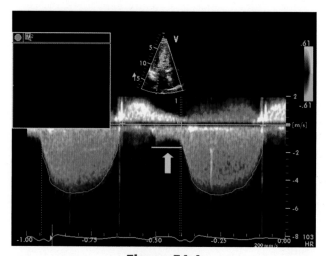

Figure 54-4

    A. Third degree heart block

    B. Acute severe aortic valve regurgitation

    C. Severe mitral valve stenosis

    D. Decompensated left ventricular (LV) low ejection fraction heart failure

ANSWER 1: A.

Aortic valve area = [(LVOT TVI) × (LVOT area)]/Ao TVI
= [(LVOT TVI) × (0.785 (LVOT D)^2]/Ao TVI
= [(20) × (3.46)]/100
= 0.69 cm^2

The evaluation of the degree of stenosis/obstruction of prosthetic valves is quite similar to the evaluation of native valves for stenosis. Just as in a comprehensive examination of a native valve, it is critical to perform a Doppler evaluation from all available transducer windows. Fifteen to twenty percent of the time, the peak signal will be obtained from a transducer location (right parasternal as in this case) other than the apex.

See *The Echo Manual, 3rd Edition,* calculation of effective prosthetic orifice area on page 231 and Table 13-1 on page 229.

ANSWER 2: D.
The calculated effective prosthetic area is severely abnormal, indicating significant obstruction of the valve. Overall, the incidence of prosthetic valve obstruction is low, ranging between 0.1% and 0.4% per year, depending on the size, type, location of the valve, and the adequacy of anticoagulation. Management decisions are based on the degree of symptoms and signs of heart failure and the underlying mechanism. Whereas the obstruction of a mitral mechanical prosthesis is caused more frequently by thrombus, the obstruction of an aortic mechanical prosthesis is caused more frequently by pannus formation. Although in this setting, the subtherapeutic INR and poor compliance with testing increase the likelihood of underlying valve thrombosis. Transesophageal echocardiography would allow better visualization of the valve leaflets to aid in the determination of pannus versus thrombus before a decision on therapeutic intervention. A hemodynamic catheterization in this setting is contraindicated because of the high risk of causing complete valve leaflet obstruction and/or embolization.[1]

ANSWER 3: A.
Thrombus. Transesophageal echocardiography demonstrates a mass on the aortic prosthesis, which measures approximately 8 by 4 mm. Although this could be consistent with vegetation, in the absence of systemic symptoms of endocarditis, and a subtherapeutic INR, the most likely pathology is thrombus on the prosthetic valve (supported by negative blood cultures).

There are a variety of available options for management of prosthetic valve thrombosis. The decision on approach to therapy of thrombus on an aortic valve prosthesis is affected by a variety of factors including, functional class, the size of the clot, and the surgical risk and need to be individualized for the patient. If patients have a large clot burden or have functional class III or IV symptoms, emergency surgery is recommended. If surgery is deemed to be high risk or not available, intravenous thrombolytic therapy is an alternative. For patients with a low clot burden and functional class I to II symptoms, thrombolytic therapy or a trial of anticoagulation may serve as an alternative to an operation.[2]

ANSWER 4: C.
Echocardiography demonstrates rocking motion of the valve prosthesis suggestive of significant dehiscence posteriorly and associated likely with severe periprosthetic aortic regurgitation. There is a large septated, echo-free space posterior to the aortic root that has free flow with unclear site of communication. This may represent an abscess, chronic pseudoaneurysm with new valve dehiscence, or less likely aortic dissection. Although recurrent thrombosis may also be present, this could not explain the aortic valve findings.

ANSWER 5: D.
There is grade 3 to 4/4 posteriorly directed mitral valve regurgitation that appears because of tethering of the posterior leaflet rather than intrinsic leaflet pathology. The likely mechanism is mitral valve annular enlargement and myocardial dysfunction because of high end-diastolic ventricular pressures.

ANSWER 6: C.
Shown here is diastolic mitral valve regurgitation. For this to occur, the LV pressures in diastole need to exceed the atrial pressures. Diastolic mitral regurgitation is commonly observed during atrioventricular (AV) block, when atrial contraction is not followed by adequately synchronized LV contraction. Under these conditions, the AV pressure gradient reverses during atrial relaxation, resulting in diastolic mitral regurgitation. In the absence of AV block, diastolic mitral regurgitation may be seen secondary to significant elevation of LV end-diastolic filling pressures in the presence of restrictive ventricular hemodynamics or severe aortic regurgitation, typically acute aortic valve regurgitation.

Blood cultures grow out *Enterococcus*. Intraoperative transesophageal echocardiography demonstrates partial dehiscence of the aortic prosthesis with severe periprosthetic regurgitation (**Videos 54-21 through 54-23**). There is a small mobile echodensity attached to the prosthetic ring that likely represents a vegetation (**Video 54-24**). These findings were confirmed at surgery where a periprosthetic abscess was debrided and a new prosthesis inserted. The patient did well.

References

1. Cannegieter SC, Torn M, Rosendaal FR. Oral anticoagulant treatment in patients with mechanical heart valves: how to reduce the risk of thromboembolic and bleeding complications. *J Intern Med.* 1999;245:369–374.

2. Bonow RO, Carabello BA, Chatterjee K, et al. 2008 focused update incorporated into the ACC/AHA 2006 guidelines for the management of patients with valvular heart disease: a report of the American College of Cardiology/American Heart Association Task Force on Practice Guidelines. *J Am Coll Cardiol.* 2008;52:e1–e142.

CASE 55

Exertional Shortness of Breath

A 52-year-old man presents for the evaluation of exertional shortness of breath.

QUESTION 1. Two-dimensional transthoracic echocardiographic images (**Video 55-1**) indicate evidence of:

A. Hypertensive heart disease complicated by an apical myocardial infarction
B. Hypertrophic cardiomyopathy (HCM)
C. Cardiac hemochromatosis
D. Eosinophilic heart disease

QUESTION 2. Which of the following 12-lead ECGs is typically associated with these echo findings?

A.

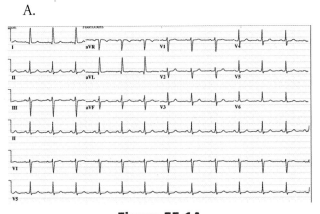

Figure 55-1A

B.

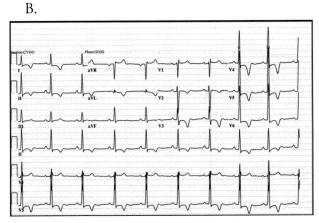

Figure 55-1B

C.

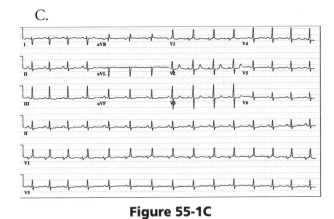

Figure 55-1C

D.

Figure 55-1D

QUESTION 3. The Doppler flow indicated by the arrow (Fig. 55-2) is related to:

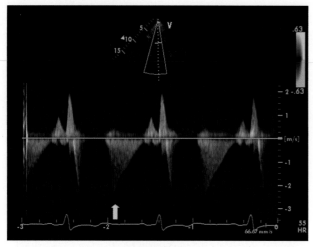

Figure 55-2

A. Late mitral valve regurgitation related to systolic anterior motion of the mitral valve apparatus

B. Dyssynchrony of myocardial relaxation related to intracavitary obstruction

QUESTION 4. Potential complications associated with this condition include:

A. Atrial fibrillation

B. Myocardial infarction

C. Sudden cardiac death

D. Heart failure

E. All of the choices

ANSWER 1: B. Parasternal and apical transthoracic echocardiographic images demonstrate massive circumferential thickening of the mid and apical left ventricular septum, with sparing of the basal segments. The apical variant of HCM is readily identified here on parasternal images with the apical images delineating the classical "ace of spades" appearance. However, some variants of this disorder will be limited to the apex and hence may be missed without a careful apical examination. Here intravenous echo contrast administration is very helpful in outlining the progressive diminution of the left ventricular cavity toward the apex with a slit-like small apical cavity. Contrast also helps separate myocardial thickening from the nonenhancing thrombus material of eosinophilic heart disease.

See *The Echo Manual, 3rd Edition*, **Figure 16-17 on page 284, and page 258.**

ANSWER 2: B. The classic 12-lead ECG associated with the apical variant of HCM is marked T-wave inversion in the precordial leads.

See *The Echo Manual, 3rd Edition*, **Figure 15-10D on page 259.**

The extensive left ventricular hypertrophy will lead to evidence of ECG criteria for left ventricular hypertrophy. Figure 55-1A is a normal ECG. Figure 55-1C demonstrates evidence of right atrial enlargement, right ventricular hypertrophy, and secondary nonspecific ST-T wave changes; findings that might be seen with right ventricular pressure overload such as with pulmonary hypertension. Figure 55-1D demonstrates a left bundle branch block that is typically associated with left ventricular dilated cardiomyopathy.

ANSWER 3: B. Brief apical flow is shown moving away from the apex in systole followed by cessation of flow. Flow is again seen during early diastole (it has a velocity of 2.5 m per second on continuous wave Doppler recording below the baseline). It is related to a moderate pressure gradient between the apex and the base of the left ventricle during early diastole. This unusual flow coming from the apex to the midcavity, starting before mitral inflow, is typical of midcavitary obstruction. During isovolumic relaxation period, there is a dyssynchrony of myocardial relaxation that results in a pressure gradient from the apex to the basal segment across the obstructed midcavity.

See *The Echo Manual, 3rd Edition*, **Figure 15-21 on page 263.**

ANSWER 4: E. All of the choices. Although the apical variant of HCM tends to have a better outcome than other forms of HCM, all of the outcomes have been reported to occur (most commonly atrial fibrillation). Although most patients with apical HCM have symptoms that can be controlled with medical management, a small proportion have progressive heart failure symptoms and for these a surgical apical myectomy is an option.[1-3]

References

1. Eriksson MJ, Sonnenberg B, Woo A, et al. Long-term outcome in patients with apical hypertrophic cardiomyopathy. *J Am Coll Cardiol.* 2002:20;39:638–645.
2. Maron MS, Finley JJ, Bos JM, et al. Prevalence, clinical significance and natural history of left ventricular apical aneurysms in hypertrophic cardiomyopathy. *Circulation.* 2008;118:1541–1549.
3. Schaff HV, Brown ML, Dearani JA, et al. Apical myectomy: a new surgical technique for management of severely symptomatic patients with apical hypertrophic cardiomyopathy. *J Thorac Cardiovasc Surg.* 2010;139:634–640.

CASE 56

Hyperlipidemia, Hypertension and Carotid Disease

A 70-year-old female patient with a history of hyperlipidemia, hypertension, carotid disease, and recent onset dizziness is referred for echocardiography to evaluate a murmur (see **Video 56-1**).

QUESTION 1. On the basis of Doppler data Figure 56-1, the calculated left ventricular stroke volume (SV) is:

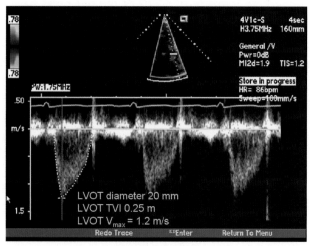

Figure 56-1

A. 55 ml
B. 78 ml

C. 126 ml
D. 157 ml

QUESTION 2. 2D and Doppler findings (Figure 56-1 through 56-4) are consistent with:

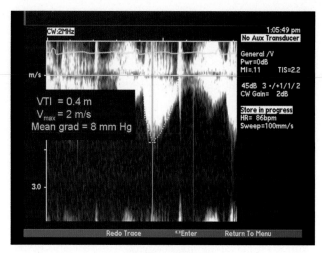

Figure 56-2

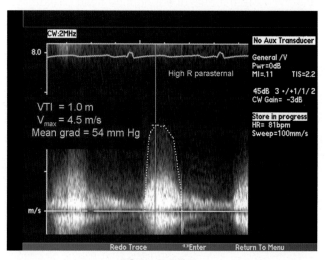

Figure 56-3

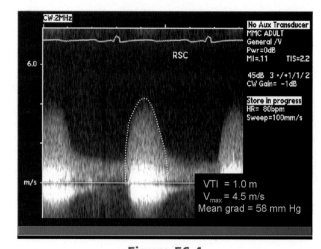

Figure 56-4

A. Aortic valve (AoV) sclerosis with trivial stenosis
B. Moderate AoV stenosis
C. Severe AoV stenosis

ANSWER 1: B. SV provides the amount of blood volume ejected with each cardiac cycle as a final product of the interaction among multiple factors and is an important measure for diagnosis and management of various cardiac conditions. Flow across a fixed orifice is equal to the product of the cross-sectional area (CSA) of the orifice and flow velocity. This is the hydraulic orifice formula, which is used in all hemodynamic calculations of flow, SV, and orifice area:

$$\text{Flow rate} = \text{CSA} \times \text{flow velocity}$$

Because flow velocity varies during ejection in a pulsatile system, such as the cardiovascular system, individual velocities of the Doppler spectrum need to be summed (i.e., integrated) to measure the total volume of flow during a given ejection period. The sum of velocities is called the time velocity integral (TVI), or velocity time integral (VTI), and is equal to the area enclosed by the baseline and Doppler spectrum. It is also equal to stroke distance (i.e., the average distance blood travels with each beat of the heart). TVI can be measured readily with the built-in calculation package in the ultrasound unit by tracing the Doppler velocity signal. After TVI has been determined, SV is calculated by multiplying TVI by CSA:

$$\text{SV} = \text{CSA} \times \text{TVI}$$

The location most frequently used to determine SV is the left ventricular outflow tract (LVOT). The CSA of the LVOT is assumed to be a circle, and it is determined from measurements of the orifice diameter (D):

$$\text{CSA} = \left(\frac{D}{2}\right)^2 \times \pi$$
$$= D^2 \times 0.785$$

Hence,

$$\text{SV} = D^2 \times 0.785 \times \text{TVI}$$

Cardiac output (CO) is obtained by multiplying SV by heart rate.

$$\text{CO} = \text{SV} \times \text{heart rate}$$

Here

$$\text{CSA} = (2/2)^2 \times \pi = \pi \text{ or } (2^2 \times 0.785)$$
$$\text{SV} = \text{CSA} \times \text{TVI} = 3.14 \text{ cm}^2 \times 25 \text{ cm}$$
$$= \textbf{78 ml}$$

Note: The unit for area and TVI is in cm.

ANSWER 2: A. The assessment of the severity of any valvular stenosis including that of the AoV should be an integrated one factoring in 2D and Doppler-derived measures including the mean systolic pressure gradient, the AoV area, and the LVOT to AoV TVI ratio (LVOT:AoV TVI). It is critical to perform a meticulous search for the maximal aortic velocity because all of these variables are derived from the peak aortic flow velocity. To obtain comprehensive hemodynamic data, a systematic and meticulous Doppler examination should be performed on all patients with valvular stenosis.

All available transducer windows should be used to obtain the Doppler signal most parallel with the direction of the stenotic jet flow, which provides the highest velocity recording. Compared with a duplex transducer, a nonimaging continuous wave Doppler transducer is smaller and thus easier to manipulate between the ribs and suprasternal notch. Color flow imaging may be helpful in aligning the continuous wave Doppler beam, so it is most parallel with the direction of blood flow.

Here, by 2D assessment, the AoV is sclerotic but the valve leaflets appear to open quite normally. The continuous wave Doppler interrogation of the AoV from the apex demonstrates a mean systolic gradient of 8 mm Hg and a calculated AoV area of 3 cm². This fits with the 2D findings. There are separate signals obtained from the right parasternal and right supraclavicular locations (see Fig. 56-4) with a much higher velocity. Here it is important not to misinterpret this as an AoV signal. The clues to this not being an aortic stenosis signal are (1) the major discrepancy between the Doppler and 2D findings and (2) the diastolic flow that is typical for arterial flow. Focused interrogation of the patient identified the location of the stenosis as the right innominate artery.

CASE 57

Progressive Exertional Shortness of Breath after Onset of Dyspnea

*A*35-year-old woman presents with progressive exertional shortness of breath. As a child, she had episodes of turning blue and underwent cardiac surgery that had included surgical repair of an atrial septal defect at the age of 5. Since then, she did well and was able to exercise quite vigorously up until the onset of dyspnea 1 year before presentation (see **Videos 57-1 to 57-17**, Fig. 57-1 through 57-6).

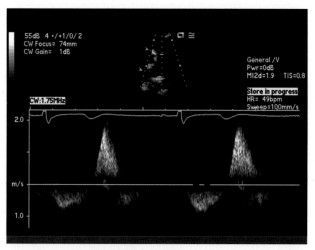

Figure 57-1

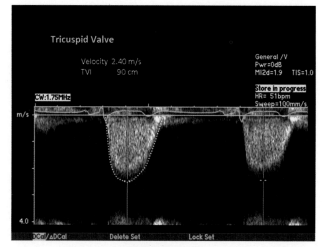

Figure 57-3

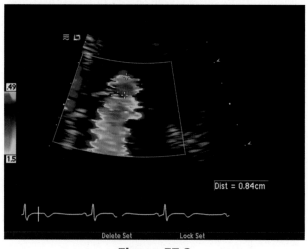

Figure 57-2

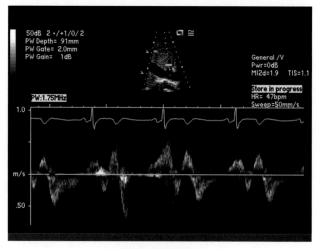

Figure 57-4

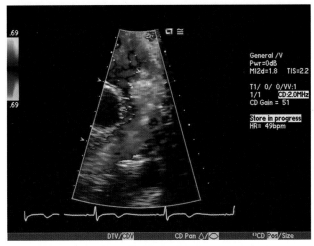

Figure 57-5

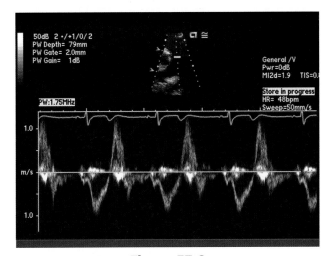

Figure 57-6

QUESTION 1. On the basis of two-dimensional echocardiography, which of the following statements is most correct?

A. Right ventricular (RV) volume overload
B. RV pressure overload
C. Combined volume and pressure overload

QUESTION 2. On the basis of his transthoracic images, the calculated tricuspid regurgitant volume by the proximal isovelocity surface area (PISA) method is:

A. 60 ml
B. 80 ml
C. 100 ml
D. 120 ml

QUESTION 3. The degree of tricuspid valve regurgitation (TR) is:

A. Trivial to mild
B. Moderate
C. Severe

QUESTION 4. The degree of pulmonary valve regurgitation is:

A. Trivial to mild
B. Moderate
C. Severe

QUESTION 5. The flow indicated by the arrows in Figure 57-7 indicates:

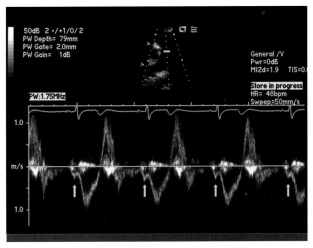

Figure 57-7

A. Evidence of RV systolic dysfunction
B. Elevated RV end-diastolic pressures
C. First-degree atrioventricular block

ANSWER 1: A. There is evidence of a D-shaped left ventricle with flattening of the intraventricular septum in diastole. However, the flattening disappears in systole unlike in a pressure overloaded RV, where septal flattening persists throughout the cardiac cycle. This is supported by the absence of Doppler findings to suggest elevated RV/pulmonary pressures.

ANSWER 2: C. 100 ml

The regurgitant flow can be calculated as follows:

Flow rate = $(r)^2$ × 6.28 × aliasing velocity × angle correction factor*
  = $(0.84 \text{ cm})^2$ × 6.28 × 49 cm per second × 220/180
  = 265 cc per second

*Unlike the mitral valve where the leaflets are flat, the tricuspid valve leaflets are funnel shaped. This needs to be accounted for when calculating PISA. The assumption of a hemispheric shape of the flow convergence needs to be corrected for by measuring the angle of the leaflets. Typically, the angle of the tricuspid leaflets is 220° rather than the 180° of the mitral valve. Without this adjustment, the additional area of flow convergence would not be accounted for if the angle of the leaflets were not measured that would lead to underestimation of the regurgitation severity.

Effective regurgitant orifice (ERO) = Flow rate/Peak TR velocity

ERO = 265 cc per second/240 cm per second = 1.1 cm²

Regurgitant volume = ERO × TR time velocity integral
  = 1.1 × 90 = 99 ml

ANSWER 3: C. There is evidence of a dense continuous wave Doppler signal with a large regurgitant area of color flow and systolic flow reversals in the hepatic veins. These features along with the quantitative findings of an ERO area >0.4 cm² and a regurgitant volume >45 ml are consistent with severe TR.

See *The Echo Manual, 3rd Edition,* pages 219 to 220 and Appendix 21 on page 414 for discussion of echo findings in severe tricuspid valve regurgitation.

ANSWER 4: C. Imaging of the pulmonary outflow tract indicates no evidence of a residual pulmonary valve with torrential pulmonary valve regurgitation. Color Doppler imaging demonstrates a wide early diastolic regurgitant flow that starts beyond the pulmonary bifurcation (Fig. 57-5). Continuous wave Doppler through the RV outflow tract demonstrates a dense early diastolic regurgitant signal that is brief with a rapid downslope consistent with severe pulmonary regurgitation and rapid equilibration of pressures between the pulmonary artery and the RV.

ANSWER 5: B. There is evidence of diastolic laminar pulmonary flow in atrial systole *(arrows)* that is indicative of restrictive RV physiology. Here a stiff RV acts as a passive diastolic conduit for flow from the right atrium to the pulmonary artery. This helps in part to offset the effect of pulmonary regurgitation increasing forward flow and RV cardiac output.[1,2]

References

1. Li W, Davlouros PA, Kilner PJ, et al. Doppler-echocardiographic assessment of pulmonary regurgitation in adults with repaired tetralogy of Fallot: comparison with cardiovascular magnetic resonance imaging. *Am Heart J.* 2004;147(1):165–172.

2. Ammash NM, Dearani JA, Burkhart HM, et al. Pulmonary regurgitation after tetralogy of Fallot repair: clinical features, sequelae, and timing of pulmonary valve replacement. *Congenital Heart Dis.* 2007;2(6):386–403.

CASE 58

Progressive Exertional Shortness of Breath with Diabetes and Systemic Hypertension

A 65-year-old man presents for further evaluation of progressive exertional shortness of breath. His medical history is notable for type 2 diabetes mellitus and systemic hypertension. He is a prior smoker. An echocardiogram at home had reportedly shown moderately increased left ventricular wall thickness and normal ejection fraction.

Physical examination is notable for a systemic blood pressure of 125/70 mm Hg and a regular pulse at 70 beats per minute. Cardiac and pulmonary examination was normal.

Twelve-lead ECG demonstrates left atrial enlargement, right bundle branch block, and left ventricular hypertrophy.

QUESTION 1. What is the least likely disorder, given clinical and reported echocardiographic findings?

- A. Cardiomyopathy secondary to hypertension and end-stage kidney disease
- B. Primary amyloidosis
- C. Hypertrophic cardiomyopathy
- D. Fabry Disease

QUESTION 2. Which associated clinical history would be compatible with the images (**Video 58-1**)?

- A. Low CD4 counts in a prior intravenous drug abuser
- B. A painful burning sensation in the hands or feet that gets worse particularly with exercise in the summertime associated with proteinuria and renal dysfunction
- C. Bilateral hilar lymphadenopathy and an elevated serum angiotensin-converting enzyme level
- D. Symmetric polyarthritis of the hand joints with joint erosions on x-ray

QUESTION 3. **Video 58-2** illustrates which of the following?

- A. Patent foramen ovale with left to right flow
- B. Patent foramen ovale with bidirectional flow
- C. Intact atrial septum with prominent superior vena cava flow

ANSWER 1: B. Many potential disorders are associated with increased left ventricular wall thicknesses. Hearts with genetic or secondary myocyte hypertrophy typically have evidence of increased QRS voltages of the left ventricular hypertrophic pattern. Thick walls related to amyloid deposition are classically associated with low QRS voltages on ECGs. Although a minority of patients with amyloidosis may have normal QRS voltage, it would be rare to have QRS voltage meeting criteria for left ventricular hypertrophy. Although Fabry's disease is an infiltrative cardiomyopathy, ECG show LVH pattern unlike cardiac amyloidosis.

See *The Echo Manual, 3rd Edition,* page 274.

ANSWER 2: B. Images demonstrate evidence of increased left ventricular wall thickness with a classic binary appearance of the left ventricular endocardial border with an endocardial stripe, seen with Fabry disease.

See *The Echo Manual, 3rd Edition,* Figure 16-4 on page 277.

Fabry disease is an X-linked chromosomal disorder leading to accumulation of sphingolipids in various tissues including the myocardium. The hypertrophy is generally homogenous and should be considered in the differential in every patient with an unexplained ventricular cardiomyopathy with thick walls. The advantage of the diagnosis is that a specific treatment is available with substitute enzyme therapy. The heart is infrequently involved in HIV/AIDS with typical manifestations being pericardial effusions, a dilated cardiomyopathy, or a pulmonary vascular arteriopathy. Cardiac sarcoidosis is frequently characterized by atypical wall motion abnormalities and diastolic dysfunction. Patients with rheumatoid arthritis are prone to episodes of pericardial disease and at increased risk for coronary disease. The appearance of left ventricular hypertrophy is not a manifestation associated with HIV infection, sarcoidosis, or rheumatoid arthritis.

Fabry disease occurs in the setting of an X-linked disorder affecting the α-galactosidase A gene, leading to enzyme deficiency and accumulation of globotriaosylceramide lipid in tissues. Clinical manifestations include neuropathy (causing a burning discomfort of the hands and feet), asymptomatic corneal dystrophy, proteinuria, and at times chronic kidney disease. The left ventricular hypertrophy is a relatively early finding in Fabry disease that generally correlates with the severity of the disease and predates renal disease.

The classic echocardiographic left ventricular finding is a thickened hyperechogenic layer (which represents intracellular deposition of glycolipid in the endocardium and the subendocardium) and a hypoechogenic layer that parallels the hyperechogenic layer (which may represent a shadowing artifact because of the intracellular lipid-rich layer).[1]

ANSWER 3: B. Seen here is a patient foramen ovale with prominent flow toward the transducer (left to right) predominantly during diastole (Fig. 58-1). After cessation of flow, there is a brief signal of flow toward the transducer (right to left) that in this clip tends to be systolic (Fig. 58-2).

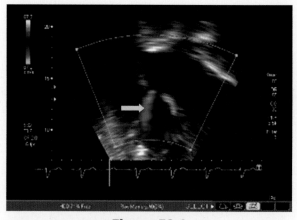

Figure 58-1

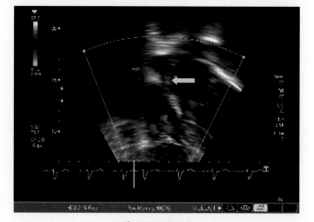

Figure 58-2

Reference

1. Pieroni M, Chimenti C, De Cobelli F, et al. Fabry's disease cardiomyopathy: echocardiographic detection of endomyocardial glycosphingolipid compartmentalization. *J Am Coll Cardiol.* 2006;47:1663–1671.

CASE 59

Transient Loss of Vision

A 45-year-old woman presents after transient loss of vision in an eye. Her history is significant for a 6-week history of a neck abscess that has failed to resolve with oral antibiotics.

On examination, her temperature is 38.3° C and she has a soft systolic murmur. Blood cultures are pending. She is referred for a transthoracic echocardiogram.

QUESTION 1. Concerning the echocardiogram (**Video 59-1**), there is evidence of:

A. Normal heart valves
B. Aortic valve endocarditis
C. Mitral valve endocarditis
D. Aortic and mitral valve endocarditis
E. Indeterminate

QUESTION 2. The most common underlying factor that predisposes to infective endocarditis is:

A. Prosthetic heart valves
B. Congenital heart disease
C. Aortic stenosis
D. Mitral valve regurgitation

QUESTION 3. Which of the following is not due to embolic complication of infective endocarditis?

A. Pulmonary infarction
B. Mycotic cerebral aneurysm
C. Janeway lesion
D. Roth spot
E. Stroke

QUESTION 4. Results obtained from blood cultures demonstrate the growth of methicillin-sensitive *Staphylococcus aureus (MSSA)*. The next appropriate step is:

A. Two-week course of intravenous antibiotics based on sensitivities
B. Six-week course of intravenous antibiotics based on sensitivities
C. Transesophageal echocardiogram
D. Repeat transthoracic echocardiogram after a 2-week course of appropriate antibiotics
E. A cardiac MRI to assess for vegetation

QUESTION 5. On the basis of the transesophageal findings (**Videos 59-2 to 59-5**), the appropriate antibiotic management would be:

A. 6 weeks of intravenous nafcillin
B. 2 weeks of intravenous gentamicin and nafcillin
C. 2 weeks of intravenous nafcillin
D. 2 weeks of intravenous gentamicin and nafcillin followed by 4 further weeks of intravenous nafcillin
E. 4 weeks of intravenous vancomycin and gentamicin

ANSWER 1: E. The characteristic echocardiographic finding of cardiac vegetation is an oscillating intracardiac mass frequently involving the proximal surface of the valve without an alternative anatomic explanation. It may involve the valve itself, the valvular apparatus, and the path of the regurgitant jet or on prosthetic material.

ANSWER 2: D. Although all these factors may predispose to infective endocarditis particularly congenital heart disease and/or prosthetic material by virtue of its incidence in the general population, the most common factor that predisposes to infective endocarditis is mitral valve regurgitation.[1]

ANSWER 3: D. Various clinical findings may be present in patients with infective endocarditis related to either embolic events or an immune complex deposition. Roth spots are hemorrhages in the retina seen on fundoscopy caused by an immune complex–mediated vasculitis. Two skin lesions may occur in endocarditis both distal, flat, and ecchymotic. Janeway lesions are flat and painless, due to microabscesses from embolization, whereas Osler nodes are raised and painful, caused by deposition of immune complexes in the skin.

ANSWER 4: C. The transthoracic echocardiogram although suggestive of valvular abnormalities was insufficient to rule in or out echocardiographic evidence of endocarditis. A transesophageal echocardiogram is the appropriate next step. A transesophageal echocardiogram is advised in patients with an equivocal transthoracic study for endocarditis as well as in patients with valvular prostheses or those suspected of having complicated endocarditis.[2]

ANSWER 5: A. The recommended treatment of left-sided MSSA endocarditis is 6 weeks of a semisynthetic penicillin such as nafcillin. Combination therapy has no advantage over monotherapy. Given the size of the vegetation, their mobility, and the fact that the patient has already had one embolic event, a cardiac surgery should see the patient with at least consideration of surgical intervention. Factors that would prompt early surgery might include enlargement of the vegetation or recurrent embolic events on antibiotic therapy.

References

1. Bonow RO, Carabello BA, Chatterjee K, et al. 2008 focused update incorporated into the ACC/AHA 2006 guidelines for the management of patients with valvular heart disease: a report of the American College of Cardiology/American Heart Association Task Force on Practice Guidelines (Writing Committee to revise the 1998 guidelines for the management of patients with valvular heart disease). *J Am Coll Cardiol.* 2008;52:e1–e142.

2. Li JS, Sexton DJ, Mick N, et al. Proposed modifications to the Duke criteria for the diagnosis of infective endocarditis. *Clin Infect Dis.* 2000;30:633–638.

CASE 60

Sharp Chest Pain

A 68-year-old man presents with 4 days of sharp chest pain. The pain is worse when lying down and improves upon sitting up. He also describes intermittent heart pounding over the last year. On examination, there is a low-pitched grade 1 to 2/6 diastolic rumble at apex and trace lower extremity edema. Chest radiograph demonstrates cardiomegaly and pulmonary venous congestion. His ECG is shown in Figure 60-1. He is referred for transthoracic echocardiogram (**Videos 60-1 through 60-4** and Fig. 60-2).

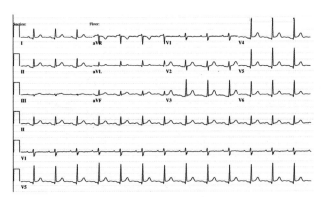

Figure 60-1

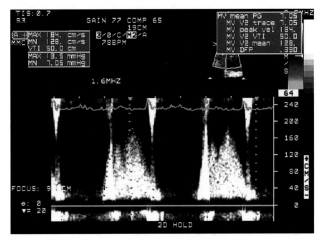

Figure 60-2

QUESTION 1. The most likely explanation for the echocardiographic findings is:

- A. Papillary fibroelastoma
- B. Thrombus
- C. Atrial myxoma
- D. Metastatic colon carcinoma

QUESTION 2. Which of the following M-modes (Fig. 60-3) do you expect to see in this patient?

A.

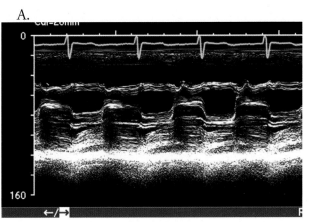

Figure 60-3A

B.

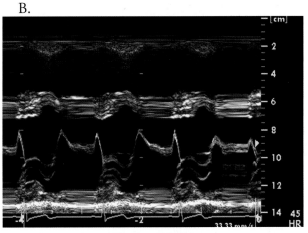

Figure 60-3B

C.

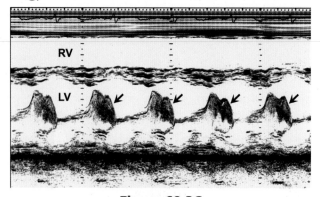

Figure 60-3C

D.

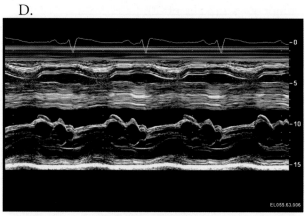

Figure 60-3D

A. Papillary fibroelastoma
B. Thrombus
C. Atrial myxoma
D. Infective endocarditis

QUESTION 5. The patient proceeded back to the operating room where a recurrent myxoma was resected. Insufficient tissue remained to support a normally functioning anterior mitral valve leaflet, and so the patient also underwent a mitral valve replacement with a mechanical prosthesis. Postoperatively, the patient went into complete heart block that required the placement of a permanent dual-chamber pacemaker. Preoperative symptoms resolved, and the patient did well for 5 years, until he again developed episodes of intermittent "heart pounding." He is referred for transthoracic echocardiogram (**Videos 60-10 through 60-13** and Figs. 60-4 through 60-7). What is the mitral valve prosthesis area?

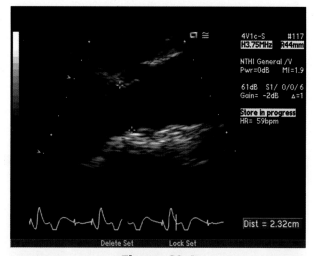

Figure 60-4

QUESTION 3. What auscultatory finding is typical for this disorder?

A. Plop
B. Click
C. Knock
D. Snap

QUESTION 4. The patient proceeded to surgical resection of the mass that was adherent to the inferior portion of the left side on the intra-atrial septum close to the base of the anterior mitral valve leaflet. It was shaved off easily, and pathology confirmed an atrial myxoma. Postbypass transesophageal images demonstrated no residual mass and normal mitral valve function. The patient did well and symptoms resolved immediately. Six months after surgical resection, the patient returns with recurrent symptoms of "heart pounding." He otherwise feels well. Review images from the repeat echocardiogram (**Videos 60-5 through 60-9**). The most likely explanation for the new echocardiographic finding is:

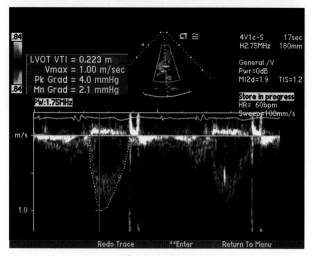

Figure 60-5

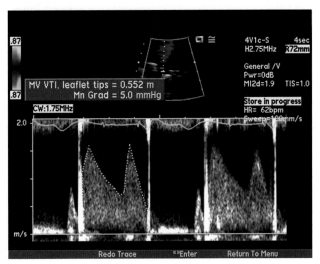

Figure 60-6

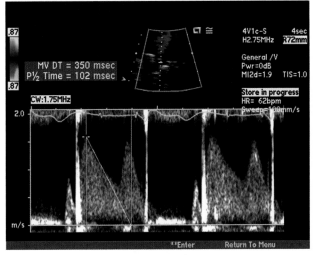

Figure 60-7

A. 1.5 cm²
B. 1.7 cm²
C. 2.2 cm²

QUESTION 6. The patient's INR is 2.5. There is no evidence of high atrial rate activity on his pacemaker interrogation to suggest atrial fibrillation. He is referred for transesophageal echocardiography (**Videos 60-14 through 60-18**). What is the most appropriate management at this time?

A. Thrombolytic therapy
B. Increase INR and repeat TEE
C. Add clopidogrel
D. Surgical removal

QUESTION 7. Which of the following statements with regard to myxomas is true?

A. Myxomas occur more commonly in men than in women
B. After the left atrium, the left ventricle is the most common site for myxomas to occur
C. Symptoms of myxomas may include fatigue, fever, and myalgias
D. Recurrence of sporadic myxomas is common, occurring in 10% to 15% of cases

QUESTION 8. Which of the following syndromes is associated with an increased risk of myxomas?

A. Turner syndrome
B. Carney syndrome
C. Shone syndrome
D. Osler–Weber–Rendu syndrome

ANSWER 1: C. There is a mobile, smooth spherical structure that appears attached by a stalk to the atrial septum at the base of the anterior mitral valve leaflet. This most likely represents an atrial myxoma. Myxoma is the most common cardiac tumor accounting for 20% to 30% of primary intracardiac tumors.

ANSWER 2: C. M-mode echocardiography of a left atrial myxoma recorded from the parasternal transducer position. During diastole, the mitral orifice is filled with increased echodensity (*arrows*) representing protruding atrial myxoma. Also shown are examples of mitral stenosis (A: the mitral leaflet is thickened, and the E–F slope is prolonged) and mitral valve prolapse (B: the mitral leaflets are thickened, and there is late systolic posterior motion [prolapse] of the posterior mitral leaflet below the C–D line) (Fig. 60-3).

ANSWER 3: A. The characteristic physical examination finding of an atrial myxoma is a tumor plop heard immediately after the second heart sound. Various explanations have been given for this sound including a sudden increase in tension on the tumor stalk or reverberation of the tumor of the intraventricular septum; however, most likely, it is related to partial obstruction to flow through the mitral valve leading to a high velocity early diastolic jet.[1]

ANSWER 4: C. The echocardiographic characteristics are very similar to those at presentation. Although thrombus or endocarditis is possible, recurrent myxoma at the site is most likely, probably, related to incomplete resection of the tumor base related to attempts at avoiding mitral valve replacement.

ANSWER 5: B. The pressure half time (PHT) method of 220/PHT useful in native mitral stenosis overestimates the effective orifice area in prosthetic valves. In the absence of clinically significant mitral or aortic valve regurgitation, the continuity method is better for calculating the area of left-sided prostheses e.g. mitral prosthesis (MP) area.

MP area = LVOT area × (LVOT TVI)/(MV TVI)
  $= (2.3)^2 \times (0.785) \times (23)/(55) = 1.73 \ cm^2$

ANSWER 6: D. Echocardiography demonstrates a new left atrial mass, concerning for recurrent tumor.

The patient returns to the operating room for the third time for resection of the mass. Pathology demonstrates no evidence of myxoma but solely organized thrombus.

ANSWER 7: C. Most myxomas are sporadic, occurring in females three times as likely as in males and are present in the left atrium in 75% of cases. Most of the remaining 15% to 20% develop in the right atrium and the remainder in either the left or right ventricle. Patients with myxomas commonly present with symptoms related to valve obstruction or embolic events however constitutional symptoms of fatigue, fever, myalgias, and weight loss.

ANSWER 8: B. Carney syndrome is an autosomal dominant disorder characterized by myxomas involving the heart and skin. The cardiac myxomas are frequently multiple and often involve chambers other than the left atrium. Overall 5% to 10% of cardiac myxomas occur in the setting of Carney syndrome. The other clinical components of the syndrome include skin hyperpigmentation and endocrine dysfunction. Turner syndrome, occurring when a woman lacks an X chromosome, is characterized by short stature, low-set ears, a webbed neck, gonadal dysfunction, hypothyroidism, and diabetes. Cardiac defects are common and may include a bicuspid aortic valve and coarctation of the aorta. The Shone complex or Shone syndrome is a group of cardiac left-sided obstructive defects including a supravalvular mitral membrane, parachute mitral valve, subaortic stenosis, and coarctation of the aorta. The Osler–Weber–Rendu syndrome is characterized by arterial-venous malformations involving the skin (telangiectasias), gastrointestinal tract, liver, and lungs. These may give rise to high-output states and/or pulmonary arterial hypertension with associated right heart dysfunction.

Reference

1. Kolluru A, Desai D, Cohen GI. The etiology of the atrial myxoma tumor plop. *J Am Coll Cardiol*. 2011;57:e371.

Transient Loss of Vision with Modest Exertional Shortness of Breath

A 25-year-old previously well woman presents for the evaluation of transient loss of vision lasting an hour on the background of new symptoms of modest exertional shortness of breath over the past 10 days. She is referred for a transthoracic echocardiogram (**Videos 61-1 to 61-16** and Figs. 61-1 and 61-2).

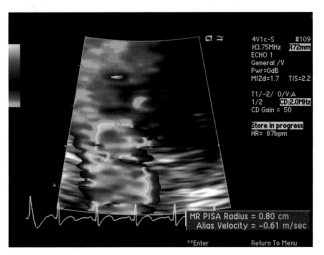

Figure 61-1

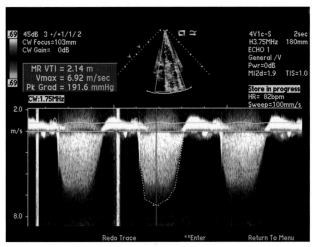

Figure 61-2

QUESTION 1. A visual estimate of the left ventricular ejection fraction is:

    A. 35% to 40%

    B. 45% to 50%

    C. 55% to 60%

    D. 65% to 70%

QUESTION 2. The quantified effective regurgitant orifice (ERO) area of the mitral valve by the proximal isovelocity surface area (PISA) method is:

    A. 0.05 cm^2

    B. 0.10 cm^2

    C. 0.15 cm^2

    D. 0.25 cm^2

    E. 0.35 cm^2

QUESTION 3. If the aliasing velocity is changed to 40 cm per second by further shifting the color baseline downward, PISA radius will become:

    A. 0.7 cm

    B. 0.8 cm

    C. 0.9 cm

    D. 1.0 cm

QUESTION 4. What is the quantified regurgitant volume of the mitral valve regurgitation (MR) by the PISA method?

A. 25 cc
B. 50 cc
C. 75 cc
D. 100 cc

QUESTION 5. The degree of MR is:

A. Trivial to mild
B. Mild to moderate
C. Moderate to severe

QUESTION 6. She undergoes a brain MRI that demonstrates bilateral scattered small subacute infarcts. Which finding on TEE (**Videos 61-17 to 61-26**) likely explains these MRI findings?

A. Patent foramen ovale with right to left shunt
B. Mitral valve endocarditis
C. Left atrial appendage thrombus
D. Aortic valve endocarditis

QUESTION 7. The blood test most likely to be abnormal in this patient is:

A. Serum eosinophil level
B. Bacterial blood culture
C. Lupus anticoagulant
D. Thyroid stimulating hormone

QUESTION 8. The appropriate treatment is/are:

A. Mitral valve repair
B. Mitral valve replacement
C. Anti-inflammatory agents
D. Systemic anticoagulation

ANSWER 1: D. Left contractility is upper normal.

ANSWER 2: E. The regurgitant flow rate across the aortic valve is obtained from the flow rate of a proximal surface area with a known flow velocity as follows:

Flow rate = $2\pi r^2$ × aliasing velocity
 Flow rate = 6.28 × $(r)^2$ × aliasing velocity
       = 6.28 × $(0.8)^2$ × 60
       = 241 cm^3 per second

   ERO = Flow rate/Peak MR velocity
       = 241 (cm^3 per second)/692 (cm per second)
       = 0.35 cm^2

ANSWER 3: D. Flow rate is still 241 cm^3 per second. If the flow rate is divided by 6.28 × 40 cm per second, $(r)^2$ is calculated. Square-root of the calculated number is the PISA radius.

See *The Echo Manual, 3rd Edition*, PISA method on page 215.

ANSWER 4: C.

Regurgitant volume = ERO × regurgitant time velocity integral
       = 0.35 cm^2 × 214 cm
       = 75 cc

See *The Echo Manual, 3rd Edition*, PISA method on page 215.

ANSWER 5: C. The quantitative data collectively indicate severe MR.

See *The Echo Manual, 3rd Edition*, Appendix 19 on page 412.

ANSWER 6: B. TEE demonstrates small vegetations on the atrial surface of the mitral valve. The aortic valve is normal and free of masses. The left atrial appendage is free of thrombus, and the foramen ovale appears closed.

ANSWER 7: C. Transesophageal echocardiography demonstrates the classic appearance of Libman–Sacks endocarditis, with verrucous valvular lesions involving the mitral valve. As is typical, the vegetations are found on the basal portion of the mitral valve, although they can extend to the chordal structure or papillary muscles. The aortic valve is not involved, which is typical. These lesions are typically associated with systemic lupus erythematosus (SLE) and the lupus anticoagulant.[1]

See *The Echo Manual, 3rd Edition*, page 286.

ANSWER 8: D. Glucocorticoid and/or cytotoxic therapy have no effect on this valve disease. Systemic anticoagulation (or antiplatelet therapy) is effective in most patients, although a few refractory patients will require definitive surgical management. After a 4-month course of anticoagulation, the patient was reevaluated and the valve abnormalities had resolved (**Videos 61-27 to 61-29**).

Reference

1. Libman E, Sacks B. A hitherto undescribed form of valvular and mural endocarditis. *Arch Intern Med.* 1924;33:701–737.

CASE 62

Fever and Back Pain

A 68-year-old man presents with fever and back pain. His medical history is significant for small cell carcinoma of the lung for which he has been undergoing radiotherapy and chemotherapy (cisplatin and etoposide).

On examination, his heart rate is 125 beats per minute and his blood pressure 90/60 mm Hg. His temperature was 39°C. He recently had an episode of *Escherichia coli* bacteremia in the setting of an urinary tract infection. He was treated with appropriate ciprofloxacin antibacterial therapy. He did well for a week and was dismissed from hospital but returns now with recurrent fever and new onset back pain.

He is referred for transesophageal echocardiography.

QUESTION 1. On the basis of the available transesophageal echocardiographic views (**Videos 62-1 and 62-2**), which of the following is true?

- A. No echocardiographic evidence of left-sided valvular endocarditis
- B. Echocardiographic evidence of aortic valve endocarditis
- C. Echocardiographic evidence of mitral valve endocarditis
- D. Echocardiographic evidence of both aortic and mitral valve endocarditis

QUESTION 2. On the basis of review of the transesophageal echocardiographic views (**Videos 62-3 and 62-4**), which of the following is true?

- A. Patent foramen ovale with left–right shunt
- B. Patent foramen ovale with right–left shunt
- C. Patent foramen ovale with bidirectional shunt
- D. Closed foramen ovale

QUESTION 3. On the basis of review of the transesophageal echocardiographic views in **Videos 62-5 to 62-11**, which of the following is present?

- A. DeBakey type I aortic dissection
- B. DeBakey type II aortic dissection
- C. DeBakey type III aortic dissection

QUESTION 4. Appropriate next step could include:

- A. Emergency cardiothoracic surgery
- B. Reinstitution of intravenous antibiotics with an indium white blood cell scan
- C. Intravenous corticosteroids

ANSWER 1: A. The echocardiographic features typical of infective endocarditis include an oscillating intracardiac mass on a valve or supporting structure. The initial attachment site to the mitral valve is usually on the atrial side, whereas an aortic valve vegetation usually starts from the ventricular surface. The sensitivity of detecting a vegetation with two-dimensional (2D) transesophageal echocardiography is 95%. Here the aortic and mitral valves although mildly thickened are otherwise normal.

ANSWER 2: A. 2D and color Doppler imaging demonstrates a small defect in the intra-atrial septum consistent with a small patent foramen ovale. Color Doppler demonstrates flow in early diastole from the left to right atrium (Fig. 62-1). There is no evidence of

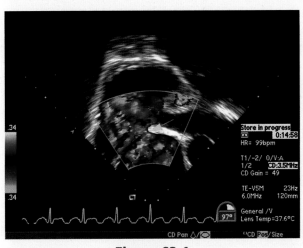

Figure 62-1

flow directed from right to left, a finding supported by the absence of agitated saline bubbles seen in the left atrium.

See *The Echo Manual, 3rd Edition,* discussion of role of agitated saline on page 99.

ANSWER 3: C. Transesophageal echocardiography demonstrates a localized aortic dissection in the lower descending thoracic aorta (starting at approximately 34 cm from the incisors). There is a mobile flap with probable thrombus in the space between the flap and the aortic wall.

See *The Echo Manual, 3rd Edition,* discussion of aortic dissection and intramural hematoma on page 324.

ANSWER 4: B. Echo images demonstrate that the surrounding aortic wall is thickened with heterogeneous soft-tissue thickening in the periaortic region at this level. In this clinical setting, the likely explanation is focal infective aortitis with secondary contained rupture. Reinstitution of antimicrobial therapy and investigation to support the clinical suspicion of infective aortitis is appropriate. Scout CT images demonstrate an irregular lateral aortic wall with a small outpouching that shows increased enhancement. There is a small amount of fluid collection along this abnormal segment of the descending aorta. Labeled white blood cell scan demonstrates intense tracer uptake along the descending aorta, corresponding to these abnormalities. These findings are very suspicious for infectious aortitis.

Unlike aortic dissection involving the ascending aorta, which is a surgical emergency, many cases of descending thoracic aortic dissection can be managed conservatively or if aortic intervention is required, this can be performed semielectively, often through a percutaneous route.

Immunosuppression with corticosteroid therapy should be avoided in light of the high concern for serious bacterial infection. Steroid therapy does play a primary role in large-vessel vasculitis of the aorta (e.g., giant cell arteritis), although this typically will present with more generalized inflammation of the vessel rather the focal finding seen in this case.

CASE 63

Diffuse ST-Segment Depression

*A*55-year-old woman is brought to the emergency department by the emergency medical service after collapsing. She was previously well without known disease. On examination, she is sedated, intubated, and unresponsive. She is tachycardic, but the remainder of her cardiac examination is normal. Twelve-lead ECG demonstrates diffuse ST segment depression.

QUESTION 1. Transthoracic echocardiography (**Videos 63-1 and 63-2**) (Apical 4 chamber images are in Mayo format with the left ventricle displayed in the left) suggests:

  A. Acute myocardial infarction because of coronary artery occlusion
  B. Stress-induced cardiomyopathy
  C. Normal findings

QUESTION 2. Potential explanations underlying the pathogenesis for this condition include:

  A. Coronary artery spasm
  B. Catecholamine excess
  C. Microvascular dysfunction
  D. All of the choices

QUESTION 3. On the basis of the 2D images and Figures 63-1 and 63-2, the diastolic function grade in this case is:

  A. Normal
  B. Grade 1
  C. Grade 2
  D. Grade 3

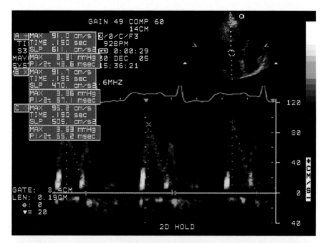

Figure 63-1

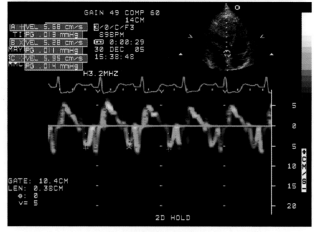

Figure 63-2

ANSWER 1: B. Transthoracic echocardiography demonstrates an unusual pattern of regional wall motion abnormalities with akinetic midventricular segments although the base and apex are hyperdynamic. This would be an unusual distribution for coronary artery disease but is a pattern that can be seen in the setting of stress-induced cardiomyopathy. An echo contrast perfusion study (see **Video 63-2**) demonstrates normal perfusion with replenishment of microbubbles even in the akinetic segments within three to five beats suggesting normal blood flow. The patient was found to have suffered a subarachnoid hemorrhage on brain CT imaging.[1,2]

See *The Echo Manual, 3rd Edition,* myocardial perfusion imaging on pages 103 to 107, and Tako-tsubo on pages 167 and 168.

ANSWER 2: D. Although the underlying pathogenesis for stress-induced cardiomyopathy remains unclear, proposed mechanisms include direct catecholamine toxicity, catecholamine-triggered coronary artery spasm, or microvascular dysfunction. Factors that suggest a central role for catecholamines include the following: (1) the onset is often triggered by a severe emotional or physical stress, (2) catecholamine levels tend to be elevated in correlation with cardiac findings, and (3) similar cardiac findings can be seen in disorders of catecholamine excess such as pheochromocytoma.

ANSWER 3: C. The ratio of early mitral filling (E) to that of late mitral filling from atrial contraction (A) suggests either normal or pseudonormal (grade 2) diastolic function. The ratio of E to the early relaxation velocity of the medial mitral annulus (e′) is 9/0.05 = 18, which is consistent with significant elevation in left ventricular filling pressure and grade 2 diastolic dysfunction.

References

1. Hurst RT, Askew JW, Reuss CS, et al. Transient midventricular ballooning syndrome: a new variant. *J Am Coll Cardiol.* 2006;48:579–583.

2. Dhoble A, Abdelmoneim SS, Bernier M, et al. Transient left ventricular apical ballooning and exercise induced hypertension during treadmill exercise testing: is there a common hypersympathetic mechanism? *Cardiovasc Ultrasound.* 2008;6:37.

CASE 64

Functional Class III Exertional Dyspnea

A 45-year-old woman presents with functional class III exertional dyspnea. She has been known to have a systolic murmur for many years.

On examination, her blood pressure is 134/80 mm Hg. Her body mass index is 40 kg per m². Her carotid pulse is diminished and delayed. She had a 3/6 mid-peaking systolic ejection murmur that did not change with Valsalva (see **Videos 64-1 through 64-4** and Figs. 64-1 through 64-3).

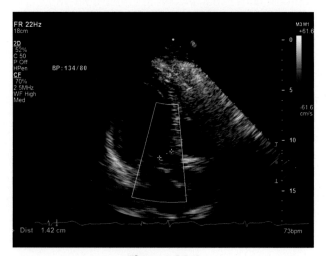

Figure 64-1

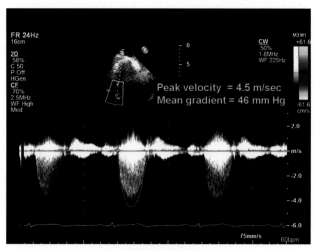

Figure 64-3

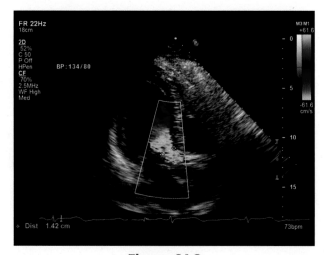

Figure 64-2

QUESTION 1. What is the diagnosis?

A. Calcific aortic valve stenosis

B. Subaortic membrane

C. Hypertrophic obstructive cardiomyopathy

D. No clear diagnosis, consider transesophageal echocardiography

QUESTION 2. What is instantaneous maximum gradient through the left ventricular outflow tract?

A. 20 mm Hg

B. 46 mm Hg

C. 49 mm Hg

D. 53 mm Hg

E. 81 mm Hg

QUESTION 3. Review the images (**Videos 64-5 through 64-9**). The appropriate management step is:

A. Repeat echocardiography in 1 year or sooner if worsening symptoms
B. Proceed with percutaneous balloon dilation
C. Proceed to surgical resection

QUESTION 4. Associated lesions to this defect may include all of the following *except*:

A. Aortic valve regurgitation
B. Left ventricular hypertrophy
C. An incidence of concomitant bicuspid aortic valve in 20% to 25%
D. Female 2:1 predominance
E. Coarctation of the aorta

ANSWER 1: D. Although there is flow turbulence in the left ventricular outflow tract corresponding to a high-pressure systolic gradient, the images are of insufficient quality to make a diagnosis to the mechanism. Further imaging is required.

ANSWER 2: E. On the basis of the modified Bernoulli equation, the maximum instantaneous

gradient = $4(v)^2 = 4(4.5)^2 = 81$ mm Hg

ANSWER 3: C. Proceed with surgical resection of the subaortic membrane. The definitive therapy for a subvalvular membrane is surgical resection. Balloon valvuloplasty is not a suitable option.

ANSWER 4: D. Subaortic valve membranes are more common in men occurring with a 2:1 male predominance. Approximately 20% to 25% of patients with a subaortic membrane have a concomitant bicuspid aortic valve. A subaortic membrane may be seen with other left-sided obstructive lesions such as coarctation of the aorta. Left ventricular hypertrophy is a common associated finding if the degree of obstruction is significant. A significant complication of a subaortic membrane is aortic regurgitation caused by the poststenotic turbulent jet striking the aortic valve leading to deformity and malfunction.

Surgical resection is recommended with a peak instantaneous gradient of 50 mm Hg or a mean systolic gradient of 30 mm Hg or if there is associated (1) progressive aortic valve regurgitation and an left ventricular ejection fraction <55%, (2) left ventricular hypertrophy, (3) planned pregnancy, or (4) plan to engage in competitive sports.[1]

Reference

1. Warnes CA, Williams RG, Bashore TM, et al. ACC/AHA guidelines for the management of adults with congenital heart disease: a report of the American College of Cardiology/American Heart Association Task Force on Practice Guidelines (writing committee to develop guidelines on the management of adults with congenital heart disease). *Circulation*. 2008;118;e714–e833.

CASE 65

Murmur with Systemic Hypertension

A 55-year-old woman is referred for transthoracic echocardiography for the evaluation of a murmur. She is asymptomatic. Her medical history is significant for systemic hypertension for which she takes hydrochlorothiazide, gastroesophageal reflux disease for which she takes omeprazole, and a right nephrectomy 8 years previously for localized renal cell carcinoma. She exercises daily without symptoms.

On examination, her heart rate is 75 beats per minute and her blood pressure 130/82 mm Hg. Her carotid pulses are normal in character and intensity. She has a 3/6 ejection systolic murmur heard best at the left sternal border that decreases on expiration and disappears with Valsalva. Both the aortic and pulmonary components of the second heart sound are preserved.

QUESTION 1. The most likely etiology of the murmur based on the clinical examination is:

A. Aortic valve stenosis
B. Pulmonary valve stenosis
C. Tricuspid valve stenosis
D. Dynamic outflow tract obstruction from hypertrophic cardiomyopathy

QUESTION 2. On the basis of review of the echocardiogram (Videos 65-1 through 65-12 and Fig. 65-1), the likely etiology of the pathology is:

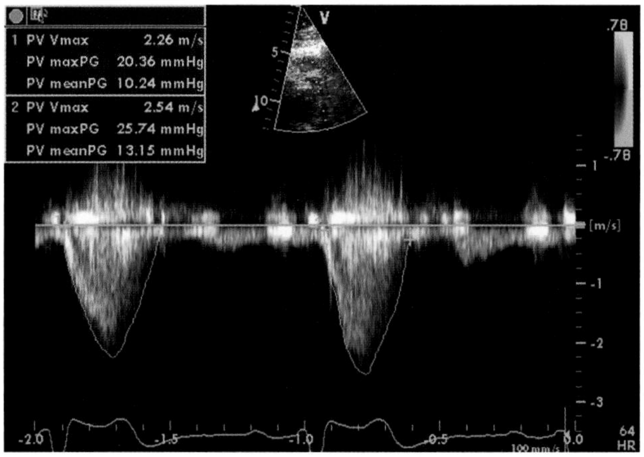

A. Hypertrophic cardiomyopathy
B. Myxoma
C. Metastatic carcinoma
D. Papillary fibroelastoma
E. Pheochromocytoma

Figure 65-1

ANSWER 1: B. Several bedside maneuvers can be performed to help clarify the type of cardiac murmur. Two of the most useful of these are assessing how the murmur quality changes with (1) respiration and (2) Valsalva. With inspiration, there is an increase in right heart filling. This leads to the clinical finding of an increase in the intensity of all murmurs from right-sided lesions with inspiration and a decrease with expiration. The reverse is true with left-sided lesions, although the changes may be less marked. During the late strain phase of the Valsalva maneuver, the decrease in venous return leads to a decrease in left ventricular (LV) filling and a decline in LV size. All murmurs will decrease in intensity apart from a dynamic outflow tract murmur that will increase in intensity because the decreased LV volume leads to an increased proximity of the septum and mitral valve and a higher gradient. Tricuspid stenosis leads to a diastolic murmur.[1]

ANSWER 2: C. Although myxomas are the most common primary cardiac tumors, they present as intracavitary tumors, most typically arising from the intra-atrial septum, and are present in the left atrium.

Papillary fibroelastomas are also intracavitary smaller tumors occurring on the endocardial lining of the heart, most typically attached to valvular apparatus. Myxomas and papillary fibroelastomas typically present with embolic symptoms, and the treatment is resection. Pheochromocytomas rarely involve the heart, but when they occur, they are well-circumscribed tumors present in the atrioventricular groove. This case demonstrates a large mass that arises from the intraventricular septum, distinct from the underlying myocardium, extending into the right ventricular cavity leading to right ventricular outflow tract obstruction, and impairing tricuspid valve function leading to eccentric moderate tricuspid valve regurgitation. Although a primary cardiac tumor is possible, statistically this is far more likely to present a metastatic malignancy. In light of the patient's prior renal cell carcinoma history, this is most likely.

Biopsy confirmed metastatic renal cell carcinoma, and the patient was commenced on sunitinib therapy. Two years later, the mass remains unchanged and the patient is asymptomatic.

See *The Echo Manual, 3rd Edition,* **tumors and masses on pages 310 to 311, and 315 to 316.**

Reference

1. Lembo NJ, Dell'Italia LJ, Crawford MH, et al. Bedside diagnosis of systolic murmurs. *N Engl J Med.* 1988;318:1572–1578.

CASE 66

Palpitations and Dyspnea

*D*oppler recordings were obtained from a 74-year-old woman with palpitations and dyspnea.

Figure 66-1 is from mitral inflow and Figure 66-2 is from the medial mitral annulus tissue Doppler recording.

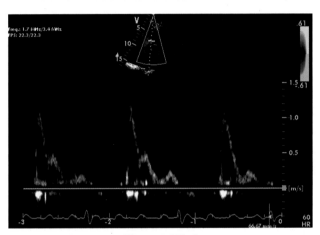

Figure 66-1

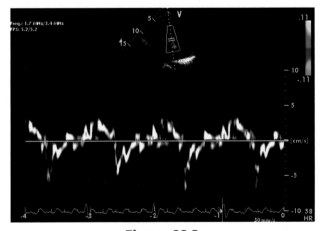

Figure 66-2

QUESTION 1. Which of the following is the correct value for the A velocity?

A. 1.4 m per second

B. 0.5 m per second

C. 0.2 m per second

D. Cannot determine

QUESTION 2. Which of the following statements is correct regarding diastolic function in this patient?

A. Myocardial relaxation is markedly delayed

B. Left ventricular (LV) filling pressure is not elevated

C. LV filling pressure cannot be estimated

D. This pattern is characteristic for cardiac amyloidosis

QUESTION 3. What is E/e' ratio?

A. >20

B. 15

C. 10

D. 5

QUESTION 4. Which of the following statements regarding LV systolic function is/are correct (Figs. 66-3 to 66-5 and **Videos 66-1 to 66-5**)?

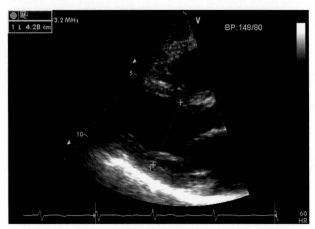

Figure 66-3

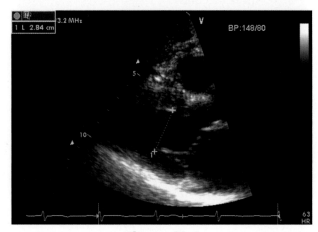

Figure 66-4

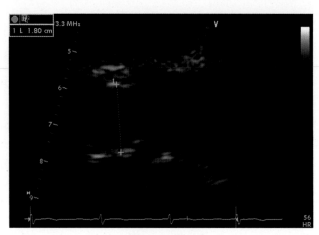

Figure 66-5

A. Using the apical correction factor, the calculated left ventricular ejection fraction (LVEF) is 64%

B. The Doppler-derived cardiac output is 3.1 L per minute

C. There are no discrete regional wall motion abnormalities

D. All of the choices

QUESTION 5. Which of the following medications would most likely improve the patient's symptoms?

A. Isosorbide mononitrate

B. Metoprolol succinate

C. Digoxin

D. Lisinopril

ANSWER 1: C. The underlying rhythm of this patient is atrial flutter. Atrial flutter is generating A velocity of 20 cm per second (or 0.2 m per second) just before the QRS. It may be better to designate the velocity as F velocity, but is analogous to A velocity in sinus rhythm. There is another velocity (0.5 m per second) between E and A (or F) velocities, and it is not related to flutter wave because A velocity produced by flutter was much lower. The velocity is "L wave" that is related to delayed myocardial relaxation.

ANSWER 2: A. Myocardial relaxation is markedly delayed.

ANSWER 3: A. The fact that E velocity is high (1.4 m per second) with a little variability from beat to beat in the setting of irregular rhythm and deceleration time is short indicates that filling pressure is elevated in this patient. That is also supported by the finding that E/e' ratio is >20 because e' velocity varies from 0.5 to 0.7 cm per second. The velocity peak right after e' velocity of mitral annulus is analogous to L wave in mitral inflow followed by a velocity generated by flutter. E/e' ratio can be used for patients with atrial fibrillation or sinus tachycardia with fusion of E and A velocities for estimation of LV filling pressure.

ANSWER 4: D. In the absence of LV regional wall motion abnormalities, the LV dimensions measured from the level of the papillary muscles can be used to calculate the LVEF as follows:

Uncorrected LVEF = $[(EDd)^2 - (ESd)^2/(EDd)^2] \times 100$
  Corrected LVEF = uLVEF + $[(100 - uLVEF) \times 15\%]$,

where uLVEF is uncorrected LVEF.

Here,

Uncorrected LVEF = $[(43)^2 - (28)^2/(43)^2] \times 100 = 58\%$
  Corrected LVEF = $58 + [(100 - 58) \times 15\%] = 64\%$

See *The Echo Manual, 3rd Edition,* page 109.

Stroke volume (SV) is calculated as the product of the cross-sectional area of the left ventricular outflow tract (LVOT) and the time velocity integral (TVI) of a pulse wave sample from the LVOT.

SV (ml) = $[(D/2)^2 \times \pi] \times$ [LVOT TVI]
      = $[(1.8/2)^2 \times \pi] \times [22]$
      = 56 ml

Cardiac output is equal to the product of SV and heart rate = $56 \times 56 = 3.1$ L per minute

See *The Echo Manual, 3rd Edition,* Figure 4-16 on page 71.

The apparent disconnect between a low cardiac output and a preserved LVEF is not an uncommon finding in patients with a restrictive cardiomyopathy.

ANSWER 5: A. This patient has diastolic heart failure with preserved ejection fraction. His LV filling and SV are relatively fixed, so that lower heart rate and afterload reduction may decrease cardiac output and blood pressure, respectively. Because increased LV filling pressure is most likely responsible for dyspnea, the patient's symptoms will improve with a preload reducer such as isosorbide mononitrate.

CASE 67

Transient Loss of Motor Function in Right Upper Extremity

A 46-year-old man is referred for a transthoracic echocardiogram with agitated saline bubble study, following a transient loss of motor function in his right upper extremity. One week previously, he underwent surgical resection of a suppurative appendicitis and is currently receiving intravenous antibiotics through a peripherally inserted central (PIC) venous catheter. Apart from the transient neurologic event, which has entirely resolved, he feels well without any systemic symptoms. He has no cardiovascular history. Examination is otherwise entirely normal (see **Video 67-1**).

QUESTION 1. What is the structure identified by the arrow (Fig. 67-1)?

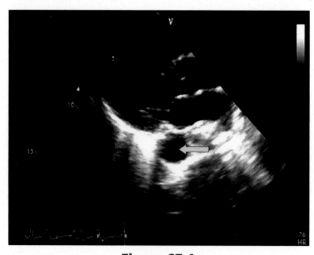

Figure 67-1

A. Descending thoracic aorta
B. Coronary sinus
C. Esophagus
D. Left pulmonary artery
E. Left inferior pulmonary vein

QUESTION 2. The appropriate next step in this patient's management is:

A. Referral for closure of patent foramen ovale or atrial septal defect
B. Referral to vascular radiology
C. Transesophageal echocardiogram to exclude thrombus/vegetation

QUESTION 3. What is the mobile structure in the right atrium?

A. Thrombus
B. Eustachian valve
C. Ventricular pacing lead
D. Myxoma

QUESTION 4. How would you estimate left ventricular ejection fraction?

A. 35%
B. 50%
C. 65%
D. 75%

ANSWER 1: A. The round structure posterior to the left atrium and outside the pericardium is the descending thoracic aorta that is of normal dimension. The coronary sinus is a smaller structure present in the posterior atrioventricular groove present within the pericardium.

See *The Echo Manual, 3rd Edition*, page 8 and Figure 2-4 on page 11.

ANSWER 2: B. The resting transthoracic echocardiogram is normal. With administration of agitated saline, bubbles are first visualized in the left ventricle, then after approximately five to seven cardiac cycles bubbles are seen in the right-sided chambers. Preceding the presence of bubbles in the left ventricle, the descending thoracic aorta (Fig. 67-2, arrow) is seen to opacify.

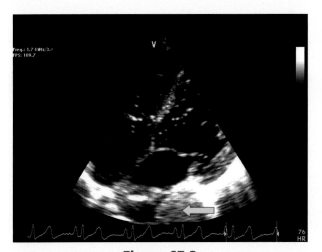

Figure 67-2

The only plausible explanation for these findings is that the PIC catheter has been misplaced with the tip lying in the arterial system. With agitated saline intravenous administration, the thoracic aorta opacifies first and related to mild aortic valve regurgitation a small amount of saline refluxes into the left ventricle. Given these findings, the appropriate next steps would include cessation of the use of the catheter, assessment of catheter location by vascular radiology, and removal. Iodinated contrast injection through the PIC catheter

confirmed that the tip was located in the mid-ascending thoracic aorta (Fig. 67-3). Intra-arterial placement occurred in the right antecubital fossa where the tip had been placed through the brachial vein into the brachial artery.

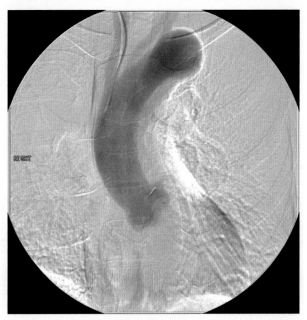

Figure 67-3

See *The Echo Manual, 3rd Edition*, the role of echocardiography in the evaluation of cardiac source of embolus on page 396.

ANSWER 3: B. In fetal life, the eustachian valve helps direct the flow of oxygenated blood from the inferior vena cava across the foramen ovale in utero. Although the eustachian valve remains after birth, it has no specific function and regresses to varying degrees. By adulthood, its typical appearance is a crescentic fold of tissue endocardium arising from the anterior rim of the orifice of the inferior vena cava. However, in some patients (as in this case), the eustachian valve persists as a highly mobile, elongated thin structure projecting several centimeters into the right atrial cavity.

ANSWER 4: B. 65%.

CASE 68

Cold Left Foot

A 60-year-old woman presents with a cold left foot. She is brought to the operating room where she undergoes embolectomy. You are asked to perform a transesophageal echocardiogram.

QUESTION 1. Which left ventricular wall segment is highlighted (**Video 68-1** and Fig. 68-1)?

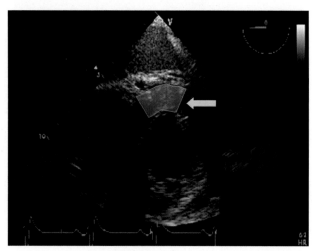

Figure 68-1

A. Mid anterior wall
B. Mid anteroseptal wall
C. Mid inferior wall
D. Mid inferolateral wall

QUESTION 2. Patients with this finding on echocardiography (**Videos 68-2 and 68-3**) are also likely to have:

A. An atrial septal defect
B. A patent foramen ovale and higher risk of stroke
C. A patent ductus arteriosus
D. A persistent left superior vena cava
E. Coarctation of the aorta

QUESTION 3. The left-sided chambers, valves, and left atrial appendage were all normal. Review **Videos 68-4 and 68-5**. Is the foramen ovale patent?

A. Yes
B. No

QUESTION 4. The next appropriate step is:

A. Aspirin
B. Clopidogrel
C. Warfarin
D. Referral for a percutaneous closure of the foramen ovale
E. Further imaging

QUESTION 5. On the basis of the images updated from the descending thoracic aorta (**Videos 68-6 to 68-8**), what is the appropriate next step?

A. Systemic anticoagulation with warfarin
B. Prednisone
C. Foramen ovale closure

QUESTION 6. Which of the following is not associated with an increased rate of atherosclerotic plaque in the thoracic aorta in patients older than 55 years?

A. Age
B. Smoking history
C. Systolic blood pressure
D. Sex
E. Location

ANSWER 1: C. Mid inferior wall. Various orientations may be used on transgastric transesophageal imaging without any clear standard. Here the right ventricle is shown on the left of the screen with the left ventricular septum between 7 o'clock and 11 o'clock. The segment illustrated in the figure between 11 and 1 o'clock is flanked by the liver and is the inferior wall of the left ventricle.

ANSWER 2: B. An atrial septal aneurysm is defined as a highly mobile atrial septum that has a maximum to minimum excursion distance of 15 mm. An atrial septal aneurysm is present in up to 3% to 4% of patients referred for transesophageal echocardiogram to assess for an embolic source. Atrial septal aneurysms are also associated with cerebral embolic events. The reason for this is unclear but may repeat to the frequent concomitant patent foramen ovale (50% to 75%). The cause and effect relationship of a patent foramen ovale in the setting of an atrial septal aneurysm and a cryptogenic embolic event remains unclear.

ANSWER 3: A. Yes. Color Doppler demonstrates a bidirectional shunt across the foramen ovale. Agitated saline demonstrated a modest amount of right-left shunting on Valsalva release.

ANSWER 4: E. An integral part of the transesophageal examination for evaluation source of embolus is a careful ultrasound examination of the thoracic aorta.

ANSWER 5: A. The transesophageal demonstrated focal areas of complex atherosclerosis with one notable highly mobile segment of atherosclerotic thrombotic plaque. There are no echo findings that suggest aortitis. Appropriate therapy should include consideration of warfarin anticoagulation. Surgical removal of the focal aortic debris should be considered in patients with recurrent embolic events.

ANSWER 6: D. In patients older than 55 years, sex is not particularly associated with the prevalence of atherosclerotic plaque in the thoracic aorta. Factors associated with risk include advancing age, smoking history, and increasing systolic blood pressure. Plaque is much more prevalent in the arch and descending aorta than in the ascending aorta.

See *The Echo Manual, 3rd Edition,* Figure 19-3 on page 324.

CASE 69

Chest Pain and ECG Changes

*A*40-year-old man nonsmoker presents with chest pain and ECG changes. He was brought emergently to the catheterization laboratory. An echocardiogram was performed.

QUESTION 1. His echocardiogram (**Videos 69-1 to 69-12** and Figs. 69-1 to 69-5) is consistent with:

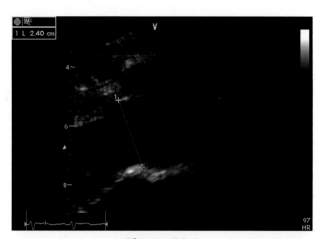

Figure 69-1

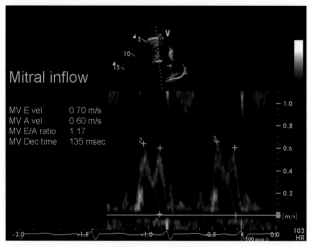

Mitral inflow

MV E vel	0.70 m/s
MV A vel	0.60 m/s
MV E/A ratio	1.17
MV Dec time	135 msec

Figure 69-2

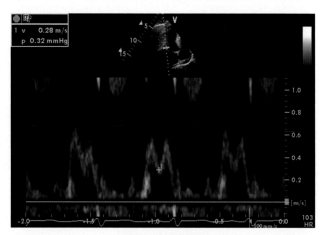

Figure 69-3

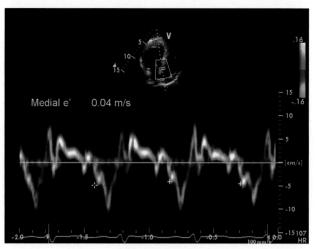

Medial e'   0.04 m/s

Figure 69-4

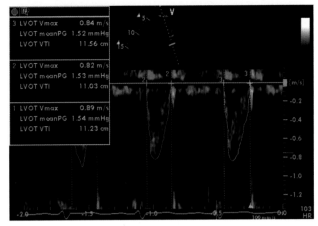

Figure 69-5

A. Acute infarction in the distribution of the left anterior descending coronary artery (LAD)
B. Acute infarction in the distribution of the left circumflex coronary artery
C. Acute infarction in the distribution of the right coronary artery
D. Apical ballooning syndrome
E. Normal echocardiogram

QUESTION 2. What proportion of the myocardium needs to be ischemic/infarcted to cause akinesis?

A. 20%
B. 40%
C. 50%
D. 80%
E. 100%

QUESTION 3. The Doppler derived stroke volume (SV) is:

A. 40 ml
B. 50 ml
C. 60 ml
D. 70 ml
E. Cannot be calculated on the basis of the available data

QUESTION 4. Which of the following is true with regard to this patient's diastolic function (left atrial volume index is 28 cc per m²)?

A. The diastolic function is normal
B. Mildly abnormal (grade 1, delayed relaxation pattern)

C. Moderate to severely abnormal
D. Indeterminate owing to tachycardia

QUESTION 5. Which of the following echocardiographic parameters is predictive of increased risk in this setting?

A. Extent of myocardial infarction
B. Left ventricular ejection fraction (LVEF) <40%
C. Restrictive diastolic filling
D. Reduced longitudinal right ventricular contractility
E. All of the choices

QUESTION 6. The patient is successfully revascularized within 90 minutes of the onset of chest pain (angiogram demonstrating single vessel disease). He is discharged from hospital 4 days later symptom free. After 3 months, he returns for echocardiography. (Videos 69-13 to 69-17 and Fig. 69-6). Implantation with a cardiac defibrillator is now appropriate.

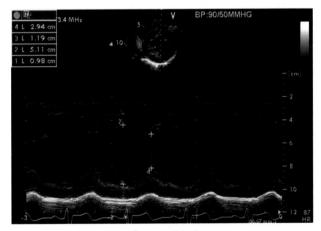

Figure 69-6

A. True
B. False

QUESTION 7. With regard to further testing which of the following is true/appropriate, assuming no change in symptoms?

A. Transthoracic echocardiogram at 1 year
B. An exercise echocardiogram at 1 year
C. A and B
D. No further testing within the first 2 years is appropriate

ANSWER 1: A. There is akinesis of the septum, anterior wall, and apex consistent with an acute myocardial infarction secondary to a proximal LAD coronary artery lesion. Apical ballooning is very unlikely in a 40-year-old man.

ANSWER 2: A. Akinesis is defined as when there is only 10% or less of an increase in wall thickness during systole. However, akinesis does not require transmural ischemia or infarction. In fact, only 20% of the myocardial thickness needs to be ischemic to lead to akinetic motion. Hence, there is potential for recovery of function (potential viability) in the setting of akinesis.

ANSWER 3: B. SV is calculated as the product of the cross-sectional area of the left ventricular outflow tract (LVOT) and the time velocity integral (TVI) of a pulse-wave sample from the LVOT.

$$SV\ (ml) = [(D/2)^2 \times \pi] \times [LVOT\ TVI]$$
$$= [(2.4/2)^2 \times \pi] \times [11]$$
$$= 4.5 \times 11$$
$$= 49.5\ ml$$

Cardiac output is the product of SV and heart rate = 49.5 × 100 = 4950 ml per minute.

See *The Echo Manual, 3rd Edition*, Figure 4-16 on page 71.

ANSWER 4: C. Here the left atrium is upper normal in size indicating that the patient has had no chronic elevation in filling pressures. However, there is evidence of an acute elevation in filling pressures with restrictive left ventricular filling pattern and a high E/e' ratio. As is commonly the case in the setting of sinus tachycardia, there is partial fusion of the E and A waves. This leads to a relative increase in the A wave velocity, leading to a relative reduction in the E/A wave ratio. One can adjust for this by subtracting the E at A velocity (Fig. 69-3) from the peak A velocity. The resulting ratio of E to corrected A is likely more representative of the true diastolic function profile. Either way the E/e' ratio (0.7/0.04) = 18 and the deceleration time of 135 milliseconds are in keeping with a restrictive pattern correlating with an elevated pulmonary capillary wedge pressure.[1,2]

ANSWER 5: E. Patients at increased risk for future cardiac events after acute myocardial infarction can be identified by (1) systolic dysfunction (LVEF <40%), (2) extensive infarction (wall motion score index ≥1.7), (3) restrictive diastolic filling (deceleration time <140 milliseconds and E/e' ≥15), (4) Left ventricular enlargement, (5) Left atrial enlargement (≥32 ml per m²), (6) mitral regurgitation with an effective regurgitant orifice of 0.2 cm² or more, (7) reduced right ventricular function (by tricuspid annular systolic plane excursion or strain), and (8) abnormal stress test findings on echocardiography.

ANSWER 6: B. Although there remains some residual anterior and apical hypokinesis, repeat echocardiography demonstrates that there has been a normalization of LVEF. The implantation of a primary prevention defibrillator is not indicated. "Stunned" myocardium takes from a few days up to a few months to improve.

ANSWER 7: D. In asymptomatic patients who have had complete revascularization within the past 2 years, stress echocardiography is not appropriate. Routine surveillance of ventricular function with known coronary artery disease and no change in clinical status or cardiac exam is also inappropriate.[3]

References

1. Nagueh S, Mikati I, Kopelen HA, et al. Doppler estimation of left ventricular filling pressure in sinus tachycardia. A new application of tissue Doppler imaging. *Circulation*. 1998;98:1644–1650.

2. Sohn DW, Kim YJ, Kim HC, et al. Evaluation of left ventricular diastolic function when mitral E and A waves are completely fused: role of assessing mitral annulus velocity. *J Am Soc Echocardiogr*. 1999;12:203–208.

3. ACCF/ASE/AHA/ASNC/HFSA/HRS/SCAI/SCCM/SCCT/ SCMR 2011 Appropriate Use Criteria for Echocardiography. A Report of the American College of Cardiology Foundation Appropriate Use Criteria Task Force, American Society of Echocardiography, American Heart Association, American Society of Nuclear Cardiology, Heart Failure Society of America, Heart Rhythm Society, Society for Cardiovascular Angiography and Interventions, Society of Critical Care Medicine, Society of Cardiovascular Computed Tomography, Society for Cardiovascular Magnetic Resonance American College of Chest Physicians. *J Am Soc Echocardiogr*. 2011;24:229–267.

CASE 70

Exertional Shortness of Breath with Systolic Blood Pressure of 110 mm Hg

A 55-year-old man presents with exertional shortness of breath. His systolic blood pressure is 110 mm Hg.

QUESTION 1. An unexpected finding on examination (see **Videos 70-1** to **70-9** and Figs. 70-1 to 70-3) would be:

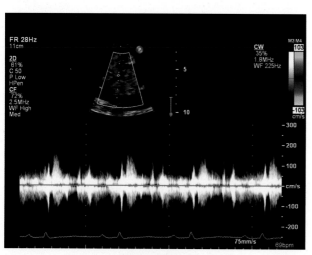

Figure 70-1

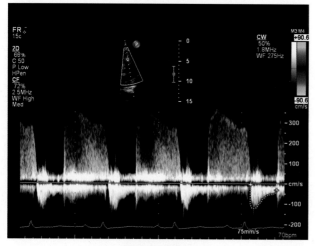

Figure 70-2

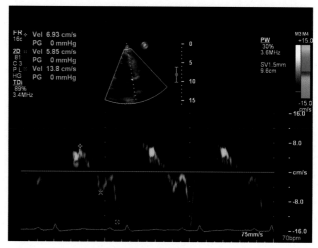

Figure 70-3

A. Cyanosis
B. Loud systolic murmur
C. Loud P2
D. Left parasternal lift
E. Digital clubbing

QUESTION 2. The estimated pulmonary artery (PA) end-diastolic pressure (based on a right atrial estimate of 10 mm Hg) is:

A. 14
B. 16
C. 46
D. 54

QUESTION 3. The estimated right ventricular systolic pressure is:

A. Elevated
B. Normal
C. Could not be estimated based on available data

QUESTION 4. On the basis of Figure 70-3, the right ventricular longitudinal contractility is:

A. Decreased
B. Normal
C. Hyperdynamic

QUESTION 5. The patient in this case is at risk for:

A. Visual disturbances
B. Iron-deficiency anemia
C. Infective endocarditis
D. Headaches
E. Syncope
F. All of the choices

QUESTION 6. Patients with Eisenmenger syndrome should take great caution/avoid all of the following *except*:

A. High altitude
B. Hot tubs
C. Pulmonary vasodilators
D. Volume depletion

QUESTION 7. Which of the following requires endocarditis prophylaxis?

A. Secundum atrial septal defect (ASD) having colonoscopy
B. Muscular ventricular septal defect (VSD) having cardiac catheterization
C. Bicuspid aortic valve, functionally normal having TEE
D. Inlet VSD having dental extraction
E. Repaired primum ASD with tissue mitral prosthesis having dental extraction

ANSWER 1: B. Echocardiography demonstrates a large membranous VSD with low velocity flow across the defect, indicative of equalization of ventricular pressures (Eisenmenger syndrome). This results in systemic PA pressures (loud P2), an enlarged right ventricle (left parasternal lift), clubbing, and central cyanosis. Unlike patients with a small, restrictive VSD that results in a loud systolic murmur, the low velocity flow across an Eisenmenger VSD is not audible. A systolic murmur may be audible if there is significant tricuspid valve regurgitation.

See *The Echo Manual, 3rd Edition,* **pages 337 to 344.**

ANSWER 2: C. PA diastolic pressure can be estimated by $4v^2$ + an estimate of right atrial pressure, where v = the end-diastolic velocity of the pulmonary regurgitant jet. Hence, PA diastolic pressure = $4(3)^2 + 10 = 46$ mm Hg

ANSWER 3: A. Although a tricuspid regurgitant jet is not displayed, there is a Doppler signal across the VSD, showing a peak systolic velocity <1.5 m per second (i.e., a gradient <9 mm Hg). Hence, the ventricular pressures are essentially equivalent. Therefore, as the left ventricular peak systolic pressure is equal to the systemic blood pressure (110 mm Hg), then the right ventricular systolic pressure is >100 mm Hg.

ANSWER 4: A. The lateral tricuspid annulus peak systolic longitudinal velocity at 6 to 7 m per second is very low indicative of a marked decrease in right ventricular longitudinal systolic function. Unlike the left ventricle, the predominance of right ventricular contractility occurs in the longitudinal plane with the basal plane moving down toward the apex with systole. The peak systolic lateral annular velocity is normally 12 to 15 m per second.

ANSWER 5: F. Owing to the erythrocytosis and resulting hyperviscosity syndrome that develops with Eisenmenger syndrome, patients may complain of headaches, visual disturbances, paresthesias, and dizziness. Patients with Eisenmenger syndrome are at risk for infective endocarditis, and other patients with severe pulmonary hypertension are at risk for syncope. Iron deficiency may develop either through bleeding or through excess phlebotomy.

ANSWER 6: C. Patients with Eisenmenger syndrome develop erythrocytosis and hyperviscosity, which can be exacerbated by high altitude, vasodilatory response in hot tubs, and volume depletion. Pulmonary vasodilators such as phosphodiesterase type 5 (PDE5) inhibitors (e.g., sildenafil), endothelin receptor antagonists (e.g., bosentan), or inhaled prostacyclin analogs (e.g., iloprost) are all potentially indicated for the treatment of the pulmonary arteriopathy that characterizes Eisenmenger syndrome. Pulmonary vascular targeted therapies improve symptoms and functional capacity and potentially may improve long-term survival.[1,2]

ANSWER 7: E. The updated guidelines (class IIa) list the following indications for antibiotic prophylaxis for dental procedures:

- Prosthetic cardiac valves
- Previous infective endocarditis
- Unrepaired and palliated cyanotic congenital heart defect (CHD) including surgically constructed shunts and conduits
- Repaired CHD with prosthetic materials for the first 6 months after procedure
- Repaired CHD with residual defects at site or adjacent to site of prosthetic patch or device (that inhibit endothelialization)

References

1. Beghetti M, Galiè N. Eisenmenger syndrome a clinical perspective in a new therapeutic era of pulmonary arterial hypertension. *J Am Coll Cardiol.* 2009;53:733–740.

2. Dimopoulos K, Inuzuka R, Goletto S, et al. Improved survival among patients with Eisenmenger syndrome receiving advance therapy for pulmonary arterial hypertension. *Circulation.* 2010;121:20–25.

CASE 71

Class III Shortness of Breath

*A*45-year-old woman with class III shortness of breath has on examination a loud first heart sound, an audible early opening snap, and a diastolic murmur. She is referred for transthoracic echocardiography (**Videos 71-1 through 71-10** and Figs. 71-1 through 71-9).

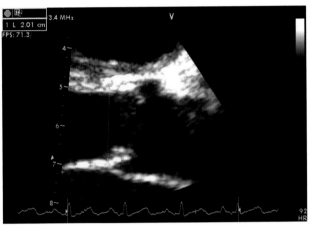

Figure 71-1

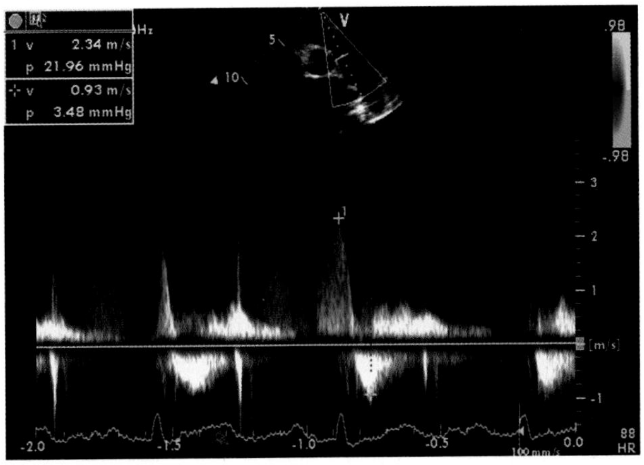

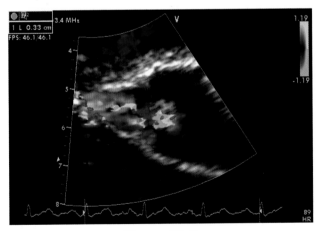

Figure 71-2

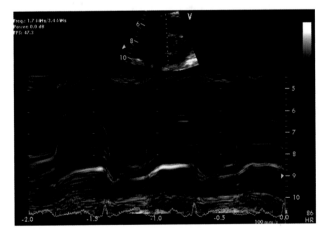

Figure 71-3

Figure 71-4

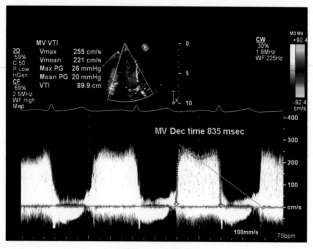

Figure 71-5

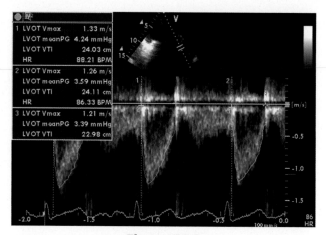

Figure 71-8

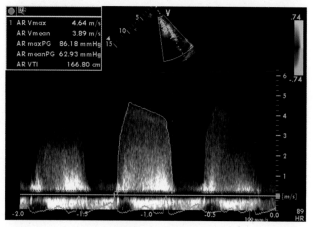

Figure 71-6

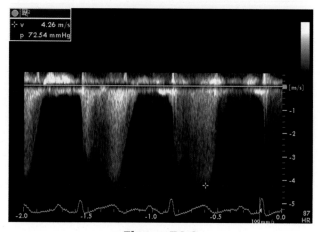

Figure 71-9

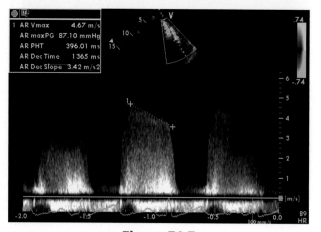

Figure 71-7

QUESTION 1. The likely pathology affecting the mitral and aortic valves is:

   A. Degenerative calcification

   B. Rheumatic disease

   C. Healed endocarditis

   D. Carcinoid heart disease

QUESTION 2. The severity of aortic valve regurgitation is:

   A. Trivial

   B. Mild–moderate

   C. Severe

QUESTION 3. The mitral valve area (MVA) based on the pressure half-time (PHT) method is:

A. 0.8 cm^2
B. 0.9 cm^2
C. 1.0 cm^2
D. 1.1 cm^2

QUESTION 4. The MVA based on the continuity equation is:

A. 0.8 cm^2
B. 0.9 cm^2
C. 1.0 cm^2
D. 1.1 cm^2

QUESTION 5. The severity of mitral valve stenosis is:

A. Mild
B. Moderate
C. Severe

QUESTION 6. The appropriate next step includes:

A. Hemodynamic catheterization
B. Coronary evaluation followed by mitral valve replacement
C. Transesophageal echocardiography
D. Mitral valve balloon valvuloplasty
E. Exercise Doppler echocardiography

ANSWER 1: B. The echocardiographic images demonstrate classic features of mitral and, to a lessor extent, aortic valve involvement of rheumatic valve disease.

See *The Echo Manual, 3rd Edition,* discussion of the typical M-mode and 2D echocardiographic features of rheumatic mitral stenosis on page 202.

ANSWER 2: B. There is concomitant rheumatic involvement of the aortic valve with thickening and calcification particularly of the noncoronary cusp. There is associated central holodiastolic aortic valve regurgitation. The jet width is relatively small with a vena contracta diameter of 3 mm and a PHT of 396 milliseconds consistent with no more than mild–moderate regurgitation. Estimating the severity of concomitant aortic valve regurgitation is particularly important in the setting of mitral valve stenosis because the presence of severe regurgitation has important diagnostic and therapeutic implications.

ANSWER 3: B. There are two steps involved in calculating the MVA by the PHT method. The first is calculating the PHT. PHT is the time interval where the peak pressure gradient falls by exactly 50%. PHT is always 29% of the deceleration time (DT), which can be rounded to 30%. Here DT is 835 milliseconds, so PHT is (835 / 0.3) = 250.

MVA = 220/PHT = 220/250 = 0.9 cm^2

This equation should not be used immediately after balloon valvuloplasty, in the setting of severe aortic valve regurgitation or in the presence of high left ventricular filling pressures as in diastolic dysfunction.

ANSWER 4: A. To determine the MVA with the continuity equation, determine the stroke volume from the left ventricular outflow tract (LVOT) diameter (D) and time velocity integral (TVI), then calculate the MVA by dividing the LVOT stroke volume by mitral valve TVI as follows:

See *The Echo Manual, 3rd Edition,* Figure 12-19 on page 205.

$$MVA = LVOT\ D^2 \times 0.785 \times \frac{TVI_{LVOT}}{TVI_{MV}} [(2)^2 \times 0.785 \times 24]/[90] = 0.8\ cm^2$$

This equation cannot be used if there is marked aortic or mitral valve regurgitation.

ANSWER 5: C. Mitral stenosis is considered severe when the resting mean transmitral pressure gradient is ≥10 mm Hg, the MVA ≤1.0 cm^2, and the PHT ≥220 milliseconds. In keeping with severe mitral stenosis, there is echocardiographic evidence of significant pulmonary hypertension (estimated pulmonary artery pressures of 83/32 mm Hg).

ANSWER 6: C. Transthoracic echocardiography is the gold standard for the diagnosis and quantification of mitral valve stenosis with the transmitral gradient by Doppler echocardiography more accurate than the gradient derived by conventional cardiac catheterization. The pressure gradient is frequently overestimated with cardiac catheterization when the pulmonary capillary wedge pressure is used to measure the transmitral pressure gradient. In the presence of a 2D echocardiogram that is in keeping with the clinical examination findings, no further hemodynamic assessment is required. When symptoms appear out of proportion to the resting hemodynamics (e.g., mild–moderate stenosis), Doppler echocardiography is appropriate to assess mitral mean diastolic gradient and pulmonary pressures.

Regarding the management of patients with severe mitral valve stenosis, a key step is to determine the mitral valve pliability and hence suitability for percutaneous treatment. In the setting of a noncalcified pliable mitral valve with little regurgitation, the outcomes from mitral valve balloon valvuloplasty are excellent and should be considered in all symptomatic patients and also in asymptomatic patients with new-onset atrial fibrillation and/or a pulmonary artery systolic pressure >60 mm Hg. Mitral valve replacement is reserved for those patients with class III or IV symptoms and a nonpliable valve or concomitant moderate or greater regurgitation.

A commonly used echocardiographic scoring system to assess valve pliability and predict the outcome after balloon valvuloplasty is the one described by Abascal et al.,[1] with a score given from 4 to 16 and a higher score indicating more severe anatomic disease and a lower score indicating the likelihood of a successful balloon valvotomy with durability.

See *The Echo Manual, 3rd Edition,* Figure 12-1 on page 190.

Simply, the absence of significant commissural calcification[2] also predicts long-term outcome after balloon valvuloplasty.

Here there is little mitral valve leaflet, subvalvular, and commissural calcification indicating a high likelihood of success with valvuloplasty. Before valvuloplasty, the patient requires a transesophageal echocardiogram (TEE) to exclude LA thrombus and significant mitral valve regurgitation.

Following TEE, the patient underwent successful valvuloplasty with an immediate reduction in mean gradient (Fig. 71-10) and an improvement in symptoms.

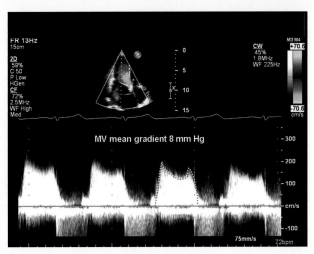

Figure 71-10

References

1. Abascal VM, Wilkins GT, Choong CY, et al. Echocardiographic evaluation of mitral valve structure and function in patients followed for at least 6 months after percutaneous balloon mitral valvuloplasty. *J Am Coll Cardiol.* 1988;12:606–615.

2. Cannan CR, Nishimura RA, Reeder GS, et al. Echocardiographic assessment of commissural calcium: a simple predictor of outcome after percutaneous mitral balloon valvotomy. *J Am Coll Cardiol.* 1997;29:175–180.

Asymptomatic Murmur

A 30-year-old man presents for the evaluation of a murmur. He exercises regularly and is asymptomatic.

Review echocardiogram (**Videos 72-1 to 72-8** and Figs. 72-1 to 72-5).

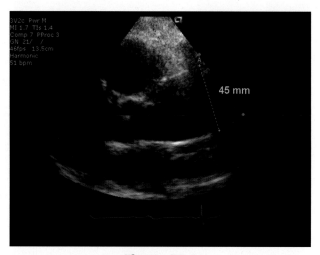

Figure 72-1

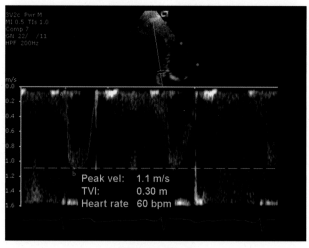

Figure 72-2

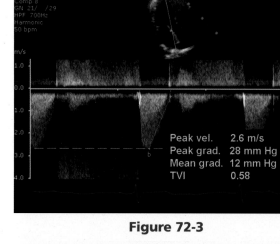

Peak vel.   2.6 m/s
Peak grad. 28 mm Hg
Mean grad. 12 mm Hg
TVI   0.58

Figure 72-3

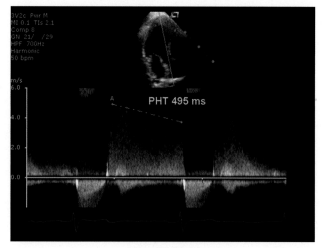

PHT 495 ms

Figure 72-4

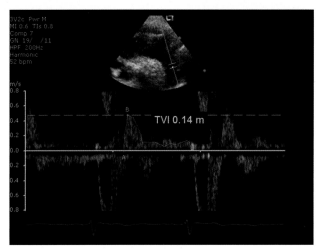

Figure 72-5

QUESTION 1. Which of the following statements concerning the left ventricle is correct?

A. The left ventricular is upper normal in size with an estimated ejection fraction of 65%

B. The left ventricle is moderately dilated with an estimated ejection fraction of 50%

C. The left ventricle is normal in size with an estimated ejection fraction of 45%

D. The left ventricle is severely dilated with an estimated ejection fraction of 70%

QUESTION 2. Given a left ventricular outflow tract (LVOT) diameter of 25 mm, the calculated cardiac output is:

A. 5.0 L per minute

B. 6.5 L per minute

C. 7.0 L per minute

D. 8.5 L per minute

E. 10 L per minute

QUESTION 3. The aortic valve pathology is:

A. Bicuspid aortic valve with moderate stenosis and moderate regurgitation

B. Bicuspid aortic valve with trivial–mild stenosis and moderate regurgitation

C. Bicuspid aortic valve with moderate stenosis and mild regurgitation

D. Bicuspid aortic valve with trivial–mild stenosis and mild regurgitation

QUESTION 4. You recommend the patient follow-up in 1 year. He presents 4 years later for reevaluation. On examination, his blood pressure is 120/70 mm Hg. His heart sounds are normal. He has an early systolic click, grade 2/6 mid to late peaking systolic ejection murmur, and a diastolic decrescendo murmur. His central venous pressure and carotid pulses are normal. He is no longer physically active but denies symptoms (**Video 72-9** and Figs. 72-6 to 72-10). Calculate the aortic valve effective regurgitant orifice (ERO).

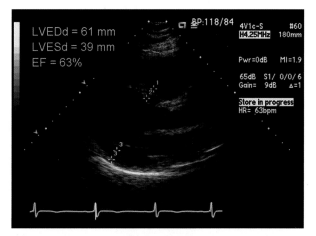

Figure 72-6

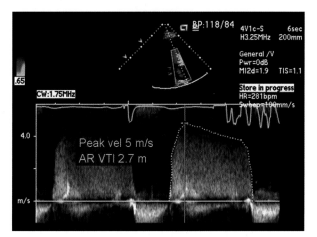

Figure 72-7

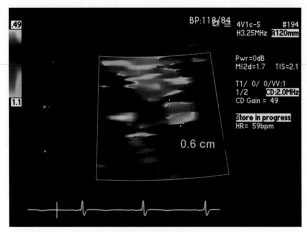

Figure 72-8

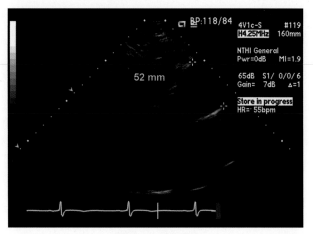

Figure 72-10

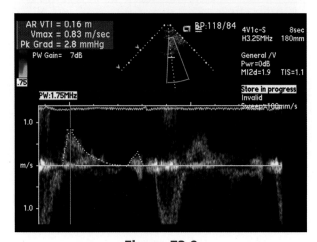

Figure 72-9

A. 0.1 cm²

B. 0.2 cm²

C. 0.3 cm²

D. 0.4 cm²

QUESTION 5. The next appropriate step is:

A. Routine follow-up

B. Consider surgical consultation for progressive aortic valve regurgitation

C. Consider surgical consultation for progressive aortic dilation

ANSWER 1: A. The left ventricle has an end diastolic dimension of 57 mm and an ejection fraction of approximately 65%.

ANSWER 2: D. The cardiac output can be calculated using the LVOT Diameter (D), the LVOT time velocity integral [TVI] and the heart rate (HR) as follows:

$$= 0.785(D^2)(LVOT\ TVI)(HR)$$
$$= 0.785(2.5^2)(30)(60)$$
$$= 8.5\ L\ per\ minute$$

See *The Echo Manual, 3rd Edition*, **pages 69 to 71 and Figure 4-16 on page 71.**

ANSWER 3: B. The aortic valve is bicuspid with mildly thickened leaflets with normal mobility. The mean transvalvular systolic gradient is 12 mm Hg with a dimensionless index over 0.5 (LVOT TVI/AV TVI of 0.3/0.58). These are all in keeping with trivial–mild stenosis. The aortic valve regurgitation is holodiastolic with a reasonable broad jet seen on both long and short axis. The pressure halftime at 495 milliseconds and the TVI in the descending thoracic aorta of 14 cm are both in the intermediate range of severity indicating a moderate degree of aortic valve regurgitation. This is supported by the mildly elevated cardiac output.

See *The Echo Manual, 3rd Edition*, **discussion of severity of aortic valve regurgitation on pages 207 to 210, and ASE guidelines in Appendix 20 on page 413.**

ANSWER 4: B. The regurgitant flow rate across the aortic valve is obtained from the flow rate of a proximal surface area with a known flow velocity as follows:

Flow rate $= 2\pi(r)^2 \times$ aliasing velocity
$= 6.28 \times (r)^2 \times$ aliasing velocity
$= 6.28 \times (0.6)^2 \times 49$
$= 111\ cm^3$ per second

ERO $=$ Flow rate/peak aortic valve regurgitation peak velocity
$= 111\ cm^3$ per second/500 cm per second
$= 0.22\ cm^2$

See *The Echo Manual, 3rd Edition*, **page 209.**

ANSWER 5: C. The general recommendations for the timing of surgical intervention for aortic valve regurgitation in the absence of cardiovascular symptoms would be a consideration if severe aortic valve regurgitation was associated with a progressive left ventricular dilation or progressive decline in left ventricular systolic function. Here the degree of aortic valve regurgitation remains moderate without a significant change in left ventricular dimensions or ejection fraction. However, the ascending aortic dilation has significantly progressed increasing from 45 mm to 52 mm over 4 years. Ascending aortic reconstruction is indicated in patients with aortic valve disease and an ascending aortic diameter exceeding 50 mm or an increase of 5 mm over a year. In the setting, consideration of surgical ascending aortic replacement with concomitant aortic valve replacement should be considered.[1]

Reference

1. Bonow RO, Carabello BA, Chatterjee K, et al. 2008 focused update incorporated into the ACC/AHA 2006 guidelines for the management of patients with valvular heart disease: a report of the American College of Cardiology/American Heart Association Task Force on Practice Guidelines. *Circulation.* 2008;118:e523.

CASE 73

Intermittent Dyspnea with Modest Exertion

*A*n 83-year-old man presents for the evaluation of new-onset dyspnea over the past 2 weeks, which occurs intermittently with modest exertion. His exercise capacity is limited by osteoarthritis of the knee.

His medications include aspirin 81 mg daily, metoprolol 50 mg twice daily, simvastatin 40 mg daily, and hydrochlorothiazide 12.5 mg daily.

On examination, his blood pressure was 120/80 mm Hg and heart rate 60 beats per minute. Cardiopulmonary examination was normal apart from a left-sided fourth heart sound.

Twelve-lead ECG is normal. He is referred for dobutamine stress echocardiography.

The patient receives a combination of dobutamine and atropine to achieve a peak heart rate of 125 beats per minute. He was asymptomatic throughout the test but did develop 1.5 mm of horizontal ST segment depression in his anterior leads with stress.

QUESTION 1. Concerning dobutamine stress echocardiography:

A. The effects of dobutamine infusion lead to an increase in contractility before effects on heart rate

B. Dobutamine infusion predictably leads to a decline in systemic blood pressure secondary to β_2-receptor–mediated systemic vasodilation

C. Dobutamine stress echocardiography is preferred to exercise stress echocardiography in patients with a pacemaker

D. Nonsustained ventricular tachycardia with stress is an uncommon but specific marker for underlying significant coronary artery disease

---

QUESTION 2. Concerning atropine use in dobutamine stress echocardiography:

A. Atropine increases the sensitivity for the detection of mild coronary artery disease in patients taking β-blockers

B. Atropine use is contraindicated in all patients with glaucoma

C. Atropine use is not associated with an increased risk of atrial fibrillation

---

QUESTION 3. Appropriate indications for the cessation of dobutamine infusion include all of the following *except*:

A. Exceeding a target heart rate of 85% of age-predicted maximum

B. Symptomatic arrhythmias such as atrial fibrillation or ventricular tachycardia

C. Two-millimeter flat/downsloping ST segment depression on 12-lead ECG in the absence of symptoms or wall motion abnormalities

D. Left ventricular dilation with 10% decline in left ventricular ejection fraction

---

QUESTION 4. Dobutamine stress echocardiography demonstrates evidence of (see **Videos 73-1 through 73-4**):

Note: Orientation in all views is as follows: *top left*, apical four chamber (displayed in the Mayo format with the left ventricle on the left); *top right*, apical long axis; *bottom left*, apical 2 chamber; *bottom right*, apical short axis.

A. Lateral wall ischemia

B. Anterior ischemia

C. No evidence of ischemia

QUESTION 5. He was managed medically. Despite this, 1 week later, the patient develops chest discomfort and then becomes acutely dyspneic and hypotensive. On examination, he is distressed secondary to dyspnea and angina and is unable to lie flat. His blood pressure is 80/50 mm Hg, and heart rate is 140 beat per minute. There is a new systolic murmur. ECG shows ST segment elevation in the inferior and lateral leads. The patient undergoes emergent transthoracic echocardiography (see **Video 73-5**). The most likely explanation for the systolic murmur is:

   A. A ventricular septal rupture
   B. A papillary muscle rupture
   C. Dynamic left ventricular outflow tract obstruction

ANSWER 1: A. Dobutamine is a synthetic catecholamine that stimulates both β_1- and β_2-adrenergic receptors but has little action on α-adrenergic receptors. The predominant action of dobutamine is a positive inotropic and chronotropic effect (β_1) with some vasodilatation (β_2). The effects are dose dependent with an augmentation in cardiac contractility occurring at lower doses and with the chronotropic effects progressively occurring at intermediate and higher doses. This dose-dependent difference in action is utilized in cases of low-output, low-gradient aortic stenosis (see Case 20). Although β_2-receptor stimulation may lead to systemic vasodilation, the effects on systemic blood pressure are offset because of the increased cardiac output seen with the β_1 effects on heart rate and contractility. Like exercise stress, dobutamine is associated with an aggravated abnormal septal motion response in patients ventricularly paced (or those who have a left bundle branch block) and may be associated with septal and apical wall motion abnormalities that are unrelated to coronary artery ischemia. Nonsustained ventricular tachycardia may occur in 3% to 5% of patients undergoing dobutamine stress echocardiography. It is generally well tolerated and is not associated with a specific risk of underlying ischemia.[1–4]

See *The Echo Manual, 3rd Edition*, page 178.

ANSWER 2: A. Use of atropine augments the capacity to reach target heart rate where dobutamine infusion is insufficient, and thereby increases the sensitivity for the detection, particularly of mild, coronary artery disease. Use of atropine is most commonly required in patients taking β-blockers. Through inhibition of the cholinergic effect in the eye, atropine leaves the sympathetically mediated dilation of the pupil unopposed. Hence, in the setting of closed-angle glaucoma, atropine is contraindicated. Use in the more common "open-angle glaucoma" is not associated with complication. By inhibiting muscarinic receptors in atrial muscle, atropine increases the risk of atrial flutter or fibrillation. Atropine does not directly increase the risk of ventricular dysrhythmia because ventricular myocardium has no cholinergic innervation.[4,5]

ANSWER 3: C. The decision on stopping a stress echocardiogram must be individualized to the patient.

Pharmacologic stress echocardiography affords the opportunity to directly monitor wall motion during the study that can aid in the decision on whether to stop a study early in a patient complaining of chest pain or who develops ECG changes. A well-tolerated small area of stress-induced ischemia does not necessarily require the early cessation of the study because this may prevent a clear demonstration of a more widespread burden of coronary artery disease. ECG evidence of either ST segment depression or elevation in the absence of typical angina or wall motion abnormalities is not specific for the presence of ischemia and does not warrant early test termination. However, in the setting of a high-risk left ventricular ischemic response, such as left ventricular dilation and/or a decline in left ventricular ejection fraction, it would be appropriate to stop the test early. In the absence of the development of any of these findings, significant limiting symptoms/signs, dobutamine stress echocardiography is typically terminated when the patient's heart rate exceeds 85% of the age-predicted maximum.[1–4]

See *The Echo Manual, 3rd Edition*, Table 11-2 on page 178.

ANSWER 4: A. Overall, the left ventricular volume decreases with an increase in left ventricular ejection fraction. At prepeak and peak doses, there is evidence of new regional wall motion abnormalities in the inferolateral wall and anterior-septum. Anterior wall contractility is normal.

ANSWER 5: B. A number of mechanical complications of acute myocardial infarction may present with a sudden clinical change and a new systolic murmur, and echocardiography can play a direct role in diagnosis. Typically associated with acute pulmonary edema and a brief early systolic murmur a papillary muscle rupture, see here with posteromedial rupture (see **Video 73-6**) typically occurs in the setting of a small infarct in the distribution of the right or circumflex coronary artery. Treatment is urgent surgical mitral valve replacement.[6]

See *The Echo Manual, 3rd Edition*, pages 162 to 165, including Table 10-2 on page 162.

References

1. Kane GC, Hepinstall MJ, Kidd GM, et al. Safety of stress echocardiography supervised by registered nurses: results of a 2-year audit of 15,404 patients. *J Am Soc Echocardiogr*. 2008;21:337.

2. Mathias W Jr, Arruda A, Santos FC, et al. Safety of dobutamine-atropine stress echocardiography: a prospective experience of 4,033 consecutive studies. *J Am Soc Echocardiogr*. 1999;12:785.

3. Mertes H, Sawada SG, Ryan T, et al. Symptoms, adverse effects, and complications associated with dobutamine stress echocardiography. Experience in 1118 patients. *Circulation*. 1993;88:15.

4. Pellikka PA, Nagueh SF, Elhendy AA, et al. American Society of Echocardiography recommendations for performance, interpretation, and application of stress echocardiography. *J Am Soc Echocardiogr*. 2007;20:1021.

5. Ling LH, Pellikka PA, Mahoney DW, et al. Atropine augmentation in dobutamine stress echocardiography: role and incremental value in a clinical practice setting. *J Am Coll Cardiol*. 1996;28:551–557.

6. Reeder GS. Identification and treatment of complications of myocardial infarction. *Mayo Clin Proc*.1995;70:880–884.

CASE 74

Exertional Shortness of Breath, Systolic Murmur and Lower Extremity Edema

A 68-year-old woman presents with exertional shortness of breath, bilateral lower extremity edema, and a systolic murmur.

QUESTION 1. On the basis of her transthoracic images (**Videos 74-1 to 74-6** and Figs. 74-1 and 74-2), her calculated mitral effective regurgitant orifice (ERO) area by the proximal isovelocity surface area method is:

A. 0.2 cm²
B. 0.3 cm²
C. 0.4 cm²
D. 0.5 cm²

QUESTION 2. The mechanism of the mitral valve regurgitation appears to be:

A. Infective endocarditis with leaflet perforation
B. Bileaflet mitral valve prolapse without evidence of flail leaflet
C. Mitral annulus dilation with secondary (functional) regurgitation
D. Inferior wall akinesis with secondary papillary muscle dysfunction

QUESTION 3. On the basis of the transthoracic images (**Videos 74-7 to 74-9** and Figs. 74-3 to 74-5), the tricuspid valve regurgitation is:

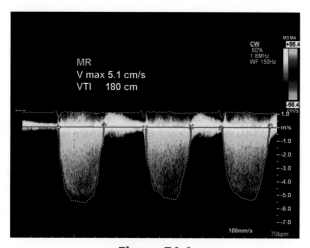

Figure 74-1

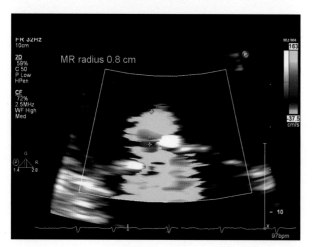

Figure 74-2

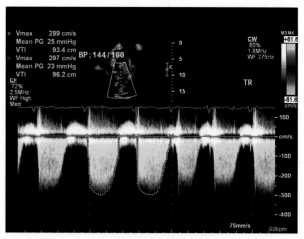

Figure 74-3

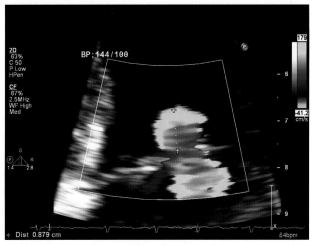

Figure 74-4

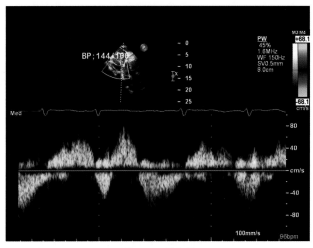

Figure 74-5

A. Mild
B. Mild–moderate
C. Moderate–severe
D. Severe

QUESTION 4. The patient is referred for transesophageal echocardiography (TEE) before direct current (DC) cardioversion (Fig. 74-6). Concerning left atrial appendage (LAA) flow velocities, which of the following is *false*?

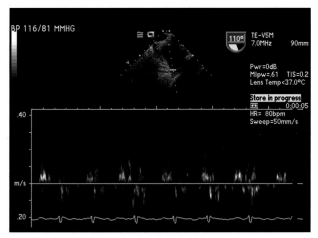

Figure 74-6

A. Typical emptying velocities in sinus rhythm are >50 cm per second
B. Emptying velocities <20 cm per second are associated with an increased risk of systemic thromboembolic disease post cardioversion
C. Emptying velocities are best recorded with continuous wave Doppler of flow through the midpoint of the LAA on TEE
D. Emptying velocities are associated with the likelihood of successful cardioversion

QUESTION 5. On the basis of the TEE (**Video 74-10**), is it safe to proceed with DC cardioversion?

A. Yes (no intracardiac thrombus present)
B. No (probable intracardiac thrombus present)

ANSWER 1: B. 0.3 cm² (see **Video 74-5**).

The regurgitant flow can be calculated as follows:

Flow rate = $(r)^2$ × 6.28 × aliasing velocity
= $(0.8 \text{ cm})^2$ × 6.28 × 38 cm per second
= 153 cc per second

ERO = Flow rate/peak mitral regurgitant velocity

= 153 cc per second/510 cm per second
= 0.3 cm²

See *The Echo Manual, 3rd Edition*, discussion of PISA method on page 215.

ANSWER 2: C. The mitral valve leaflets are mildly thickened with some nodular calcification. However, the predominant pathology leading to the regurgitation is not related to the valve structure but rather a dilation of the mitral annulus. Leaflet perforation leads to the presence of valvular regurgitation that passes through a defect in a valve leaflet rather than through the central orifice. Mitral valve prolapse is defined as late (or holosystolic) systolic bowing of one or both the valve leaflets into the left atrium below the valve plane (not present here). Papillary muscle dysfunction is also a mechanism of "functional" regurgitation. Seen here on the apical two-chamber view (**Video 74-5**), the inferior wall contractility is preserved and the regurgitant jet is central rather than the eccentrically directed jet that would be expected with papillary muscle dysfunction.

See *The Echo Manual, 3rd Edition*, discussion of mechanisms of mitral valve regurgitation on pages 210 to 212.

ANSWER 3: D. Several factors present here suggest the presence of severe tricuspid valve regurgitation. These include:

1. Color flow regurgitant jet area ≥30% of the right atrial area
2. Dense continuous wave Doppler signal
3. Annulus dilatation (≥4 cm) or inadequate cusp coaptation
4. Systolic flow reversals in the hepatic vein
5. ERO ≥0.4 cm²
6. Regurgitant volume ≥45 mL

The regurgitant flow can be calculated as follows:

Flow rate = $(r)^2$ × 6.28 × aliasing velocity
= $(0.9 \text{ cm})^2$ × 6.28 × 41 cm per second
= 209 cc per second

ERO = Flow rate/peak MR velocity

= 209 cc per second/300 cm per second
= 0.70 cm²

Regurgitant volume = ERO × regurgitant TVI
= 0.70 cm² × 95 cm
= 66 cc

See *The Echo Manual, 3rd Edition*, discussion of PISA method on page 215, and of tricuspid valve regurgitation on pages 219 and 220.

ANSWER 4: C. Emerging data point toward the utility of quantifying LAA function by assessing LAA emptying flow velocities. Contraction and relaxation of the LAA produce flow velocities that can be detected by pulse wave Doppler at the mouth of the appendage (i.e., at the entry to the main body of the left atrium). The velocities are normally >50 cm per second, but with the loss of sinus rhythm, they become less. Studies have indicated that patients with LAA velocities <20 cm per second are more likely to develop LAA thrombus or systemic thromboembolism (or both) than those with a higher velocity. Also, cardioversion to or maintenance of sinus rhythm is less likely in these patients.[1]

ANSWER 5: A. TEE demonstrates a dilated severely hypokinetic (emptying velocities <20 cm per second) LAA without thrombus. A small amount of pericardial fluid is seen around the appendage. On further imaging, a small round bright mass is seen in this pericardial fluid posterior to the ascending aorta. A small rounded amount of pericardial fat is not uncommonly seen in this location of transesophageal imaging. It is located outside the cardiac chambers and is of no consequence (it is in the oblique sinus in the pericardial sac, not the intracardiac cavity). If the operator is not confident based on the available images, the use of echo contrast (although not usually required) will confirm the extracardiac nature of the "mass" (**Video 74-11**) and that the appendage is free of thrombus (**Video 74-12**).

Reference

1. Antonielli E, Pizzuti A, Pálinkas A, et al. Clinical value of left atrial appendage flow for prediction of long-term sinus rhythm maintenance in patients with nonvalvular atrial fibrillation. *J Am Coll Cardiol.* 2002;39:1443–1449.

CASE 75

Murmur on Routine Physical Examination

A 40-year-old asymptomatic man without prior cardiac history is referred for echocardiography to evaluate a murmur heard on routine physical examination.

QUESTION 1. On the basis of the images (**Videos 75-1 through 75-16** and Figs. 75-1 and 75-2), what is the appropriate next step?

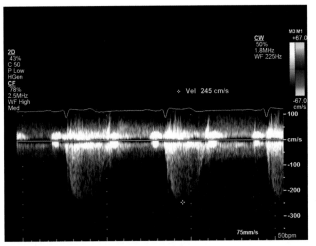

Figure 75-1

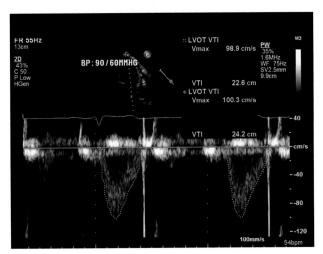

Figure 75-2

A. Reassurance
B. Agitated saline injection
C. Transesophageal echocardiography
D. CT scan

QUESTION 2. Patients with this finding most typically present:

A. In infancy
B. With symptoms in adulthood
C. Without symptoms

QUESTION 3. Presentations of this condition in adulthood may include:

A. Ischemic cardiomyopathy
B. Mitral valve regurgitation
C. Sudden death
D. Ventricular dysrhythmias
E. All of the choices

QUESTION 4. Management in this case should include:

A. Observation
B. Surgical repair

ANSWER 1: D. Transthoracic echocardiography demonstrates normal left and right chamber sizes and function without significant valvular disease. However, there are abnormal flow patterns seen on Doppler imaging. There appears to be aneurysmal dilation of the right coronary artery (**Videos 75-2, 75-4, 75-7, and 75-8**, and Fig. 75-3, yellow arrow). In addition, there are dilated structures (presumably vessels) with continuous flow seen coursing from right to left particularly prominent in the interventricular septum (**Video 75-12** and Fig. 75-3, green arrow) and an abnormal flow profile into the proximal posterior pulmonary artery (**Videos 75-17 and 75-18**). Agitated saline (useful for assessing right-sided chambers, venous flow, and right-left shunts) will not help delineate these structures. Although transesophageal echocardiography may provide better images of the coronary ostia, contrast CT will delineate the coronary anatomy (Figs. 75-4 and 75-5).

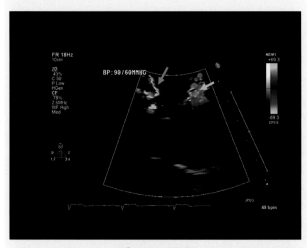

Figure 75-3

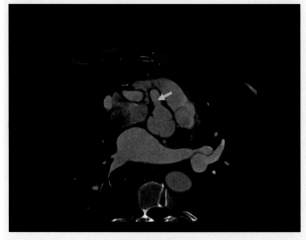

Figure 75-4

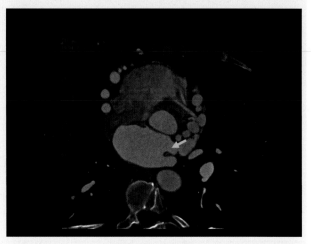

Figure 75-5

ANSWER 2: A. Cardiac CT confirms the echo findings that are highly suspicious for the syndrome of anomalous origin of the left main coronary artery from the pulmonary artery (ALCAPA) with a dilated right coronary artery arising from the right coronary cusp (Fig. 75-4) with extensive collaterals to the left circulation. The left coronary artery arises (Fig. 75-5) from the posterior proximal main pulmonary artery. ALCAPA is a rare congenital anomaly that typically presents in infancy with heart failure, arrhythmias, or sudden death. Far less commonly, patients may present in adulthood with symptoms. Presentation, as in this patient, without symptoms or signs of heart disease is very rare.

ANSWER 3: E. If patients survive childhood, presentation in early adulthood is common. Typical features may include angina, ischemic cardiomyopathy, mitral valve regurgitation, ventricular dysrhythmias, or sudden death.

ANSWER 4: B. The recommendations are that all patients diagnosed with ALCAPA[1,2] even if asymptomatic are referred for surgical repair with implantation of left coronary artery into the ascending aorta. The patient described here was referred for surgery and did well.

References

1. Yang YL, Nanda NC, Wang XF, et al. Echocardiographic diagnosis of anomalous origin of the left coronary artery from the pulmonary artery. *Echocardiography*. 2007;24:405–411.

2. Yau JM, Singh R, Halpern EJ, et al. Anomalous origin of the left coronary artery from the pulmonary artery in adults: a comprehensive review of 151 adult cases and a new diagnosis in a 53-year old woman. *Clin Cardiol*. 2011;34:204–210.

CASE 76

Atypical Chest Pain

A 55-year-old woman presents for the evaluation of atypical chest pain. Previously well, her medical history is only notable for an episode of transient visual loss lasting an hour that occurred 1 month ago. Her examination is unremarkable. She is referred for transthoracic echocardiogram (**Videos 76-1 to 76-6** and Figs. 76-1 to 76-3).

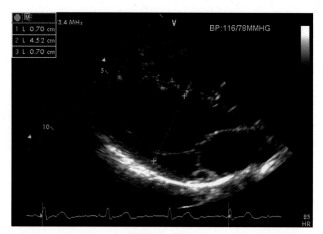

Figure 76-1

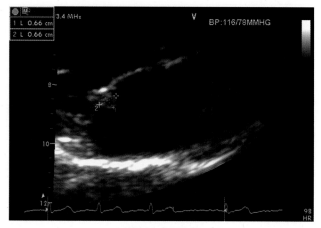

Figure 76-3

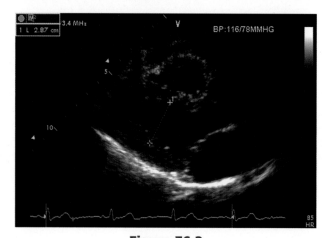

Figure 76-2

QUESTION 1. Assuming normal left ventricular (LV) apical function, what is the calculated left ventricular ejection fraction (LVEF)?

A. 36%

B. 48%

C. 58%

D. 64%

E. 70%

QUESTION 2. The most likely diagnosis is:

A. Vegetation from bacterial endocarditis

B. Myxoma

C. Lambl excrescence

D. Papillary fibroelastoma (PFE)

QUESTION 3. The patient is referred for transesophageal echocardiogram (**Videos 76-7 to 76-10**). To which scallop of the anterior mitral valve leaflet is the mass attached?

    A. A1
    B. A2
    C. A3

QUESTION 4. Which of the following management steps is appropriate?

    A. Surgical resection
    B. No treatment, annual echocardiogram, and clinical follow-up
    C. Systemic anticoagulation, no further follow-up unless symptoms develop

QUESTION 5. Which of the following statements is correct regarding this abnormality?

    A. It is always attached to the valve
    B. It occurs as a single lesion
    C. Its frequency increases in patients with radiation
    D. It becomes malignant if not excised

ANSWER 1: D. LVEF can be calculated from M-mode or two-dimensional images from the midventricular papillary muscle level as follows:

$$LVEF = (\%\Delta D^2) + [(1 - \Delta D^2)\,(\%\Delta L)],$$

where

$$\%\Delta D^2 = \frac{(LV\ end\text{-}diastolic\ dimension)^2 - (LV\ end\text{-}systolic\ dimension)^2}{(LV\ end\text{-}diastolic\ dimension)^2} \times 100\%$$

ΔL is the percentage fractional shortening of the long axis, mainly related to apical contraction: 15% for normal, 5% for hypokinetic apex, 0% for akinetic apex, −5% for dyskinetic apex, and −10% for apical aneurysm.

There are two components in the equation. The first component is actually a percentage change in the LV area or fractional shortening of the square of the LV short axis. If it is assumed that the apical long-axis dimension remains the same during systolic contraction, the percentage area change or fractional area change is equal to the percentage volume change. Because the apical long axis shortens 10% to 15% with systole, an apical correction factor, the second component, is added. This factor varies with the contractility of the apex.

$$Here\ \%\Delta D^2 = \frac{(45)^2 - (29)^2}{(29)^2} = 58\%$$

$$LVEF = 58 + (42 \times 15\%) = 64\%$$

ANSWER 2: D. The transthoracic echocardiogram demonstrates a small mass on the atrial surface of the distal aspect of the anterior mitral valve leaflet. The appearance with a stippled edge with a shimmer or vibration at the tumor–blood interface is characteristic for the appearance of a papillary fibroelastoma (PFE). Typically present on either surface of the aortic or mitral valve, PFEs are benign intracardiac tumors. Myxomas, while rarely associated with atrioventricular valves, are typically attached to the intra-atrial septum typically by a stalk. Lambl excrescences are thinner strand-like structures. Although infective endocarditis is in the differential of a valvular mass in the absence of systemic symptoms of infection, a bacterial vegetation is unlikely to be the cause in this case.

ANSWER 3: B. Each of the mitral valve leaflets can be divided in three scallops (1) lateral, (2) middle, and (3) medial. Identification of which scallop is involved by the pathology is best performed in a two-step process by transesophageal echocardiography (TEE). *Step 1*: at 0° with a multiplane TEE, one can easily identify whether

the involved leaflet is anterior, posterior, or bileaflet. Here on **Video 76-7**, the mass clearly is attached to the anterior leaflet. However, at 0°, because you are cutting across the valve from anterior to posterior, it is difficult to determine which part of the leaflet is involved. To decide which of the three scallops is affected, the probe needs to be rotated to about 60° to 75° (the commissural view; Video 7-25). Here all three scallops are seen: (1) lateral scallop (closest to left atrial appendage), (2) the middle scallop, and (3) the medial scallop. Here from **Video 76-8**, it is clear that the mass is attached to the middle (A2) scallop. Three-dimensional echo imaging of the atrial surface of the mitral valve (**Video 76-11**) also clearly demonstrates a mass attached to the middle scallop of the anterior leaflet (Fig. 76-4).

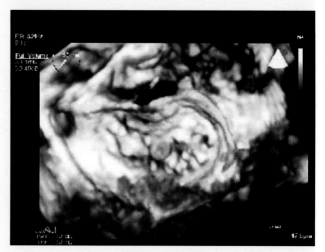

Figure 76-4

See *The Echo Manual, 3rd Edition,* **Figures 21-11 and 21-12 on pages 374 and 375, respectively.**

ANSWER 4: A. PFEs are benign tumors—typically about 10 mm in size—that have a central avascular collagenous core of dense connective tissue covered with hyperplastic endocardial cells. If found and the patient has a history of unexplained thromboembolic event (as in this case), the management is surgical removal, almost always with valve-sparing surgery. If a left-sided PFE is found incidentally, options include surgery or anticoagulation (typically with antiplatelet therapy) with close follow-up.

ANSWER 5: C. A PFE may occur when there is endocardial damage as in patients with hypertrophic cardiomyopathy and radiation. Occasionally in this setting we see multiple PFEs.[1–3]

References

1. Klarich KW, Enriquez-Sarano M, Gura GM, et al. Papillary fibroelastoma: echocardiographic characteristics for diagnosis and pathologic correlation. *J Am Coll Cardiol.* 1997;30:785.

2. Gowda RM, Khan IA, Nair CK, et al. Cardiac papillary fibroelastoma: a comprehensive analysis of 725 cases. *Am Heart J.* 2003;146:404.

3. Ngaage DL, Mullany CJ, Daly RC, et al. Surgical treatment of cardiac papillary fibroelastoma: a single center experience with eighty-eight patients. *Ann Thorac Surg.* 2005;80:1712–1718.

CASE 77

Dilated Cardiomyopathy

A 32-year-old male patient with dilated cardiomyopathy returns for reevaluation (see **Videos 77-1 through 77-7** and Figs. 77-1 through 77-9).

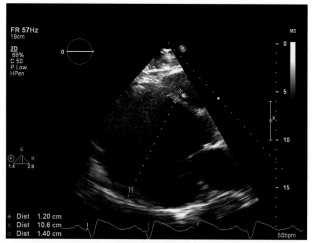

Figure 77-1

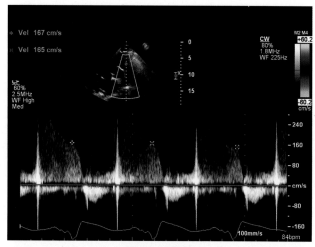

Figure 77-3

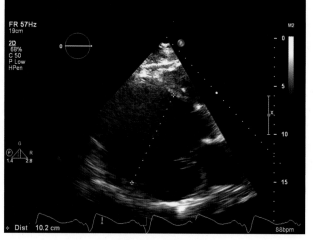

Figure 77-2

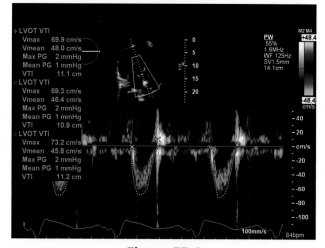

Figure 77-4

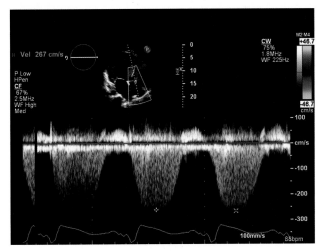

Figure 77-5

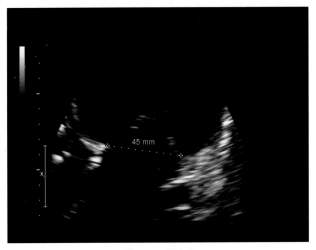

Figure 77-8

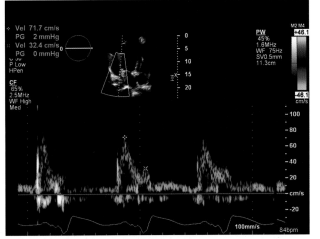

Figure 77-6

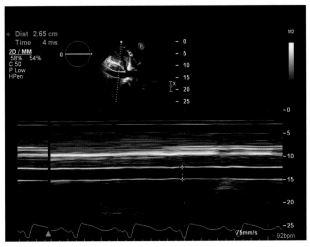

Figure 77-9

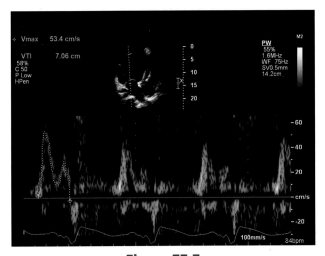

Figure 77-7

QUESTION 1. The patient's left ventricular ejection fraction (LVEF) is:

A. <5%

B. 5% to 15%

C. 16% to 25%

D. 26% to 35%

E. 36% to 45%

QUESTION 2. The patient's Doppler-derived cardiac output based on a left ventricular outflow tract (LVOT) diameter of 26 mm is:

    A. 2.4 L per minute
    B. 4.9 L per minute
    C. 5.5 L per minute
    D. 6.2 L per minute
    E. 6.8 L per minute

QUESTION 3. Which of the following statements regarding the sphericity index (see Fig. 77-10) is correct?

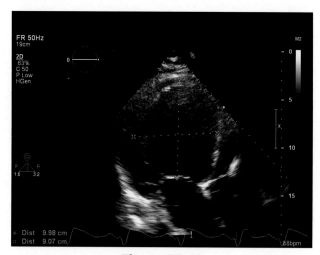

Figure 77-10

    A. Sphericity index is an important parameter to determine diastolic function of left ventricle
    B. Sphericity index correlates with severity of MR better than the mitral tenting area
    C. Sphericity index is prognostic in patients after acute myocardial infarction
    D. Surgical obliteration of dysfunctional apex improves the sphericity index in ischemic cardiomyopathy

QUESTION 4. The calculated mitral valve regurgitant fraction based on the volumetric method is:

    A. 37%
    B. 43%
    C. 49%
    D. 54%
    E. 60%

QUESTION 5. Doppler estimates of the pulmonary artery (PA) (systolic/diastolic) pressures are:

    A. 29/12 mm Hg
    B. 39/22 mm Hg
    C. 39/32 mm Hg
    D. 49/32 mm Hg
    E. 49/43 mm Hg

QUESTION 6. On the basis of the echocardiographic images, a next step in investigation or management might include:

    A. Agitated saline intravenous infusion
    B. Myocardial echo contrast intravenous infusion
    C. Initiation of warfarin anticoagulation to goal International Normalized Ratio (INR) of 2 to 3
    D. Nothing further required

ANSWER 1: B. Visually, there is marked global severe hypokinesis with a visual ejection fraction of 10% or less. This is supported by the calculated ejection fraction by the simple Quinone's method where $LVEF = (EDd^2 - ESd^2)/EDd^2$

Here $LVEF = (106^2 - 102^2)/106^2 = 0.07 = 7\%$

See *The Echo Manual, 3rd Edition*, page 116.

ANSWER 2: B. Stroke volume (SV) is calculated from the LVOT as a product of the LVOT area (LVOT diameter × 0.785) and the LVOT time velocity integral (VTI).

Here $SV = (2.6 \text{ cm})^2 \times 0.785 \times 11 \text{ cm} = 58 \text{ ml}$ at a heart rate of 84 bpm = 4.9 L per minute

See *The Echo Manual, 3rd Edition*, Figure 4-16 on page 71.

ANSWER 3: C. End-diastolic sphericity index is calculated as the ratio of the minor to the long (or major) axis of the left ventricle at end diastole and is an easy marker of abnormal left ventricular remodeling. The more spherical the ventricle, the worse the patient's outcome following myocardial infarction.

ANSWER 4: E. Mitral regurgitant volume is calculated by subtracting the LVOT stroke volume (here 58 ml, calculated in answer to Question 2) from the mitral inflow SV.

The mitral inflow SV is calculated using similar steps to the calculation of the LVOT SV.

Mitral inflow SV = product of the mitral valve area (mitral annulus diameter × 0.785) and the mitral inflow VTI.

Here mitral inflow $SV = (4.5 \text{ cm})^2 \times 7.1 \text{ cm} = 144 \text{ ml}$

Mitral regurgitant volume = Mitral inflow SV − LVOT SV = 144 − 58 = 86 ml

Mitral valve regurgitant fraction = Regurgitant volume/mitral inflow SV = 86/144 = 60% (which is severe).

ANSWER 5: D. PA pressures may be calculated based on data derived from the tricuspid (TR) and pulmonary regurgitant (PR) pulse-wave Doppler signals and an estimate of right atrial pressure (RAP). Here the inferior vena cava is enlarged (>25 mm) with no change in size with inspiration, suggesting the RAP is very high (20 mm Hg).

Right ventricular systolic pressure = PA systolic pressure = $4(\text{peak TR vel})^2 + RAP = 4(2.7)^2 + RAP = 49$ mm Hg

PA diastolic pressure $= 4(\text{end PR vel})^2 + RAP = 4(1.7)^2 + RAP = 32$ mm Hg

PA pressures $= 49/32$ mm Hg

ANSWER 6: B. Echo apical images demonstrate a severely hypokinetic/akinetic apex with an indistinct shadow in the apical region on all views. Although it is not definitive for an apical thrombus (and hence insufficient to warrant anticoagulation) and may represent an artifact, the available images are unable to exclude a thrombus. To provide left ventricular opacification, a myocardial echo contrast agent is required. After administration (see **Videos 77-8 through 77-10**), there was complete opacification of the apex indicating indeed the "mass" seen on the 2D images is an artifact and no thrombus is present.

CASE 78

Three Months of Progressive Exertional Dyspnea

A 59-year-old man is referred for transthoracic echocardiogram. His history is notable for bioprosthetic mitral and aortic valve replacements performed elsewhere 6 years before after an episode of infective endocarditis. He presents now with 3 months of progressive exertional dyspnea (**Videos 78-1 to 78-5** and Figs. 78-1 and 78-2).

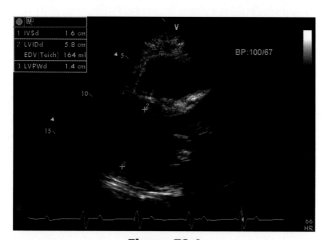

Figure 78-1

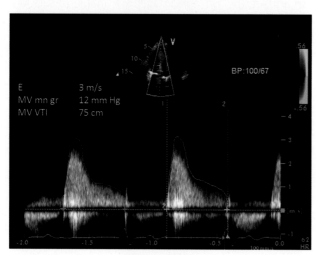

Figure 78-2

QUESTION 1. On the basis of the options in Figure 78-3, calculate the pressure halftime of the mitral bioprosthesis.

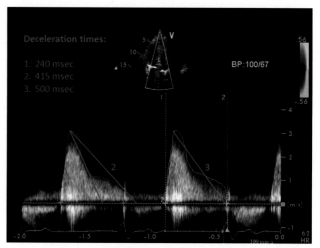

Figure 78-3

A. 70 milliseconds

B. 120 milliseconds

C. 145 milliseconds

QUESTION 2. There appears to be echocardiographic evidence of:

A. Significant mitral valve prosthetic obstruction

B. Significant mitral valve prosthetic regurgitation

C. Normal mitral valve prosthetic function

QUESTION 3. On the basis of review of **Videos 78-6 to 78-9** and Figures 78-4 to 78-7, the estimated right atrial pressure is:

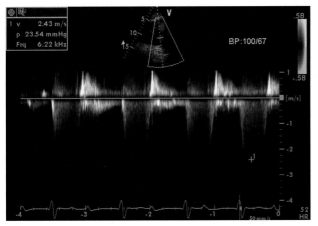

Figure 78-4

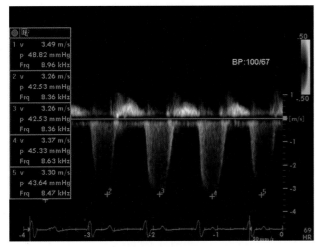

Figure 78-5

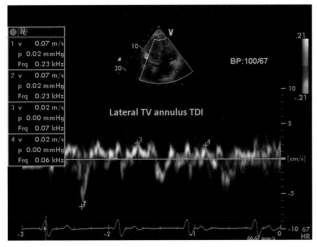

Figure 78-6

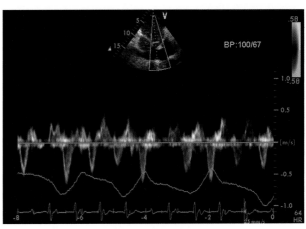

Figure 78-7

A. 3 mm Hg
B. 10 mm Hg
C. 20 mm Hg

QUESTION 4. The likely explanation for the hepatic vein flow patterns seen on Figure 78-7 is:

A. Severe tricuspid valve regurgitation
B. Severe right ventricular dysfunction
C. Constriction

QUESTION 5. The next step in the assessment of this patient's dyspnea should include:

A. Hemodynamic catheterization
B. Cardiac magnetic resonance scan
C. Transesophageal echocardiogram
D. Left ventriculogram

QUESTION 6. Following review of **Videos 78-10 to 78-12** and Figure 78-8, there is evidence of two regurgitant jets (one prosthetic and one periprosthetic). To quantitate the degree of mitral valve regurgitation (MR) by the PISA technique, how should one handle the two PISA radii (Figs. 78-9 to 78-11)? The combined radius is equal to:

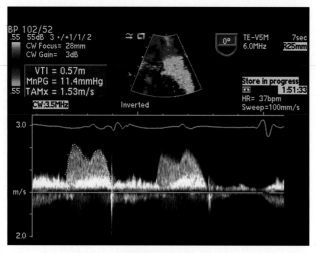

Figure 78-8

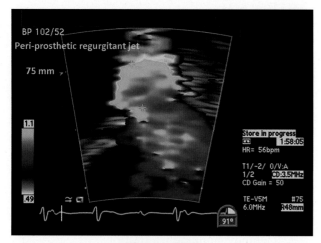

Figure 78-9

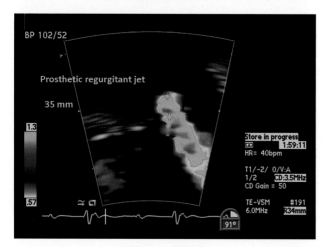

Figure 78-10

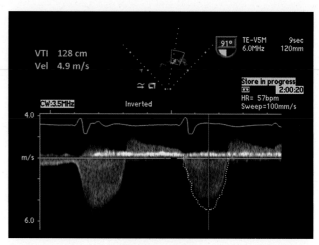

Figure 78-11

A. 0.75 + 0.35

B. $(0.75)^2 + (0.35)^2$

C. $(0.75 + 0.35)/2$

D. $\sqrt{[(0.75)^2 + (0.35)^2]}$

E. Unable to use PISA if two jets

QUESTION 7. The combined effective regurgitant orifice (ERO) by the PISA method is:

A. 0.4 cm^2

B. 0.5 cm^2

C. 0.6 cm^2

D. 0.7 cm^2

QUESTION 8. The appropriate treatment is:

A. Medical management

B. Percutaneous mitral valve periprosthetic leak closure

C. Surgical re-replacement of the mitral prosthesis and tricuspid valve repair

D. Surgical re-replacement of the mitral prosthesis

ANSWER 1: A. The pressure halftime is calculated as 0.29 times the deceleration time. The appropriate deceleration time is indicated in number 1, which is the time interval from the peak of the early filling velocity (E) to its extrapolation to the baseline.

Here pressure halftime = 240 × 0.29 = 70 milliseconds.

ANSWER 2: B. There is evidence of increased flow velocities across the mitral valve with a super evaluation in early (E) peak velocity at 3 m per second and an elevated mean gradient at 12 mm Hg. Although flow velocities and mean gradient may be elevated in both prosthetic obstruction and regurgitation, the pressure halftime is prolonged in the former but not in the latter. Here a normal pressure halftime suggests a regurgitant rather than an obstructive etiology. This is despite the absence of an obvious regurgitant jet on color Doppler, likely obscured by annular shadowing.

See The Echo Manual, 3rd Edition, pages 229 and 230.

ANSWER 3: C. An echocardiographic estimate of right atrial pressure can be based on the size and collapsibility of the inferior vena cava and the information on forward flow patterns in the hepatic veins. Seen here the inferior vena cava is dilated and does not collapse, and the only forward flow in the hepatic veins is in diastole. These are all features suggestive of a high right atrial pressure.

ANSWER 4: B. Pulsed wave Doppler of the hepatic veins demonstrates evidence of systolic flow reversals. There is diastolic forward flow. In general, systolic flow reversals in the hepatic veins may be related to severe tricuspid valve regurgitation (which tends to be late peaking) or right heart failure (which tends to be early peaking). Color Doppler imaging (**Videos 78-6 and 78-7**) fails to show evidence of more than mild tricuspid valve regurgitation, and the continuous wave Doppler signal is weak, incomplete, and round

(Figs. 78-7 and 78-8), suggesting mild regurgitation. However, visually the right ventricle has severe decrease in contractility with a peak systolic annular velocity of only 2 cm per second (severely reduced, normal 12 cm per second or higher)[1]. These features and the fact that the systolic reversals tend to be early peaking suggest right ventricular dysfunction rather than tricuspid valve regurgitation as the mechanism. The classic feature of constrictive hemodynamics and expiratory diastolic flow reversals is not seen here (see Case 16).

ANSWER 5: C. As discussed in answers to Question 2, the transthoracic echocardiogram shows evidence of mitral bioprosthesis dysfunction, most likely related to MR. The best test to better characterize mitral valvular function/dysfunction is a transesophageal echocardiogram.

ANSWER 6: D. The combined radius of multiple different regurgitant jets is equal to the square root of the sum of the individual radii squared. In this case, the combined radius = 0.83.

ANSWER 7: B. The regurgitant flow can be calculated as follows:

Flow rate = $(r)^2$ × 6.28 × aliasing velocity
= $(0.83 \text{ cm})^2$ × 6.28 × 57 cm per second
= 246 cc per second

ERO = Flow rate/peak MR velocity

= 246 cc per second/490 cm per second
= 0.5 cm^2

See The Echo Manual, 3rd Edition, discussion of PISA method on page 215.

ANSWER 8: D. There is evidence of severe symptomatic MR. Percutaneous perivalvular leak closure would fail to address the significant prosthetic regurgitation. There is little evidence of tricuspid valve regurgitation.

Reference

1. Rudski LG, Lai WW, Afilalo J, et al. Guidelines for the echocardiographic assessment of the right heart in adults: a report from the American Society of Echocardiography endorsed by the European Association of Echocardiography, a registered branch of the European Society of Cardiology, and the Canadian Society of Echocardiography. J Am Soc Echocardiogr. 2010;23:685–713.

CASE 79

Exertional Dsypnea following Bypass Grafting

A 67-year-old man who presents with stable functional class II exertional dyspnea. He denies angina, orthopnea, or edema. He has a history of four-vessel coronary artery bypass grafting 2 years before. He was referred for transthoracic echocardiography.

QUESTION 1. On transthoracic imaging (**Video 79-1** and Figs. 79-1 and 79-2), the left ventricle is:

A. Normal in size with left ventricular ejection fraction (LVEF) 55% to 60%
B. Moderately dilated with LVEF 35%
C. Severely dilated with LVEF 35%
D. Severely dilated with LVEF 25%
E. Moderately dilated with LVEF 25%

QUESTION 2. The inferior wall:

A. Has normal contractile function
B. Is hypokinetic
C. Is akinetic
D. Is dyskinetic

QUESTION 3. After 12 months, Mr. CD returns for a repeat echocardiogram to reassess LVEF and response to medical therapy. He has no new symptoms. See **Video 79-2.** Figure 79-3 shows a still frame of the apical two-chamber view. The structure identified by the triangle is:

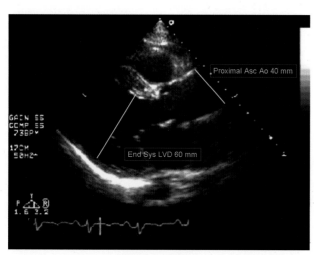

Figure 79-1

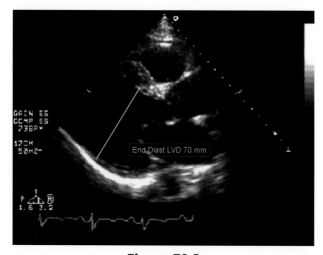

Figure 79-2

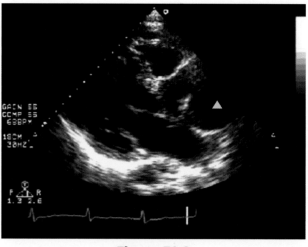

Figure 79-3

252

A. Right main pulmonary artery
B. Ascending thoracic aorta
C. Right atrium
D. Dilated left atrial appendage
E. Esophageal hernia

A. Dilated left lower pulmonary vein
B. Inferior vena cava
C. Dilated coronary sinus
D. Left atrial appendage
E. Aneurysm on the left circumflex graft

QUESTION 4. The structure identified by the circle (Fig. 79-4) is:

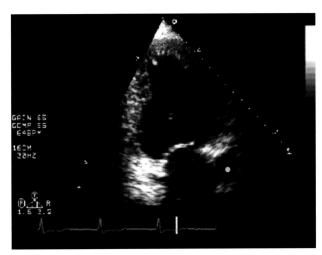

Figure 79-4

ANSWER 1: D. The left ventricle is severely dilated with an LVEF 25%. Quantification of cardiac chambers and assessment of ventricular systolic function are essential parts of all echocardiography examinations. The left ventricular end-diastolic (LVEDD) and end-systolic (LVESD) dimensions are measured at the level of the mitral valve leaflet tips as the largest and smallest dimensions, respectively. Satisfactory delineation of the endocardial border is critical for reliable chamber quantification. The normal range for LVEDD for men is 42 to 59 mm. A left ventricle (LV) is severely dilated when the LVEDD is ≥69 mm.

See *The Echo Manual, 3rd Edition*, Appendix 3 on page 403.

LVEF can be calculated from the LVEDD and LVESD. In this case, the LVEDD is 70 mm and the LVESD 60 mm. The LVEF is calculated as follows:

$$LVEF = [LVED\ D^2 - LVES\ D^2] / LVED\ D^2$$

This equation actually calculates the area change because the dimensions are squared. Assuming that the long axis of the left ventricle remains the same with systolic contraction, which is not always the case, the fractional area change is same as the volumetric change. For this patient with no significant contractile apical function, it is reasonable to use this area change calculation as a volume change to calculate ejection fraction. In cases with apical contractility, a correction fraction is used. Because LVEDD^2 is 4900 and LVESD^2 is 3600, the LVEF is 27%. The normal range for LVEF for men is ≥55%. A LVEF is severely reduced when <30%.

See *The Echo Manual, 3rd Edition*, ejection fraction on pages 115 and 116.

ANSWER 2: C. The inferior wall is akinetic. Normally, LV free wall thickness increases >40% during systole. In normal people, the percentage of thickening of the ventricular septum is somewhat less than that of the free wall of the LV. Hypokinesis is defined as systolic wall thickening <30%, and akinesis is defined as systolic wall thickening <10%. Dyskinesis is defined as a myocardial segment moving outward during systole, usually in association with systolic wall thinning.

See *The Echo Manual, 3rd Edition*, page 119 and Figure 7-14 on page 118.

ANSWER 3: B. The structure identified by the triangle is the ascending thoracic aorta. The parasternal long-axis image demonstrates a dilated ascending aorta with an apparent aneurysm or pseudoaneurysm. When compared with the comparative image from the transthoracic study 12 months before, there has been a striking interim change. Given the history of prior coronary artery bypass grafting 3 years before and an already dilated ascending aorta (40 mm) on the prior echo, the finding is most consistent with a chronic type A aortic dissection with a secondary ascending aortic aneurysm. The major identified risk factors for type A aortic dissection are aortic disease (e.g., Marfan syndrome or arteriopathy associated with bicuspid aortic valve), systemic hypertension, and prior cardiac surgery. Dissections occurring related to prior surgery are typically more stable, frequently presenting with few or no symptoms and occurring on average 3 to 4 years postoperatively. Suggested etiologies include injury at the time of cross-clamp, graft sites, and associated factors of long-standing systemic hypertension and/or atherosclerosis of the aorta. Patients identified to have a chronic type A aortic dissection should be referred for open surgical repair.

Figure 79-5 demonstrates type A thoracic aortic dissection seen on thoracic CT angiography, and Figure 79-6 demonstrates site of proximal dissection seen on intraoperative transesophageal echocardiography.[1,2]

See *The Echo Manual, 3rd Edition*, Figure 19-6 on page 325.

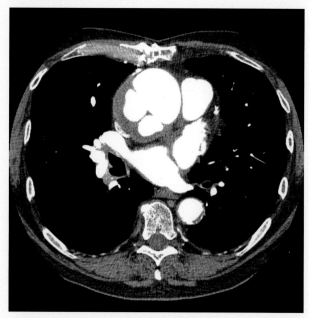

Figure 79-5

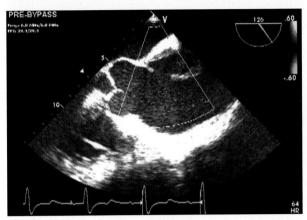

Figure 79-6

ANSWER 4: D. The structure identified by the circle is the left atrial appendage. The image demonstrates a dilated left atrial appendage in the setting of a dilated left atrium, likely reflecting a chronic elevation in left atrial pressures. The left atrial appendage may also be visualized from transthoracic echocardiography from parasternal short-axis views at the base and is typically only seen well in patients with dilated appendages. To confidently exclude appendage thrombus, a trans-esophageal study is required.

References

1. Hagl C, Ergin MA, Galla JD, et al. Delayed chronic type A dissection following CABG: implications for evolving techniques of revascularization. *J Card Surg*. 2000;15:362–367.

2. Hirose H, Svensson LG, Lytle BW, et al. Aortic dissection after previous cardiovascular surgery. *Ann Thorac Surg*. 2004;78:2099–2105.

CASE 80

Exertional Shortness of Breath with History of Lymphoma

A 38-year-old man presents with exertional shortness of breath. His medical history is significant for lymphoma when a teenager. He remains in remission.

On examination, his heart rate is 75 beats per minute, blood pressure 116/70 mm Hg, and body mass 40 kg per m². Left ventricular apical impulse is nondisplaced. There is a 2/6 systolic ejection murmur and a third heart sound. There is a trace pedal edema (**Videos 80-1 to 80-7** and Figs. 80-1 to 80-6).

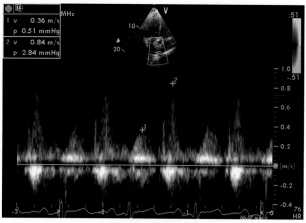

Figure 80-1

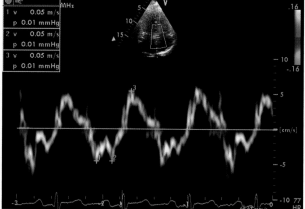

Figure 80-2

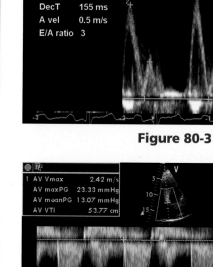

Figure 80-3

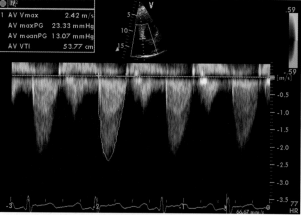

Figure 80-4

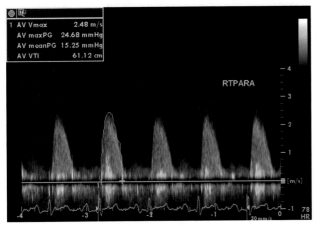

Figure 80-5

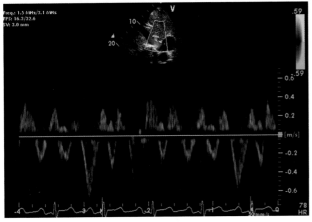

Figure 80-6

QUESTION 1. Left ventricular diastolic function is:

A. Normal
B. Grade 1 (delayed relaxation) dysfunction
C. Grade 2 (pseudonormal) dysfunction
D. Grade 3 (restrictive) dysfunction

QUESTION 2. Diastolic flow reversal in hepatic vein occurs predominantly during which of respiratory phase?

A. Inspiration
B. Expiration
C. Apnea

QUESTION 3. Right atrial (RA) pressure based on hepatic vein velocity (Fig. 80-6) is:

A. Normal
B. Increased
C. Decreased
D. Not able to be determined

QUESTION 4. On the basis of the M-mode (Fig. 80-7) and tissue Doppler (Fig. 80-8) assessment of the tricuspid annulus, right ventricular longitudinal systolic function is:

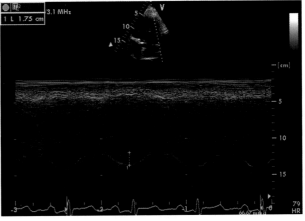

Figure 80-7

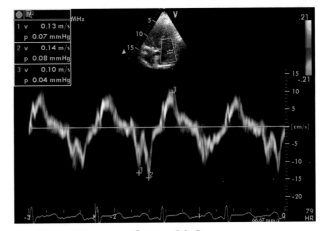

Figure 80-8

A. Normal
B. Reduced

QUESTION 5. Which of the following therapies most likely explains the constellation of echocardiographic findings?

A. Anthracyclines
B. Thoracic radiation
C. Rituximab
D. Imatinib

ANSWER 1: D. The constellation of Doppler findings is consistent with a significant elevation in left atrial pressure and grade 3, restrictive diastolic filling. Pulmonary vein flow (Fig. 80-1) demonstrates a reduction in systolic forward flow velocity because of a combination of higher left atrial pressure and a reduction in left atrial compliance. There is a marked reduction in myocardial relaxation characterized by very low diastolic tissue velocities with a medial annulus E' of 5 cm per second (Fig. 80-2). The high left atrial pressure results in a high initial transmitral gradient (high E velocity, Fig. 80-3) with an associated short deceleration time caused by the rapid equalization of left atrial and ventricular pressures. The high E/A ratio of 3 and the high E/e' ratio of 30 further underscore the marked diastolic dysfunction grade.

ANSWER 2: A. With inspiration, forward flow velocity in hepatic vein increases, and with expiration, it decreases. Predominant diastolic flow reversal which increases with inspiration is characteristic for myocardial disease This is in contrast to diastolic flow reversals that increase with expiration in constriction.

ANSWER 3: B. Systolic forward velocity is lower than diastolic forward velocity indicating increased RA pressure.

ANSWER 4: B. Unlike the left ventricle, the predominance of myocardial fibers in the lateral wall of the right ventricle is in the longitudinal plane. Therefore, there is a greater contribution of longitudinal contractility to overall ventricular function on the right side. Quantification of longitudinal right ventricular motion can be performed through measurement of the degree of the tricuspid annular plane systolic excursion (TAPSE) by M-mode or the peak systolic velocity of the tricuspid annulus assessed by tissue Doppler. Both the M-mode and systolic velocities are reduced from what would be expected in 38-year-old patient (TAPSE ≥22 mm and systolic velocity ≥14 cm per second).[1]

ANSWER 5: B. Manifestations of radiation-induced cardiac disease include myocardial fibrosis leading to diastolic dysfunction and heart failure and fibrotic changes leading to valvular dysfunction. Other manifestations not seen in this case include coronary, pericardial, and conduction system disease. Anthracycline chemotherapy–induced cardiac disease is typically a systolic dysfunction. No long-term cardiac toxicity has been reported with rituximab therapy. Although uncommon, left ventricular systolic dysfunction has occurred in response to imatinib chemotherapy.

Radiation-induced valvular disease occurs less frequently in the current era than in the past in large part to better anatomical targeting of the radiotherapy and the use of cardiac shielding. However, valvular disease related to mediastinal radiation is slowly progressive and commonly may not present clinically for decades. Hence, serial clinical assessment is required long term in patients who have received thoracic, particularly left-sided or mediastinal, radiotherapy. Left-sided valves appear to be more commonly affected, probably because of the concomitant increased hemodynamic stresses of higher left-sided pressures with the typical characteristic of a thickened proximal anterior portions of valves (e.g., anterior more commonly than posterior mitral valve leaflet) more likely to be injured as radiotherapy is typically given from an anterior portal.[2–4]

References

1. Innelli P, Esposito R, Olibet M, et al. The impact of ageing on right ventricular longitudinal function in healthy subjects: a pulsed tissue Doppler study. *Eur J Echocardigr.* 2009:10;491–498.

2. Heidenreich PA, Hancock SL, Lee BK, et al. Asymptomatic cardiac disease following mediastinal irradiation. *J Am Coll Cardiol.* 2003;42:743–749.

3. Wethal T, Lund MB, Edvardsen T, et al. Valvular dysfunction and left ventricular changes in Hodgkin's lymphoma survivors. A longitudinal study. *Br J Cancer.* 2009;101:575–581.

4. Galper SL, Yu JB, Mauch PM, et al. Clinically significant cardiac disease in patients with Hodgkin lymphoma treated with mediastinal irradiation. *Blood.* 2011;117:412–418.

CASE 81

Severe Chronic Obstructive Pulmonary Disease

A 76-year-old woman with a medical history of severe chronic obstructive pulmonary disease (forced expiratory volume in one minute (FEV1) 1.0 L), paroxysmal atrial fibrillation, diabetes mellitus, and chronic kidney disease (glomerular filtration rate 25 cc/min/m²) is diagnosed with lung cancer. She has a history of chest pain and limiting exertional dyspnea at 100 feet. Her 12-lead ECG is normal.

QUESTION 1. With regard to preoperative evaluation, which of the following tests is most appropriate?

A. Adenosine sestamibi

B. Treadmill exercise stress ECG

C. Treadmill exercise stress echocardiography

D. Dobutamine-atropine stress echocardiography

E. Any of these tests are appropriate

F. All of these tests are inappropriate

QUESTION 2. Based on the review of images (**Videos 81-1 and 81-2**, Figures 81-1 to 81-3), the patient's mitral inflow pattern is consistent with:

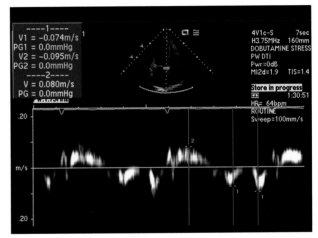

Figure 81-2

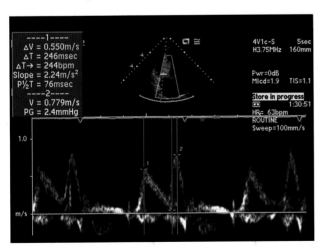

Figure 81-1

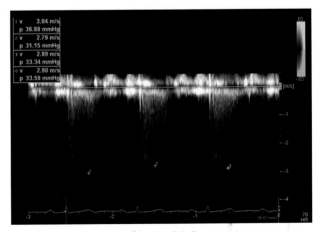

Figure 81-3

A. Normal diastolic function
B. Grade 1 (mild) diastolic dysfunction
C. Grade 2 (moderate) diastolic dysfunction
D. Grade 3 (severe) diastolic dysfunction

QUESTION 3. In a patient with severe chronic obstructive pulmonary disease and a tricuspid regurgitant velocity of 3 m per second, the use of echo contrast is contraindicated for endocardial definition.

A. True
B. False

QUESTION 4. Based on the review of the images (**Videos 81-3 to 81-6***), which of the following is correct?

*All images are displayed in quad format with rest images (**top left**), low dose (**top right**), prepeak stress (**lower left**), and peak stress (**lower right**). Please note also that the apical four-chamber views are displayed in the Mayo format with the left ventricle on the left and the right ventricle on the right.

A. Findings are indeterminate
B. There is evidence of resting ischemia/infarction
C. There is evidence of inducible ischemia
D. There is no evidence to suggest coronary disease

QUESTION 5. One hour after the test, the patient is seen by her physician. She is confused and remembers little of the events of the day. Apart from the altered mental status, examination is normal. The likely cause for the patient's confusion is:

A. Echo contrast received during the stress study
B. Dobutamine received during the stress study
C. Atropine received during the stress study
D. An embolic event occurring after an episode of paroxysmal atrial fibrillation during dobutamine infusion
E. Anoxia triggered by dobutamine-induced bronchospasm

ANSWER 1: D. The patient has a limited exercise capacity with multiple comorbidities and is being considered for a surgical procedure that comes with an intermediate risk for a cardiovascular event. The scenario is further complicated by the history of chest pain, which in an elderly woman with diabetes, chronic kidney disease, and a presumed smoking history comes with an increased pretest probability for coronary disease. Although in general, for patients of moderate risk being considered for intermediate risk surgery pretreatment with a β-blocker, without stress evaluation, is reasonable, this approach comes with increased risk of harm, given the severity of the patient's obstructive lung disease. Hence, consideration of a stress evaluation is appropriate; however, given the exercise limitation, exercise as a stress is inappropriate. This leaves the options of an adenosine perfusion study or dobutamine-atropine stress echocardiography. Given the potential for adenosine to exacerbate bronchoconstriction, dobutamine-atropine stress echocardiography is preferred here.[1]

ANSWER 2: B. The mitral inflow pattern demonstrates an early (E) diastolic wave velocity that is less than the later atrial (A) wave with a prolonged deceleration time. A pattern consistent with a "delayed relaxation," Grade 1 diastolic dysfunction pattern. The E/e' ratio of 0.6/0.07 (i.e., 8.6 cm per second) is also consistent with a Grade 1 pattern with low left ventricular filling pressures.

ANSWER 3: B. Although there are theoretical safety concerns of microbubble administration to patients with pulmonary hypertension, extensive clinical data have failed to demonstrate an increased predisposition to adverse events of this cohort. Certainly, data would indicate that patients with upper normal and modest elevations of right ventricular systolic pressure (tricuspid regurgitant velocity of 3 m per second) have no additional risk and hence echo contrast should not be avoided.[2,3]

ANSWER 4: C. Two-dimensional images aided by the use of echo contrast at rest show normal left ventricular regional and global contractility. With prepeak and particularly peak stress, there is midseptal hypokinesis and apical akinesis. Findings consistent with left anterior distribution coronary ischemia.

ANSWER 5: C. Atropine administration is commonly required as an adjunct to dobutamine to achieve an adequate chronotropic stress response. However, atropine also increases the risk of adverse systemic effects. Particularly in elderly patients, atropine-related cerebral toxicity is an important complication to recognize with confusion occurring within the minutes to hours after atropine administration. The parasympathomimetic physostigmine may be both diagnostic and therapeutic in this situation. Alternatively, the patient may be monitored while the effects of atropine wear off over a number of hours. The adverse effects of the sympathomimetic, dobutamine include palpitations, rhythm disturbances (including atrial fibrillation), headaches, nausea, and dysuria. Echo contrast, although generally very well tolerated, has been associated with back pain. The likelihood of a thromboembolic event occurring with a brief episode of atrial fibrillation is extremely low, but regardless, would present with focal neurologic findings rather than generalized confusion. Dobutamine is a β-agonist and hence is safe in obstructive lung disease as if will tend toward bronchodilatation rather than bronchoconstriction.

References

1. ACCF/ASE/AHA/ASNC/HFSA/HRS/SCAI/SCCM/SCCT/SCMR 2011 appropriate use criteria for echocardiography. A Report of the American College of Cardiology Foundation Appropriate Use Criteria Task Force, American Society of Echocardiography, American Heart Association, American Society of Nuclear Cardiology, Heart Failure Society of America, Heart Rhythm Society, Society for Cardiovascular Angiography and Interventions, Society of Critical Care Medicine, Society of Cardiovascular Computed Tomography, Society for Cardiovascular Magnetic Resonance American College of Chest Physicians. *J Am Soc Echocardiogr.* 2011;24:229–267.

2. Mulvagh SL, Rakowski H, Vannan MA, et al. American Society of Echocardiography Consensus Statement on the Clinical Applications of Ultrasonic Contrast Agents in Echocardiography. *J Am Soc Echocardiogr.* 2008;21(11):1179–1201.

3. Abdelmoneim SS, Bernier M, Scott CG, et al. Safety of contrast agent use during stress echocardiography in patients with elevated right ventricular systolic pressure: a cohort study. *Circ Cardiovasc Imaging.* 2010;3(3):240–248.

4. Wuthiwaropas P, Wiste JA, McCully RB, et al. Neuropsychiatric symptoms during 24 hours after dobutamine-atropine stress testing: a prospective study in 1,006 patients. *J Am Soc Echocardiogr.* 2011;21(11):367–373.

CASE 82

Systolic and Diastolic Murmurs

A 65-year-old man presents for an echocardiogram to evaluate systolic and diastolic murmurs (see Videos 82-1 to 82-6 and Figs. 82-1 to 82-3).

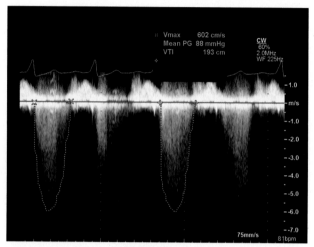

Figure 82-1

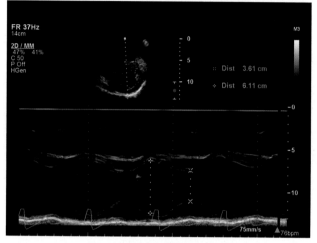

Figure 82-3

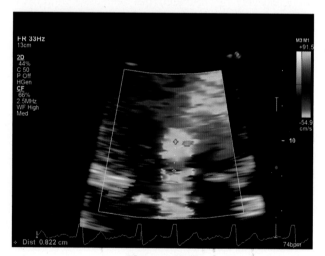

Figure 82-2

QUESTION 1. By the PISA method, what is the calculated severity of the mitral valve regurgitation (MR)?

A. (Grade 1/4) Mild

B. (Grade 2/4) Mild to moderate

C. (Grade 3/4) Moderate to severe

D. (Grade 4/4) Severe

QUESTION 2. Which of the following parameters is useful for assessing the severity of the aortic valve regurgitation (AR) in this setting?

A. The left ventricular (LV) size

B. The continuity/stroke volume method

C. The ratio of the AR jet width the left ventricular outflow tract diameter

D. The E-wave velocity

QUESTION 3. What is the severity of the aortic valve regurgitation (see **Videos 82-3, 82-4, 82-6** and Figs. 82-4 to 82-7)?

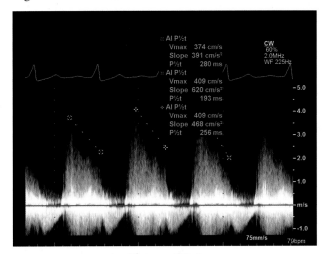

Figure 82-4

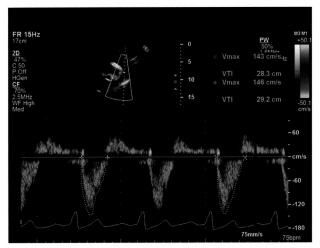

Figure 82-5

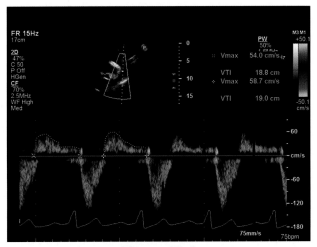

Figure 82-6

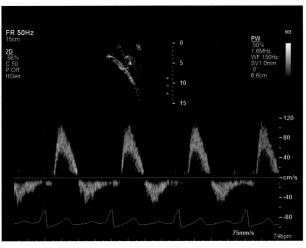

Figure 82-7

A. Mild
B. Moderate
C. Severe

QUESTION 4. Which of the following lesions/findings may give rise to holodiastolic flow reversals in the descending thoracic aorta?

A. Blalock–Taussig (B-T) shunt
B. Severe aortic valve regurgitation
C. Patent ductus arteriosus (PDA)
D. Aortic coarctation
E. Descending thoracic aortic aneurysm

QUESTION 5. The most likely etiology of the other abnormal finding on the images further illustrated on **Videos 82-7 to 82-9** is (note it does not opacify after administration of agitated saline by either the left or right extremity):

A. Pericardial cyst
B. Paraganglioma
C. Loculated pleural effusion

QUESTION 6. Complications of a coronary aneurysm include:

A. Ischemia
B. Rupture
C. Chamber compression
D. All of the choices

QUESTION 7. After 6 months, the patient returns now complaining of exertional dyspnea. In anticipation of surgical valve replacements, he undergoes coronary angiography. His right coronary angiogram is shown in **Videos 82-11 and 82-12** and demonstrates a large saccular right coronary aneurysm that corresponds to the cystic mass seen on echo. The patient proceeded with aortic and mitral valve replacement and excision of the right coronary aneurysm. He did very well. Three years later, he returns with a new systolic murmur. He eventually undergoes transesophageal echocardiography (**Videos 82-13 to 82-17**). What is the location of the mitral valve periprosthetic regurgitation?

   A. Anterior
   B. Anterolateral
   C. Posterior
   D. Posteromedial

ANSWER 1: D. There is anterior mitral valve leaflet prolapse with MR that by PISA quantifies in the severe range.

The regurgitant flow can be calculated as follows:

Flow rate = $(r)^2 \times 6.28 \times$ aliasing velocity
$= (0.82 \text{ cm})^2 \times 6.28 \times 55 \text{ cm per second}$
$= 232 \text{ cc per second}$

Effective regurgitant orifice (ERO) = Flow rate/peak MR velocity
$= 232 \text{ cc per second}/600 \text{ cm per second}$
$= 0.39 \text{ cm}^2$

Regurgitant volume = ERO × MR time velocity integral
$= 0.39 \times 193 = 75 \text{ cc}$

This implies the degree of MR is in the severe range by ERO and regurgitant volume.

See *The Echo Manual, 3rd Edition,* **discussion of PISA method on page 215.**

ANSWER 2: C. An LV diastolic dimension >75 mm, a restrictive mitral inflow pattern with high E-wave velocity, and a high ERO/regurgitant volume by the continuity method may all suggest the presence of severe AR, but are not necessarily accurate in the setting of concomitant severe MR. Hence, in the setting of significant MR, one must rely on other parameters of severity including vena contracta width and other measures of AR jet size along with PISA measures and indicators of aortic diastolic flow reversals.

ANSWER 3: C. The color flow Doppler demonstrates a broad jet of aortic valve regurgitation (**Video 82-4**), with a short pressure halftime (Fig. 82-4) and aortic diastolic flow reversals that are almost two-thirds of the forward flow (Figs. 82-5 and 82-6).

See *The Echo Manual, 3rd Edition,* **discussion of severity of aortic valve regurgitation on pages 207 to 209.**

ANSWER 4: D. Holodiastolic flow reversals are not isolated to severe AR. Any shunt into the aorta during diastole, for example, PDA in pulmonary hypertension or a B-T shunt, may give a similar finding. Alternatively, diastolic flow reversals may also be seen in a descending thoracic aortic aneurysm.

See *The Echo Manual, 3rd Edition,* **Figure 12-24 on page 209.**

ANSWER 5: A. All of the options are in the differential for an apparent mass in the right atrioventricular groove. A paraganglioma would be expected to have a more solid component appearance (e.g., **Video 82-10**). A pleural effusion would be located outside the pericardial lining.

ANSWER 6: D. Coronary aneurysms[1] are rare particular as large as was seen in this case. These most commonly occur in adult patients in the setting of coronary atherosclerosis. Other etiologies may include Kawasaki disease, arteritis, or injury from an attempted percutaneous revascularization procedure. Ischemia may develop secondary to the poor sluggish flow that may develop. Rupture, although reported, is exceedingly rare. Rarely the cardiac atria may be compressed affecting myocardial blood flow. The management is not standardized and depends on whether the aneurysm is associated with any of the above complications.

ANSWER 7: D. In the era of the ability of percutaneous leak closure with occluder devices, the ability to accurately locate these defects is of critical importance, from the standpoint of establishing feasibility and planning closure. Useful landmarks for location include the left atrial appendage (opposite the anterolateral portion of the mitral annulus), the aortic valve (the anterior portion of the mitral annulus), and the intra-atrial septum (medial aspect). In the two-chamber view (**Video 82-16**), one visualizes the anterolateral aspect (left atrial appendage) and opposite to this the posteromedial aspect of the annulus.

Reference

1. Syed M, Lesch M. Coronary aneurysm: a review. *Prog Cardiovasc Dis.* 1997;40(1):77–84.

CASE 83

Slowly Progressive Exertional Shortness of Breath

A 42-year-old woman presents with slowly progressive exertional shortness of breath. See **Videos 83-1 to 83-12** and Figure 83-1.

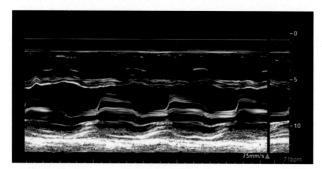

Figure 83-1

QUESTION 1. The most likely etiology for the valvular findings is:

- A. Congenital
- B. Rheumatic
- C. Radiation
- D. Prior diet-drug use (fen-phen)

QUESTION 2. The likely timing between the second heart sound and the opening snap in this patient is:

- A. 65 milliseconds
- B. 135 milliseconds
- C. It is very likely that no opening snap will be present

QUESTION 3. Which perspective is the three-dimensional (3D) image of the mitral valve (**Video 83-12**) viewed?

- A. Atrial perspective
- B. Ventricular perspective
- C. Aortic perspective
- D. Posterior perspective

QUESTION 4. With regard to assessing the degree of mitral stenosis by the PISA method, which direction do you need to shift the color zero-line?

- A. Upward toward the apex
- B. Downward away from the apex
- C. Either direction will work
- D. PISA does not work for mitral stenosis

QUESTION 5. The mitral valve area (MVA) by 3D planimetry is 0.6 cm². Calculate the MVA also by the PISA method and the continuity method (the left ventricular outflow tract [LVOT] velocity is 21 mm). On the basis of your results, which of the following statements concerning the MVA is correct (a consistent result is within 0.1 cm²)? See Figures 83-2 to 83-5.

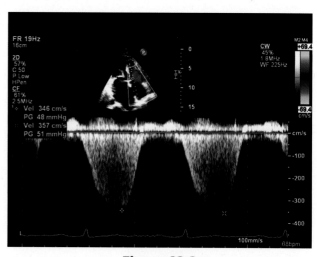

Figure 83-2

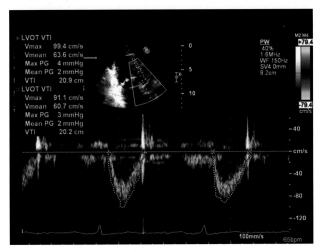

Figure 83-3

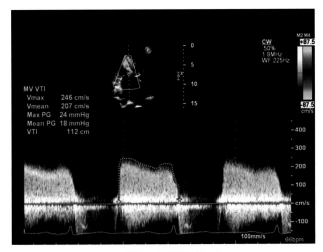

Figure 83-4

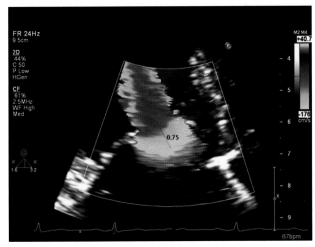

Figure 83-5

A. Planimetry MVA consistent with PISA MVA and continuity MVA

B. Planimetry MVA consistent with PISA MVA but not continuity MVA

C. Planimetry MVA consistent with continuity MVA but not PISA MVA

D. The continuity MVA consistent with PISA MVA but neither consistent with planimetry MVA

QUESTION 6. The mitral valve pressure halftime (PHT) should be:

A. 300 milliseconds

B. 370 milliseconds

C. 430 milliseconds

D. 500 milliseconds

QUESTION 7. Based on your calculation of the Abasacal score, this patient is likely to have which of the following outcomes after mitral balloon valvuloplasty?

A. A high risk of severe mitral valve regurgitation

B. A high likelihood of a durable success

C. A low future risk of atrial fibrillation

QUESTION 8. The patient proceeded with transesophageal echocardiography to exclude left atrial thrombus and then percutaneous balloon valvuloplasty. Which of the following measures of severity should not be used to evaluate response?

A. MVA by planimetry

B. Catheter-derived mean gradient between the left atrium and left ventricle

C. MVA by pressure halftime

D. Mean diastolic Doppler gradient

E. MVA by the continuity method

QUESTION 9. Can a transmitral pressure halftime of 120 milliseconds exclude the presence of severe mitral stenosis?

A. Yes

B. No

ANSWER 1: B. The two-dimensional images demonstrate the typical echocardiographic features of rheumatic mitral stenosis with thickened and calcified mitral leaflets and subvalvular apparatus and a "Hockey-stick" appearance of the anterior mitral leaflet in diastole (long-axis view). In the short-axis view, the mitral valve has a "Fish-mouth" orifice.

ANSWER 2: A. In mitral stenosis, the presence of an opening snap is associated with a valve that has pliability. The shorter the interval between the second heart sound and the opening snap, the more severe the stenosis (related to higher left atrial pressure). Typically, a mildly stenotic valve will have an interval greater than 110 milliseconds with an interval less than 70 milliseconds consistent with severe stenosis.

ANSWER 3: B. The 3D image of the mitral valve shows the ventricular perspective.

ANSWER 4: A. The zero baseline for the color map should be shifted upward (toward the apex) to an aliasing velocity between 30 and 45 m per second.

ANSWER 5: A. To determine the MVA with the continuity equation, determine the stroke volume from the LVOT diameter (D) and time velocity integral (TVI) and then calculate the MVA by dividing the LVOT stroke volume by mitral valve TVI.

See *The Echo Manual, 3rd Edition,* **Figure 12-19 on page 205.**

This equation cannot be used if there is marked aortic or mitral valve regurgitation.

$$\text{MVA} = \text{LVOT D}^2 \times 0.785 \times \frac{\text{TVI}_{LVOT}}{\text{TVI}_{MVI}}$$

$$= 2.1^2 \times 0.785 \times 20/112$$

$$= 0.62 \text{ cm}^2$$

MVA by the PISA method (one does not need to use an angle correction here as the bottom surface of the hemispheric PISA is relatively flat [$\alpha = 180°$])

$$\text{MVA} = \frac{6.28 \times r^2 \times \text{aliasing velocity}}{\text{Peak}_{\text{Mitral stenosis velocity}}} \times \frac{\alpha°}{180°}$$

$$= \frac{6.28 \times 0.75^2 \times 41}{246} \times \frac{180°}{180°}$$

$$= 0.59 \text{ cm}^2$$

ANSWER 6: B.

MVA = 220/PHT

That is, PHT = 220/MVA

PHT = 220/0.6 = 370 milliseconds

See *The Echo Manual, 3rd Edition,* **Column 2 on page 202 (steps 1 through 6: the most reliable way to determine the severity of mitral stenosis).**

ANSWER 7: B. The Abasacal echocardiographic score was derived from an analysis of mitral leaflet mobility, valvular and subvalvular thickening, and calcification, and is graded from 0 (normal) to 4 according to the above criteria. This gave a total score of 0 to 16.

In this case, the valve mobility remains quite normal with only the leaflet tips being restricted (for mobility a score of 1/4). The subvalvular apparatus has modest thickening that extends to one-third of the chordal length (for subvalvular thickening a score of 2/4). The entire leaflet is thickened (for thickening score of 3/4). Total score = 7.

A score less than 8 tends to favor a greater likelihood of durable success of balloon valvuloplasty with a lower rate of complications including severe mitral valve regurgitation.

See Table 83.1 and associated discussion.

TABLE 83-1. Echocardiographic Score Used to Predict the Outcome of Mitral Balloon Valvuloplasty[a]

Grade	Mobility	Subvalvular Thickening	Thickening	Calcification
0	Normal leaflet mobility	No subvalvular thickening	No leaflet thickening	No areas of valvular calcification
1	Highly mobile valve with only leaflet tips restricted	Minimal thickening just below the mitral leaflets	Leaflets near normal in thickness (4–5 mm)	A single area of increased echo brightness
2	Leaflet mid and base portions have normal mobility	Thickening of chordal structures extending up to one-third of the chordal length	Midleaflets normal, considerable thickening of margins (5–8 mm)	Scattered areas of brightness confined to leaflet margins
3	Valve continues to move forward in diastole, mainly from the base	Thickening extending to the distal third of the chords	Thickening extending through the entire leaflet (5–8 mm)	Brightness extending into the midportion of the leaflets
4	No or minimal forward movement of the leaflets in diastole	Extensive thickening and shortening of all chordal structures extending down to the papillary muscles	Considerable thickening of all leaflet tissue (>8–10 mm)	Extensive brightness throughout much of the leaflet tissue

[a] The total echocardiographic score was derived from an analysis of mitral leaflet mobility, valvular and subvalvular thickening, and calcification, which were graded from 0 (normal) to 4 according to the above criteria. This gave a total score of 0 to 16.

ANSWER 8: C. Pressure halftime is an unreliable measure of MVA in the acute setting following mitral valvotomy as it is also strongly dependent on chamber compliance and the peak transmitral gradient, which are variables that change dramatically with valvotomy.[1]

ANSWER 9: B. Although the pressure halftime in mitral stenosis is typically prolonged (>220 milliseconds) in patients with severe mitral stenosis, some patients with marked symptoms and a very high left atrial pressure may have a shorter pressure halftime. The diastolic pressure gradient in this setting will be high.

Reference

1. Thomas JD, Wilkins GT, Choong CY, et al. Inaccuracy of mitral pressure half-time immediately after percutaneous mitral valvotomy. Dependence on transmitral gradient and left atrial and ventricular compliance. *Circulation.* 1988;78(4):980–993.

CASE 84

Exertional Fatigue, Lower Extremity Edema, and New Murmur

A 28-year-old previously well male patient presents with exertional fatigue, lower extremity edema, and a new murmur. He is referred for transthoracic echocardiography (TTE).

QUESTION 1. Based on your review of Figures 84-1 and 84-2, which lesions are in your differential?

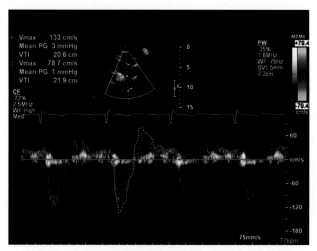

Figure 84-1

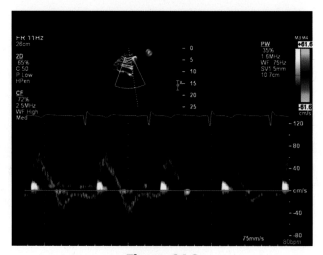

Figure 84-2

A. Severe aortic valve regurgitation

B. Coarctation of the aorta

C. Severe supra-aortic valve stenosis

D. Normal finding

QUESTION 2. Based on your review of the TTE (**Videos 84-1 to 84-16** and Figs. 84-1 to 84-6), the diagnosis is:

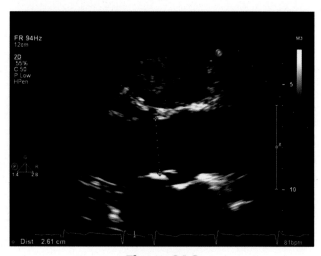

Figure 84-3

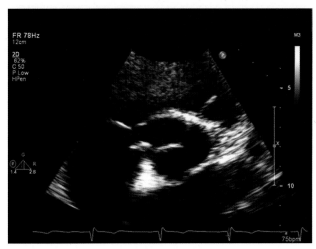

Figure 84-4

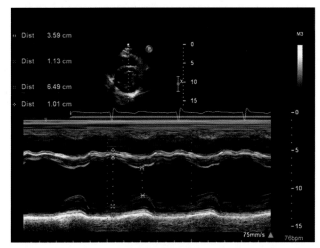

Figure 84-5

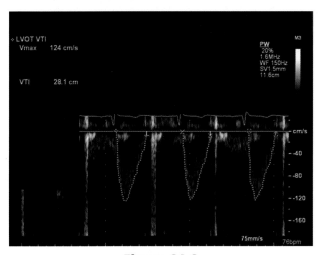

Figure 84-6

A. Isolated severe aortic valve regurgitation
B. Membranous ventricular septal defect
C. Ruptured sinus of Valsalva aneurysm
D. Primum atrial septal defect

QUESTION 3. Calculate the Doppler-derived cardiac output.

A. 7 L per minute
B. 8 L per minute
C. 9 L per minute
D. 10 L per minute
E. 11 L per minute

QUESTION 4. Which sinus is involved?

A. Right coronary sinus
B. Left aortic sinus
C. Noncoronary sinus

QUESTION 5. The patient proceeded also to TEE (**Videos 84-17 to 84-20**). What is the severity of aortic valve regurgitation?

A. Mild
B. Moderate
C. Severe

QUESTION 6. Which sinus is most commonly involved?

A. Left aortic sinus
B. Right coronary sinus
C. Noncoronary sinus

QUESTION 7. All of the following are predisposing factors to sinus of Valsalva aneurysms *except*:

A. Syphilis
B. Female sex
C. Endocarditis

ANSWER 1: A. There is evidence of marked diastolic flow reversals in both the descending thoracic aorta and the abdominal aorta, indicating a shunt from the aorta back into a lower pressure chamber during diastole. The most common cause for this is severe aortic valve regurgitation. The typical finding in coarctation of the aorta is a prolonged time to peak velocity and persistent forward diastolic flow. Large diastolic flow reversals are a feature of a patent ductus arteriosus or severe aortic regurgitation. Severe aortic stenosis typically will have a blunted peak systolic velocity with a decreased time to peak. A normal Doppler profile is demonstrated in Figure 2-8 (Case 2) and an example seen in aortic coarctation in Figure 5-2 (Case 5).

ANSWER 2: C. There is an outpouching of the aortic sinus with abnormal flow from the aorta into the right atrium just at the base of the tricuspid valve leaflet (**Video 84-10**). There is associated aortic valve regurgitation; the severity of which is indeterminate. The diastolic flow reversals in the descending thoracic aorta (Fig. 84-1) relate to a combination of abnormal diastolic flow (a proportion into the right atrium through the ruptured sinus of Valsalva aneurysm and a proportion across the aortic valve).

ANSWER 3: E. Stroke volume (SV) is calculated from the left ventricular outflow tract (LVOT) as a product of the LVOT area (LVOT diameter^2 × 0.785) and the LVOT time velocity integral (VTI).

Here SV = (2.6 cm)^2 × 0.785 × 28 cm = 149 ml at a heart rate of 76 beats per minute = 11.3 L per minute (high output state).

See *The Echo Manual, 3rd Edition*, Figure 4-16 on page 71.

ANSWER 4: A. The defect (seen well on **Video 84-11**) is in the right coronary sinus at the level of the tricuspid valve with rupture into the right atrium.

ANSWER 5: C. Although suspected on the TTE images, TEE confirms that there is severe aortic valve regurgitation, related to prolapse of the aortic valve leaflet through the defect with eccentric regurgitation. There likely has been chronicity to the aortic valve regurgitation given the dilation of the left ventricle that is present. Many patients with sinus of Valsalva aneurysms may have significant aortic valve regurgitation even in the absence of rupture due to distortion of the aortic valve leaflets.

ANSWER 6: B. The right coronary sinus is most commonly affected followed by the noncoronary sinus. Typically, the aneurysm ruptures into the right ventricular outflow tract with a resulting shunt from aorta to right ventricle.

ANSWER 7: B. Sinus of Valsalva aneurysms are most commonly congenital in origin and occur in men three times more commonly than they occur in women. However, similar defects may be caused by endocarditis, trauma, or syphilis.

CASE 85

Diabetic Nephropathy

A 35-year-old man with diabetic nephropathy on dialysis is considered for renal transplantation. Prior to recently sustaining a knee injury, he complained of functional class III dyspnea. He is referred for dobutamine stress echocardiography.

QUESTION 1. Based on the images obtained at rest (**Videos 85-1 and 85-2** and Fig. 85-1), what is the left ventricular ejection fraction (LVEF) at rest?

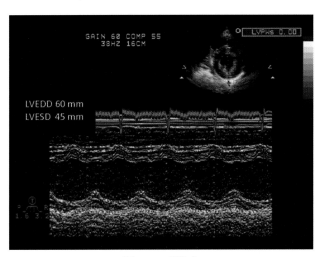

Figure 85-1

A. 20% to 25%
B. 30% to 35%
C. 40% to 45%
D. 50% to 55%
E. 60% to 65%

QUESTION 2. Based on the comparison of the rest images (**Video 85-1***) with the images taken at low dose, prepeak, and peak stress (**Videos 85-3* to 85-6***), is there echocardiographic evidence of ischemia?

*Please note that the apical four-chamber view in both the rest (**Video 85-1**) and stress images (**Video 85-5**) is in the Mayo Clinic image orientation with the left ventricle displayed on the left and the right ventricle on the right.

A. No echocardiographic evidence of ischemia
B. Evidence of ischemia in one coronary territory
C. Evidence of multivessel coronary ischemia

QUESTION 3. Ultimately, it was decided not to proceed with transplantation at this time, and the patient remained on hemodialysis. Two years later, the patient suddenly became unresponsive. He was brought to the emergency department where he was noted to have a systolic blood pressure of 90/50 mm Hg, a heart rate of 100 beats per minute, and a temperature of 100°F. He was modestly responsive to verbal commands only. An emergency noncontrast head CT scan was negative.

A lumbar puncture demonstrated high white cell count and blood cultures were positive for *Staphylococcus aureus*. He was given fluids and broad spectrum antibiotics, and heart rate and blood pressure normalize. Cardiac examination is normal. An MRI scan demonstrated "new focal lesions with associated restricted water diffusion within the cerebral hemispheres and cerebellar hemispheres bilaterally with meningeal hyper-enhancement." Which of the following statements is correct?

A. No echocardiographic imaging is required
B. Transthoracic echocardiography is indicated and if negative no further testing
C. Transesophageal echocardiography is indicated

QUESTION 4. Based on your review of **Videos 85-7 to 85-17**, there is:

A. No echocardiographic evidence of endocarditis
B. Echocardiographic evidence of vegetation on the anterior mitral valve leaflet with mild regurgitation
C. Echocardiographic evidence of vegetation on the posterior mitral valve leaflet with mild regurgitation
D. Echocardiographic evidence of vegetation on the mitral, aortic, and tricuspid valve leaflets with trivial-mild regurgitation

QUESTION 5. Which of the following factors has not been found to be associated with a higher clinical embolization risk in infective endocarditis?

A. *S. aureus* as the pathogen
B. Left- versus right-sided location
C. Fungal versus bacterial endocarditis
D. Lesion size >10 mm
E. Mitral valve versus aortic valve endocarditis
F. Patients taken chronic aspirin at diagnosis

QUESTION 6. The patient makes slow and steady improvement from a neurologic perspective on appropriate antibiotic therapy. One week later, a transthoracic echocardiogram is repeated (**Video 85-18 and 85-19**).

A further 2 weeks later, all neurologic symptoms have resolved, but now he develops worsening dyspnea, and therefore a repeat echocardiogram is performed (**Videos 85-20 to 85-24** and Fig. 85-2). There is now evidence of:

A. Mitral valve posterior leaflet prolapse with significant valvular regurgitation
B. Malcoaptation of the mitral valve leaflets secondary to the mobile vegetation
C. Anterior mitral leaflet perforation
D. Posterior mitral leaflet perforation
E. No significant change

QUESTION 7. Assume a mitral regurgitant peak velocity of 5 m per second. What is the calculated effective regurgitant orifice?

A. 0.25
B. 0.34
C. 0.39
D. 0.44
E. 0.52

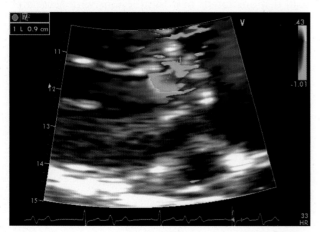

Figure 85-2

ANSWER 1: C. There is evidence of generalized reduction in left ventricular contractility with global hypokinesis worst in the inferior wall. The estimated LVEF is 40% to 45%. On the basis of the two-dimensional guided M-mode of the LVEF at the papillary muscle level, the end diastolic left ventricular dimension is 60 mm and the end systolic dimension 45 mm.

$$\text{LVEF} = \frac{60^2 - 45^2}{60^2} = 44\%$$

ANSWER 2: A. With dobutamine stress, there is modest global improvement in contractility without evidence of ischemia.

ANSWER 3: C. The patient has bacteremia with an organism that has a high propensity for causing left-sided endocarditis. In addition, there is clinical and radiographic evidence suggestive of infective embolic events to the brain. The suspicion for *S. aureus* infective endocarditis is very high. Although a transthoracic echocardiogram would be a reasonable initial investigation, a negative transthoracic study would not be sufficient to exclude the clinical diagnosis given the high clinical pretest probability.

ANSWER 4: C. On transesophageal echocardiography, there is evidence of large vegetation on the posterior mitral leaflet involving the middle and lateral scallops and extending to the atrial surface. The tricuspid and aortic valves (and pulmonary—not shown) have no echocardiographic features of endocarditis.

ANSWER 5: F. Embolization can be a devastating complication in infective endocarditis and can occur long after appropriate antimicrobial therapy has been instituted. Embolization can be a feature of both left- and right-sided endocarditis; however; events that are

clinically significant are much more common from left-sided infection and occur in 10% to 40% of patients with left-sided endocarditis. Clinical characteristics that impart a higher risk of embolization include the bacterial pathogens such as *S. aureus* and *Staphylococcus bovis* and fungal pathogens. The risk tends to fall with the duration of appropriate antimicrobial therapy. Patients previously on aspirin that is continued tend to have a lower risk of events; however, the institution of aspirin is not advantageous and may in fact increase the risk. Echocardiographically, the bigger the risk, the higher the risk with the mitral lesions a higher risk that aortic lesions. There is some evidence that vegetation on the anterior mitral valve leaflet have a higher embolic risk than those on the posterior mitral valve.

ANSWER 6: D. There is new severe mitral regurgitation directed anteriorly. Close-up views demonstrate a perforation of the posterior leaflet (**Videos 85-21 and 85-22**).

See *The Echo Manual, 3rd Edition*, **discussion of complications of endocarditis on pages 246 to 248.**

ANSWER 7: D.

$$\text{ERO} = \frac{6.28 \times r^2 \times \text{aliasing velocity}}{\text{Peak MR velocity}}$$

$$\text{ERO} = \frac{6.28 \times 0.9^2 \times 43}{500} = 0.44 \text{ cm}^2$$

An ERO >0.4 indicates mitral regurgitation in the severe range.

See *The Echo Manual, 3rd Edition*, **discussion of PISA method on page 215.**

The patient proceeded to the operating room where a successful mitral valve replacement was performed and he did well.

References

1. Bayer AS, Bolger AF, Taubert KA, et al. Diagnosis and management of infective endocarditis and its complications. *Circulation*. 1998;98:2936–2948.

2. Rohmann S, Erbel R, Görge G, et al. Clinical relevance of vegetation localization by transoesophageal echocardiography in infective endocarditis. *Eur Heart J*. 1992;13:446–452.

3. Sanfilippo AJ, Picard MH, Newell JB, et al. Echocardiographic assessment of patients with infectious endocarditis: prediction of risk for complications. *J Am Coll Cardiol*. 1991;18:1191–1199.

4. Thuny F, Di Salvo G, Belliard O, et al. Risk of embolism and death in infective endocarditis: prognostic value of echocardiography: a prospective multicenter study. *Circulation*. 2005;112:69–75.

5. Anavekar NS, Tleyjeh IM, Anavekar NS, et al. Impact of prior antiplatelet therapy on risk of embolism in infective endocarditis. *Clin Infect Dis*. 2007;44:1180–1186.

CASE 86

Recurrent Episodes of Left Heart Failure

A 55-year-old woman is referred for a transthoracic echocardiogram. She has a prior history of aortic and mitral valve replacements for rheumatic disease. She presents now with recurrent episodes of left heart failure.

QUESTION 1. Video 86-1 demonstrates which of the following:

- A. Left pleural effusion
- B. Right pleural effusion
- C. Posterior pericardial effusion

QUESTION 2. The transmitral prosthetic valve diastolic mean gradient (**Videos 86-4 to 86-8** and Figs. 86-1 to 86-3) is consistent with:

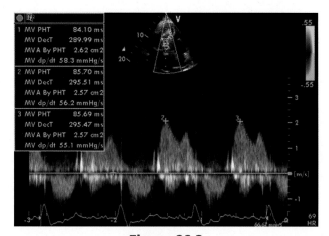

Figure 86-2

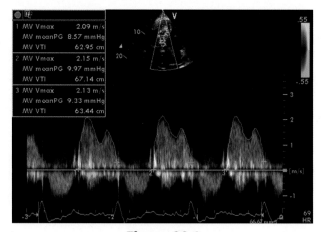

Figure 86-1

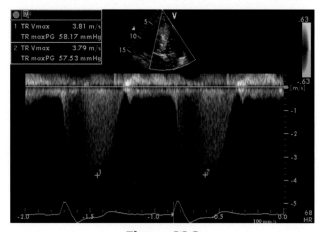

Figure 86-3

A. Normal mitral bioprosthetic function
B. Significant prosthetic dysfunction likely related to leaflet stenosis or obstruction
C. Significant prosthetic dysfunction likely related to regurgitation

QUESTION 3. What is the significance of the finding in Figure 86-3?

A. Pulmonary hypertension
B. Severe tricuspid valve regurgitation
C. Tricuspid valve stenosis
D. Normal finding

QUESTION 4. The next step in the assessment of this patient's dyspnea should include:

A. Hemodynamic catheterization
B. Cardiac magnetic resonance scan
C. Transesophageal echocardiogram

QUESTION 5. Following review of **Videos 86-9 to 86-13**, the mitral valve prosthetic gradient appears related to:

A. Normal mitral prosthetic function
B. Significant mitral valvular regurgitation
C. Significant mitral valvular obstruction

QUESTION 6. Based on **Video 86-14** and Figures 86-4 and 86-5, calculate the periprosthetic effective regurgitant orifice (ERO) by the PISA method.

A. 0.3 cm^2
B. 0.4 cm^2
C. 0.5 cm^2
D. 0.6 cm^2

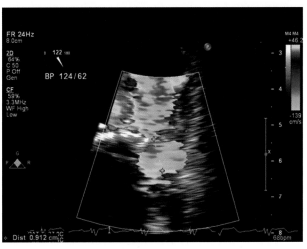

Figure 86-4

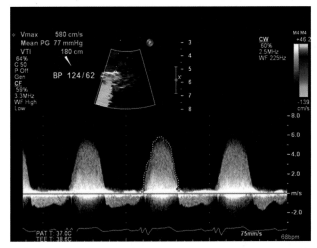

Figure 86-5

QUESTION 7. The location of the periprosthetic leak is:

A. Medial
B. Lateral

QUESTION 8. The lesion identified by the arrow in **Video 86-15** is most likely:

    A. Vegetation
    B. Suture material
    C. A papillary fibroelastoma
    D. An atrial myxoma
    E. Artifact

QUESTION 9. The finding in **Video 86-16** is associated with a higher risk of:

    A. Ventricular septal defect
    B. Anomalous pulmonary venous drainage of the right upper pulmonary vein
    C. A patent foramen ovale (PFO) and a higher risk of stroke
    D. An atrial septal defect
    E. Patent ductus arteriosus

QUESTION 10. The likely success rate of percutaneous repair of the perivalvular leak is:

    A. 20% to 40%
    B. 40% to 60%
    C. 60% to 80%
    D. >90%

ANSWER 1: A. Left-sided pleural effusions are seen posterior to the heart on left parasternal long-axis imaging. They appear as an echo-free space that can be distinguished from pericardial fluid by (1) the presence (although not always present) of atelectatic lung and (2) its location, that is, posterior (**Video 86-2**) rather than anterior (**Video 86-3**) to the descending thoracic aorta (indicated by yellow triangle in clips).

ANSWER 2: C. There is evidence of increased flow velocities across the mitral valve with an early (E) peak velocity of 2 m per second. Increased flow velocities may be related to flow acceleration related to valve obstruction, or increased quantity of flow related to valvular regurgitation. A useful indicator to help separate these mechanisms is the pressure halftime. The pressure halftime is prolonged in valvular obstruction but not in regurgitation. Here a pressure halftime of 85 milliseconds suggests there is no leaflet obstruction but rather a degree of mitral valve regurgitation that is not appreciated on color Doppler interrogation of the valve. This is likely related to echo shadowing mediated by the prosthetic material of the aortic and mitral prostheses.

See *The Echo Manual, 3rd Edition*, pages 229 and 230.

ANSWER 3: A. The peak tricuspid regurgitant velocity at 3.8 m per second (pressure gradient 58 mm Hg) is consistent with significant pulmonary hypertension that is presumably due to, and further underscores, the significance of the mitral valvular dysfunction.

ANSWER 4: C. The transthoracic echocardiogram suggests mitral prosthesis dysfunction, more likely related to valvular regurgitation and secondary pulmonary hypertension. The best test in this setting to better characterize mitral valvular function/dysfunction is a transesophageal echocardiogram.

ANSWER 5: B. Transesophageal echocardiogram demonstrates normal prosthetic leaflet mobility but partial dehiscence with periprosthetic regurgitation.

ANSWER 6: B. The regurgitant flow can be calculated as follows:

Flow rate $= (r)^2 \times 6.28 \times$ aliasing velocity

$$= (0.91 \text{ cm})^2 \times 6.28 \times 46 \text{ cm per second}$$

$$= 239 \text{ cc per second}$$

ERO $=$ Flow rate/peak MR velocity

$$= 239 \text{ cc per second}/580 \text{ cm per second}$$

$$= 0.41 \text{ cm}^2$$

See *The Echo Manual, 3rd Edition*, discussion of PISA method on page 215.

ANSWER 7: B. Transesophageal echocardiogram demonstrates an isolated lateral perivalvular defect. The defect seen at four degrees in the midesophagus is beside the inferolateral aspect of the sewing ring.

ANSWER 8: B. The lesion identified is in the typical location for a surgical suture placed at the time of valve insertion. Commonly misinterpreted as a pathologic finding, this is one of a series of independent surgical suture knots present circumferentially around the annular ring (**Video 86-17**). Three-dimensional (3D) echocardiography highlights this well-correlating well with the findings present at the time of surgery (Fig. 86-6).

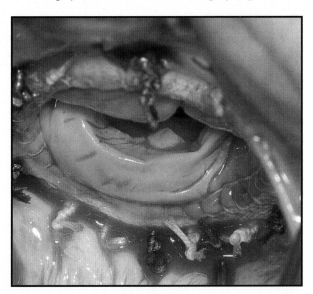

Figure 86-6

ANSWER 9: C. Approximately 20% of patients with atrial septal aneurysms have a PFO. Therefore, if one identifies an atrial septal aneurysm, it is important to carefully look for PFO, particularly if the patient has suffered a neurologic/embolic event.

ANSWER 10: C. Transesophageal echocardiogram demonstrates an isolated lateral perivalvular defect. This is a defect that appears quite approachable percutaneously and has a high likelihood of successful repair.[1] Transesophageal echocardiography plays a critical role in guiding percutaneous closure of mitral perivalvular leaks, with 3D imaging playing an important role in defining the defect size, location, and relationship to adjoining structures including the valve leaflets.

Reference

1. Sorajja P, Cabalka AK, Hagler DJ, et al. Percutaneous repair of paravalvular prosthetic regurgitation: acute and 30-day outcomes in 115 patients. *Circ Cardiovasc Interv*. 2011;4(4):314–321.

Exertional Shortness of Breath in a 68-Year-Old Woman

A 68-year-old woman is referred for an echocardiogram to evaluate exertional shortness of breath (**Videos 87-1 to 87-6** and Figs. 87-1 to 87-4).

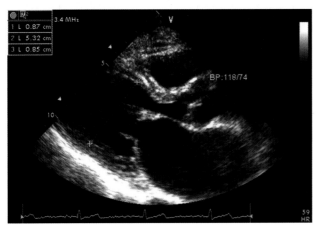

Figure 87-1

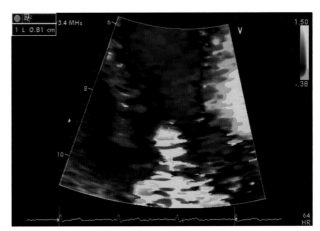

Figure 87-3

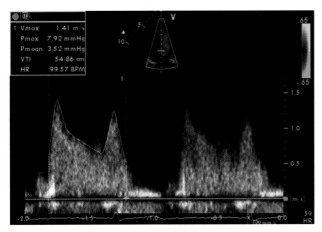

Figure 87-2

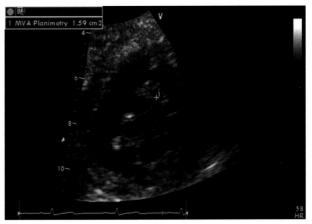

Figure 87-4

QUESTION 1. The mechanism of the mitral valve disease is likely:

A. Rheumatic disease
B. Leaflet prolapse
C. Functional (ischemia)

QUESTION 2. As the aliasing velocity was set about 40 cm per second, what simple equation can be used to calculate the effective regurgitant orifice (ERO) with respect to mitral valve regurgitation?

A. $ERO = r^2$
B. $ERO = r^2/2$
C. $ERO = r/2$
D. $ERO = 2r^2$

QUESTION 3. A TEE confirmed moderate to severe mitral valve regurgitation and mild to moderate stenosis. In the setting of functional class III shortness of breath, the patient was referred for mitral valve replacement and did well. Postoperatively, she was referred for transthoracic echocardiography (**Videos 87-7 and 87-8**, and Figs. 87-5 and 87-6). Which of the flowing factors will least impact the interpretation of the Doppler interrogation of the mitral valve prosthesis?

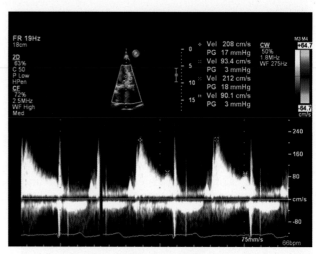

Figure 87-6

A. Heart rate
B. Gender
C. Systemic blood pressure
D. Left ventricular outflow tract (LVOT) time velocity integral

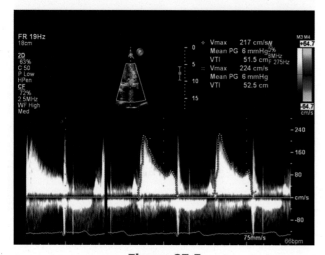

Figure 87-5

QUESTION 4. Two years later, she presents for repeat echocardiographic evaluation. She now describes functional class III shortness of breath. A diastolic murmur is heard. She is referred for transthoracic echocardiography (**Videos 87-9 to 87-13** and Fig. 87-7) and subsequently transesophageal echocardiography (**Videos 87-14 and 87-15**). What is your recommended treatment?

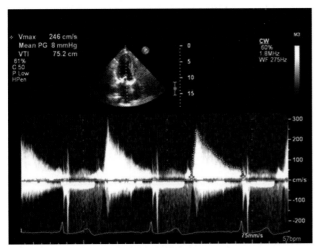

Figure 87-7

A. Intravenous heparin and warfarin to a goal INR of 2 to 3
B. Intravenous thrombolytics
C. Emergency surgery

QUESTION 5. Which of the following management strategies is appropriate to prevent a bioprosthetic thrombosis?

A. Mitral tissue prosthesis, sinus rhythm, left ventricular ejection fraction (LVEF) 35%—aspirin
B. Mitral tissue prosthesis, atrial fibrillation, LVEF 60%—aspirin and warfarin
C. Mitral tissue prosthesis, sinus rhythm, LVEF 75%—no therapy required

ANSWER 1: A. Transthoracic echocardiography demonstrates the typical echocardiographic changes of rheumatic mitral valve disease. The typical findings include thickening and calcification of the leaflets and subvalvular apparatus with commissural calcification. The anterior mitral valve leaflet in long axis has the typical "Hockey-stick" appearance in diastole with immobility of the posterior leaflet.

ANSWER 2: B.

$$ERO = 6.28 \ (r^2) \times \frac{\text{aliasing velocity}}{\text{MR velocity}}$$

If the aliasing velocity is about 40 cm per second and the mitral valve regurgitation velocity is assumed to be 500 cm per second, then

$$ERO = \frac{6.28 \times r^2 \times 40 \text{ cm per second}}{500 \text{ cm per second}} = \frac{251 \times r^2}{500} = \frac{r^2}{2}$$

ERO becomes half of the r^2 value.

ANSWER 3: B. Transvalvular gradients are very dependent on heart rates. A mean diastolic gradient of 8 to 10 mm Hg across a tissue mitral prosthesis would be quite abnormal at a heart rate of 60 beats per minute (bpm), but might be quite normal at a heart rate of 120 bpm. Although systemic blood pressure does not greatly affect diastolic gradients, mitral valve regurgitation is very dependent on blood pressure, tending to increase as the blood pressure increases. Should the patient have a high output state, for example, anemia, fever, and the transvalvular gradients will be elevated. This can be separated from abnormality by a similar degree of elevation in the LVOT flow. Gender has no impact on valve gradients.

ANSWER 4: C. TTE demonstrates a large mobile thrombus attached to one of the prosthetic leaflets prolapsing from the left atrium into the left ventricle with each heartbeat. Given its size and mobility there is a high risk of embolization. The guidelines would recommend, given its size and the degree of symptoms, the patient is referred for emergency surgery. Intravenous thrombolytic therapy is preferred for right-sided thrombotic valves, smaller clots, and patients who are felt to be too high risk for surgery.

Bioprosthetic valves are widely used as an alternative to mechanical prostheses for end-stage mitral valve disease, and following the initial healing phase after valve implantation, the risks of tissue bioprosthetic valve thrombosis or related embolism are generally considered very low, thus long-term systemic anticoagulation can typically be avoided. The potential for bioprosthetic valve thrombosis and dysfunction, although low, is still elevated compared with natural valves and is increased by the concomitant existence of atrial fibrillation or left ventricular dysfunction.

ANSWER 5: B. Bioprosthetic valves are often chosen in preference to the structurally more durable mechanical valves based solely on the absence of a requirement for mandatory warfarin anticoagulation and a consequent reduced risk of bleeding complications, particularly in elderly patients. Although a variety of strategies have been described in the early postoperative period, a universal antithrombotic strategy is not clear. Recent guidelines by the American Heart Association/American College of Cardiology recommend the use of aspirin in all patients receiving bioprosthetic heart valves and to consider warfarin in the initial 3 months and/or the presence of risk factors. Indeed, emerging data point toward the potential benefits of antiplatelet therapy in preventing thrombotic complications post bioprosthetic valve replacement. Patients with atrial fibrillation and/or left ventricular systolic dysfunction should receive both aspirin and warfarin.[1-3]

References

1. Stein PD, Alpert JS, Bussey HI, et al. Antithrombotic therapy in patients with mechanical and biological prosthetic heart valves. *Chest.* 2001;119(1)(suppl):220S–227S.

2. Bonow RO, Carabello BA, Chatterjee K, et al. ACC/AHA 2006 guidelines for the management of patients with valvular heart disease: a report of the American College of Cardiology/American Heart Association Task Force on Practice Guidelines (writing committee to develop guidelines for the management of patients with valvular heart disease). American College of Cardiology Web Site. http://www.acc.org/clinical/guidelines/valvular/index.pdf. Accessed.

3. Colli A, Verhoye J-P, Leguerrier A, et al. Anticoagulation or antiplatelet therapy of bioprosthetic heart valves recipients: an unresolved issue. *Eur J Cardio Surg.* 2007;31:573–577.

History of Symptomatic Paroxysmal Atrial Fibrillation

A 68-year-old woman is referred for a transthoracic echocardiogram (**Videos 88-1 to 88-3** and Figs. 88-1 to 88-6). She has a history of symptomatic paroxysmal atrial fibrillation.

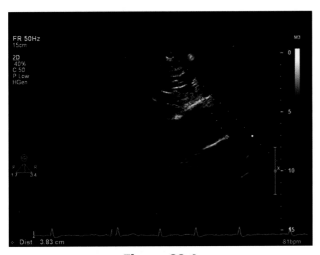

Figure 88-1

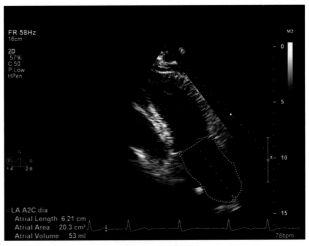

Figure 88-3

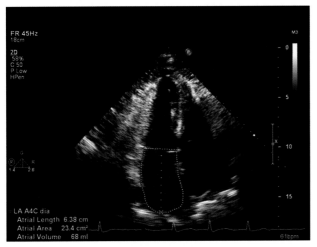

Figure 88-2

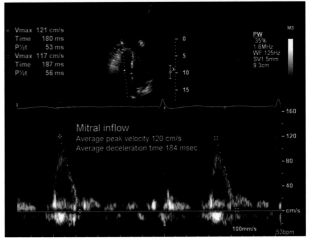

Figure 88-4

A. Normal diastolic function
B. Grade 3 diastolic dysfunction (restrictive filling)
C. Elevated left ventricular filling pressures
D. Normal left ventricular filling pressures
E. Indeterminate left ventricular filling pressures

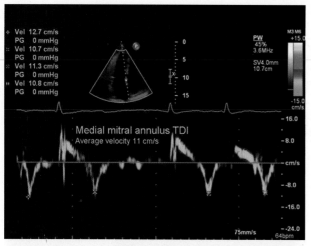

Figure 88-5

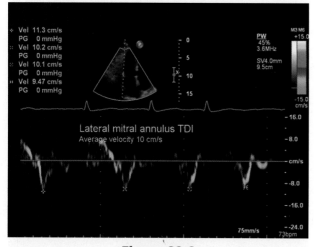

Figure 88-6

QUESTION 1. Based on a calculation of the left atrial volume by the area-length method (assume a body surface area of 2.1 m²), the patient's left atrial size is:

A. Normal
B. Mildly enlarged
C. Moderately enlarged
D. Severely enlarged

QUESTION 2. Based on the available data, which of the following statements correctly describes an assessment of diastolic function and left ventricular filling pressures?

QUESTION 3. The patient is considered for left atrial radiofrequency ablation. Before this she is referred for transesophageal echocardiography. Based on images (**Videos 88-4 and 88-5** and Fig. 88-7), which statement is correct?

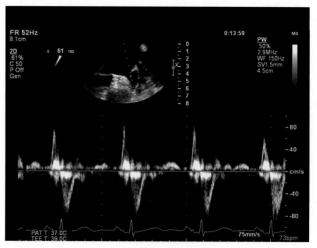

Figure 88-7

A. Direct current cardioversion is not indicated
B. The left atrial appendage (LAA) emptying velocities indicate a low likelihood of successful cardioversion
C. The LAA emptying velocities indicate an increased risk of future LAA thrombus
D. There is echocardiographic evidence of LAA thrombus

QUESTION 4. The patient undergoes successful radiofrequency wide area circumferential left atrial ablation. The day following the procedure, she is in sinus rhythm, but complains of mild sharp chest pains particularly when lying down. She is referred for transthoracic echocardiogram. Based on the available images

Video 88-6 through 88-9 and Figures 88-8 and 88-9, which of the following statements is correct?

A. Acute pericarditis is excluded based on the echocardiographic findings
B. There is evidence of a new anterior pericardial effusion
C. The mitral inflow and inferior vena cava are highly suggestive of constrictive physiology
D. A gated CT scan of the chest allows assessment of both the pericardium and pleural spaces.

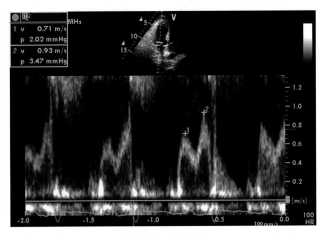

Figure 88-8

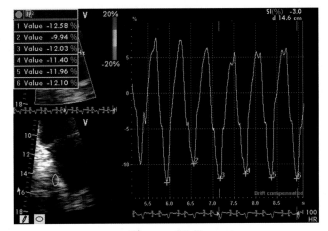

Figure 88-9

QUESTION 5. Which of the following statements is correct?

A. There is Doppler evidence of mildly reduced left atrial contractility
B. There is evidence of delayed relaxation (grade 1) left ventricular filling pattern
C. There is evidence of electrical but not mechanical left atrial function

QUESTION 6. The patient was dismissed on a combination of colchicine and indomethacin, but returned 1 week later with persistent chest pain and new shortness of breath. A repeat transthoracic echocardiogram was performed. Based on the images (**Videos 88-10 to 88-12**), which test will most likely be diagnostic?

A. A transesophageal echocardiogram
B. A repeat CT scan of the chest
C. A coronary angiogram
D. A 12-lead ECG

ANSWER 1: B. The left atrial volume should be measured based on four measurements at ventricular end systole: the area and the length in two orthogonal views (apical four-chamber and apical two-chamber views). The length is measured from the rear atrial wall to the valve plane in both views and averaged. A normal left atrial volume indexed to BSA is 22 ± 6 cc per m^2, a mildly enlarged LA 29 to 33 cc per m^2, a moderately dilated LA 34 to 39 cc per m^2, and a severely dilated LA ≥40 cc per m^2.

Here LA volume $= [(0.85)(A_1)(A_2)]/(L)$
$\qquad\qquad\quad = [(0.85)(23.4)(20.3)]/(6.2)$
$\qquad\qquad\quad = 65.1$ cc

LA volume index $= 65.1/2.1 = 31$ cc per m^2

See *The Echo Manual, 3rd Edition,* discussion of atrial size and volume on pages 110 and 112, and Appendix 8 on page 405.

ANSWER 2: E. The usual assessment of left ventricular diastolic function cannot be applied in the setting of atrial fibrillation. However, in some patients with atrial fibrillation, an estimate of left ventricular filling pressures may be made. A number of studies have suggested that an elevated E/e′ ratio particularly in the setting of a short deceleration time correlates well with elevated left ventricular filling pressures. However, here the constellation of findings is indeterminate. The E/e′ ratio of 10 to 12 is neither normal nor high but in the indeterminate range. The deceleration is also not particularly shortened. Hence, one is unable to confidently estimate left ventricular filling pressures in this situation.

ANSWER 3: A. There is clear evidence of electrical atrial activity (P waves) on ECG with evidence of normal LAA function on Doppler imaging, and hence cardioversion is not indicated. Normal LAA velocities are greater than 50 cm per second (here 70 to 80 cm per second).

See *The Echo Manual, 3rd Edition,* discussion of left atrial appendage flow velocities on page 394.

ANSWER 4: D. Although patients with acute pericarditis may display evidence of a pericardial effusion or constrictive physiology, many patients have a normal echocardiogram. There is a heterogeneously echo dense space anterior to the heart that represents fat rather than fluid. It was present also on preablation images. The classic findings of a restrictive mitral inflow pattern (high E-wave velocity that increases with expiration) and dilated IVC are not present. A CT chest does potentially allow assessment of both the pericardial and pleural spaces, although it can be difficult to separate a small amount of pericardial fluid from pericardial thickening.

As the patient has persistent pericardial pain, a CT chest was performed that was also unremarkable (**Video 88-13**).

ANSWER 5: A. Left atrial systolic strain assessment is emerging as high fidelity measure of left atrial contractility with a normal level more negative than −15%. Although the A-wave velocity is greater than the E-wave velocity, this does not represent a grade 1 diastolic dysfunction pattern but rather a "false" elevation because of a partly fused signal. Typically, if the E velocity is greater than 20 cm per second at the onset of the A wave (E at A, here 40 cm per second), both the A velocity and the E/A ratio may be affected.

ANSWER 6: B. Unlike the previous studies, there are now very poor apical images. Given this finding and in the setting of ongoing chest pain and new dyspnea and the sense of also on subcostal imaging of poor echo penetrance beyond the anterior pericardium, a pneumopericardium should be considered. A CT chest would be diagnostic in this situation.

Indeed, a CT chest (**Video 88-14**) confirms air in the pericardial space implicating a leak between the esophagus and the pericardial space as a delayed complication of the atrial ablation procedure. The patient was brought to the operating room where an abnormal communication was identified and repaired.

References

Pappone C, Oral H, Santinelli V, et al. Atrio-esophageal fistula as a complication of percutaneous transcatheter ablation of atrial fibrillation. *Circulation.* 2004;109(22):2724–2726.

Antonini-Canterin F, Nicolosi GL, Mascitelli L, et al. Direct demonstration of an air–fluid interface by two-dimensional echocardiography: a new diagnostic sign of hydropneumopericardium. *J Am Soc Echocardigr.* 1996;9(2):187–189.

CASE 89

Fever and Dyspnea with History of Severe Pancreatitis

*A*45-year-old man with a medical history of severe pancreatitis and pancreatic pseudocyst treated with a prolonged course of total parenteral nutrition. He had made a recovery with normal diet resumed 3 weeks prior. He now presents with fever and dyspnea. He is referred for transesophageal echocardiography (**Videos 89-1 to 89-17** and Figure 89-1).

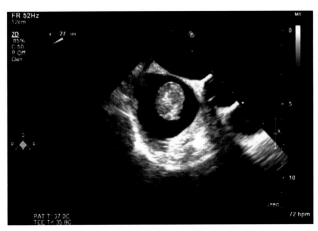

Figure 89-1

QUESTION 2. What is the incidence of thrombus formation in patients who have an indwelling central venous catheter?

  A. 1%
  B. 10%
  C. 30%
  D. 50%

QUESTION 1. What is the likely cause of the finding seen?

  A. Thrombus
  B. Atrial myxoma
  C. Tumor spread from renal cell carcinoma
  D. Papillary fibroelastoma

ANSWER 1: A. TEE demonstrates a large mobile mass attached to the upper right atrial wall and lower superior vena cava. Although an atrial myxoma is possible, approximately 90% of myxomas are attached to the intra-atrial septum. Thrombus is bar far the most likely and presumably is related to the central venous catheter that was recently in place for the parenteral nutrition. Tumor extension from a renal cell carcinoma would enter the right atrium from the inferior vena cava (**Video 89-18**).

ANSWER 2: B. The incidence of thrombus in either the superior vena cava or right atrium in patients with an indwelling central venous catheter has been reported to be between 2% and 17%.[1-3]

References

1. Merrer J, De Jonghe B, Golliot F, et al. French Catheter Study Group in Intensive Care. Complications of femoral and subclavian venous catheterization in critically ill patients: a randomized controlled trial. *JAMA*. 2001;286:700–707.

2. Timsit JF, Farkas JC, Boyer JM, et al. Central vein catheter-related thrombosis in intensive care patients: incidence, risks factors, and relationship with catheter-related sepsis. *Chest*. 1988;114:207–213.

3. Ghani MK, Boccalandro F, Denktas AE, et al. Right atrial thrombus formation associated with central venous catheters utilization in hemodialysis patients. *Intensive Care Med*. 2003;29:1829–1832.

CASE 90

Laterally Displaced Apical Impulse

A 22-year-old man is referred for an echocardiogram to evaluate 12 months of atypical chest pain. On examination, his apical impulse is displaced laterally and a soft mid-systolic murmur is audible.

QUESTION 1. Based on the echocardiographic images (Videos 90-1 to 90-7 and Figures 90-1 to 90-3), the most likely diagnosis is:

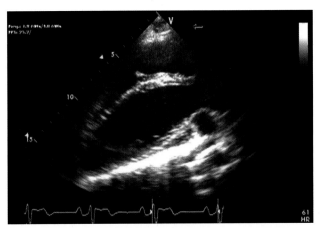

Figure 90-1

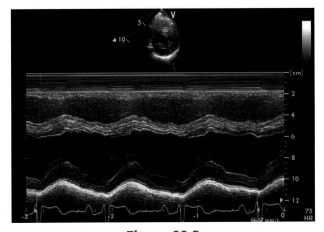

Figure 90-2

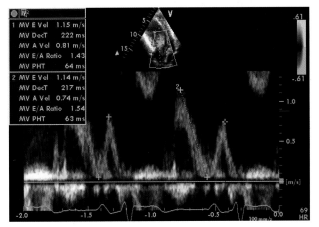

Figure 90-3

A. Pulmonary hypertension
B. Aortic valve stenosis
C. Ventricular septal defect
D. Congenital absence of the pericardium

QUESTION 2. The pulmonary vein pattern (Fig. 90-4) is:

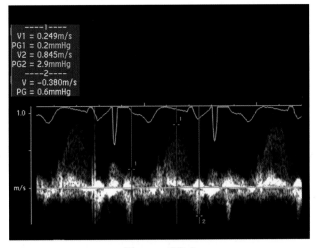

Figure 90-4

A. Suggestive of high left atrial pressure
B. Is to be expected in this condition
C. Suggestive of associated severe mitral valve regurgitation
D. Normal

QUESTION 3. Which of the following conditions has been associated with congenital absence of the pericardium?

A. Atrial septal defect
B. Bronchogenic cysts
C. Bicuspid aortic valve
D. All of the choices

ANSWER 1: D. The congenital complete absence of the left-sided pericardium is associated with a shift of the heart leftward and laterally with the right ventricle appearing bigger as more is seen in the standard parasternal images with an overall unusual orientation of the heart. The short-axis view demonstrates a paradoxical systolic anterior motion of the ventricular septum with vigorous left ventricular posterior wall movement. The apical four-chamber view of the heart has exaggerated mobility with a "swinging heart" and a displaced apex.

See *The Echo Manual, 3rd Edition,* **pages 289 to 290.**

ANSWER 2: B. Pulsed wave Doppler interrogation of the pulmonary vein indicates minimal systolic forward flow but rather filling of the left atrium during diastole. The typical indication for this is an elevation in left atrial pressure. However, it must be remembered that one of the physiologic components of normal atrial filling is the contribution of a decrease in pericardial pressure during ventricular ejection that is conferred to the atria and augment systolic atrial filling. This component will be lost in absence of the pericardium and hence is an expected finding in this case.

ANSWER 3: D. Congenital absence of the pericardium is associated with a high incidence of the listed abnormalities.

CASE 91

Ventricular Tachycardia with Rapid Palpitations

*A*35-year-old man with frequent episodes of ventricular tachycardia presents for his first echocardiogram. He was well until the previous 6 months when he began to develop episodes of rapid palpitations. Apart from a slow pulse rate (40 beats per minute), cardiovascular examination was normal.

QUESTION 1. What is the average left ventricular outflow tract (LVOT) diameter for men measured by echocardiography?

- A. 19 mm
- B. 21 mm
- C. 23 mm
- D. 25 mm
- E. 27 mm

QUESTION 2. Based on **Video 91-1** and Figure 91-1 (note the LVOT diameter is 23 mm), the calculated cardiac output is:

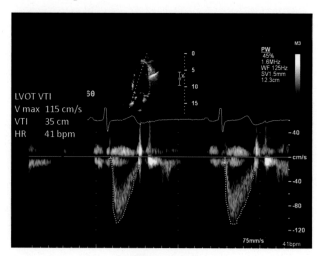

Figure 91-1

- A. 4.2 L per minute
- B. 5.3 L per minute
- C. 4.8 L per minute
- D. 5.9 L per minute
- E. 6.3 L per minute

QUESTION 3. Based on **Videos 91-2 and 91-3** and Figure 91-2, the pulmonary artery (PA) end-diastolic pressure is:

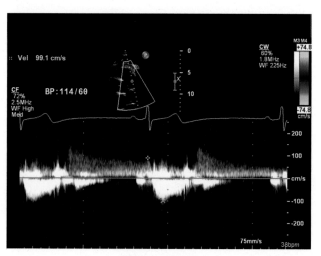

Figure 91-2

- A. Normal
- B. Mildly elevated
- C. Severely elevated

QUESTION 4. Based on the review of **Videos 91-4 to 91-13** and Figures 91-3 to 91-6, which of the following is the most likely process related to the right ventricular (RV) free wall?

- A. Artifact
- B. Pericardial cyst
- C. Benign primary cardiac tumor
- D. Aneurysm with thrombus

294

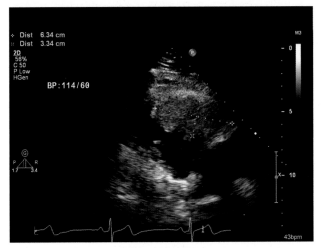

Figure 91-3

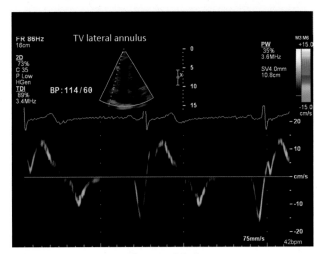

Figure 91-6

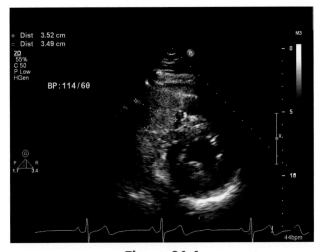

Figure 91-4

QUESTION 5. Based on the tricuspid annular tissue peak velocity, which of the following tricuspid annular plane systolic excursion (TAPSE) values would be expected?

  A. 2 mm

  B. 12 mm

  C. 22 mm

  D. 52 mm

QUESTION 6. The patient proceeds with surgical exploration (see **Videos 91-14 to 91-16** and Figure 91-7). Explain the type of artifact commonly experienced when imaging in the operating room.

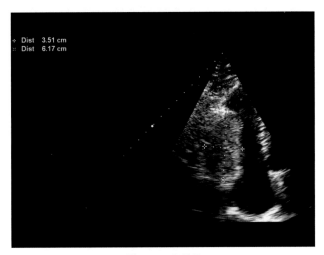

Figure 91-5

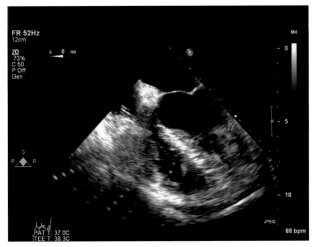

Figure 91-7

  A. Acoustic shadowing artifact

  B. Reverberation artifact

  C. Noise artifact

  D. Near-field clutter artifact

ANSWER 1: B. The mean LVOT diameter for men is 21 mm and for women 19 mm.

ANSWER 2: D. The cardiac output can be calculated as follows:

$$= 0.785 \text{ (LVOT diameter)}^2\text{(LVOT TVI)(HR)}$$
$$= 0.785 \, (2.3)^2(35)(41)$$
$$= 5.9 \text{ L per minute}$$

See *The Echo Manual, 3rd Edition*, discussion of stroke volume on page 116.

ANSWER 3: A. The PA end-diastolic pressure can be estimated by the sum of the peak pulmonary regurgitant jet velocity gradient and an estimate of right atrial pressure. Here the end PR velocity is quite normal at 1 m per second (i.e., a gradient of 4 mm Hg). Here the inferior vena cava is of normal size and collapses with inspiration, suggesting a normal right atrial pressure. This is a finding supported by normal physical examination findings.

ANSWER 4: C. Echocardiography demonstrates a large RV mass within the RV free wall, which appears well demarcated and separate from the surrounding myocardium and pericardium. Given the demarcation this suggests a benign rather than malignant process, although further testing is required.

ANSWER 5: C. Despite the RV free wall mass, the tricuspid annular systolic motion remains normal with a peak velocity of 15 to 16 cm per second. Hence, a normal TAPSE would be expected (likely in the range of 20 to 30 mm).

ANSWER 6: D. Commonly encountered in the operating room as illustrated in Figure 91-7 is noise artifact caused by electromagnetic interference from the use of cautery. Shadowing artifact is when there is apparent dropout beyond a highly reflective structure, such as the mitral sewing ring in **Video 91-17**. Reverberation artifact occurs when the ultrasound bounces backward and forward (reverberates) between two highly reflective surfaces. The artifact appears as multiple parallel lines situated in the far field extending away from the transducer (e.g., see Fig. 91-8). Near-field clutter, seen when structures particularly close to the transducer are characterized poorly, is due to high-amplitude oscillations of the piezoelectric elements in the transducer. An example of a near-field clutter artifact is shown in **Video 91-18**, where the apex of the left ventricle appears to have an indistinct endocardial border that to an untrained eye may suggest thrombus. The use of echo contrast confirms that, indeed, this is an artifact rather than thrombus (**Video 91-19**).

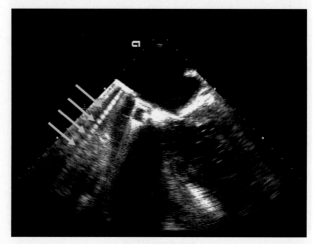

Figure 91-8

The patient proceeded to resection of the mass. Pathology confirmed it to be a hemangioma.

Cardiac hemangiomas[1] are rare benign primary cardiac tumors and have been reported to occur in almost every cardiac location. Often asymptomatic, clinical presentation will depend on size and location. Myocardial tumors as in this case may present with rhythm disturbances. Sudden death has been reported.

Reference

1. Mongal LS, Salat R, Anis A, et al. Enormous right atrial hemangioma in an asymptomatic patient: a case report and literature review. *Echocardiography*. 2009;26:973–976.

Chest Pain in a 52-Year-Old Woman

A 52-year-old woman presents for a transthoracic echocardiogram performed because of an episode of chest pain (**Videos 92-1 to 92-12** and Figs. 92-1 to 92-5).

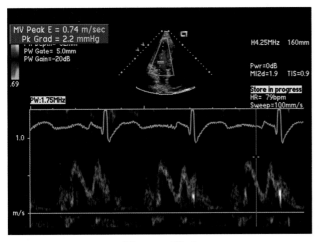

Figure 92-1

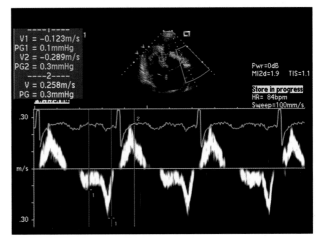

Figure 92-3

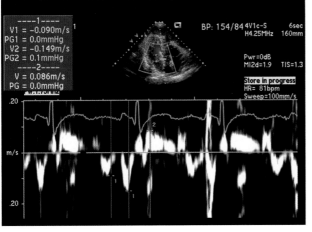

Figure 92-2

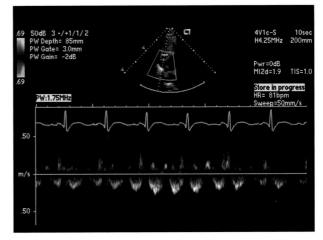

Figure 92-4

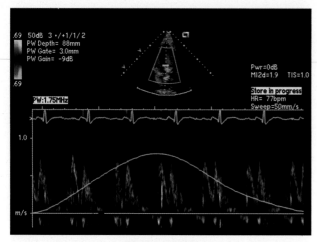

Figure 92-5

QUESTION 1. Findings are consistent with:

A. Pericardial effusion
B. Pericardial clot
C. Pericardial tumor
D. Pericardial cyst
E. Loculated pleural effusion with a normal pericardium

QUESTION 2. There are two-dimensional (2D) and Doppler features of constriction/tamponade.

A. True
B. False

QUESTION 3. Which of the following statements concerning the use of echo contrast is false (**Videos 92-13 and 92-14**)?

A. Echo contrast in this case confirms prominent vascularity
B. Echo contrast in this case confirms the presence of intrapericardial clot
C. Echo contrast in this case suggests a benign mass

QUESTION 4. Pericardial tumors are most commonly:

A. Benign primary tumors
B. Malignant primary tumors
C. Malignant secondary metastatic tumors

QUESTION 5. The patient underwent surgical removal. Pathology confirmed a leiomyosarcoma. Which of the following pieces of medical history is likely present?

A. Asbestos exposure
B. AIDS infection
C. Prior radiation for breast cancer
D. Prior Epstein–Barr virus infection

ANSWER 1: C. 2D imaging demonstrates a large irregular (9 × 3 cm) mass within the pericardial space adjacent to the cardiac apex (primarily the right ventricle). The pericardium is thickened, and there is an associated fluid collection.

ANSWER 2: B. Despite the large pericardial process, there is little to suggest hemodynamic significance. The mitral inflow is normal without respirophasic change. The septal motion is normal. The inferior vena cava is normal in size.

ANSWER 3: A. Echo contrast administration can be useful in the assessment of intracardiac masses where opacification is consistent with a vascular supply. The relatively rapid and complete opacification of the mass in this case (**Video 92-14**) implicates prominent vascularity.

ANSWER 4: C. As is the case with all cardiac tumors, metastatic tumors are by far the most common group. Of primary cardiac tumors, benign tumors are approximately twice as common as malignant tumors.

ANSWER 5: C. Leiomyosarcoma is a very rare primary cardiac malignancy derived from smooth muscle cells. Unlike many primary cardiac tumors, they commonly arise on the left side particularly in the left atrium. This tumor was likely stimulated in this patient by prior radiation therapy. Other rare cardiac tumors include mesothelioma (typically associated with prior asbestos exposure). AIDS is associated with Kaposi's sarcoma and lymphoma. Epstein–Barr virus is associated with lymphomas.

CASE 93

Soft Systolic Murmur after Fainting Episode

A 19-year-old college athlete is referred after a fainting episode while playing basketball on a hot humid day. A soft systolic murmur is heard on physical examination. He is referred for transthoracic echocardiography.

QUESTION 1. Which of the following constellations of findings is not a contraindication to participation in competitive athletics?

A. A low normal sized left ventricle (LV) with an ejection fraction (EF) of 70%, a ventricular diastolic septal diameter of 19 mm, and a global average peak systolic longitudinal strain of −14%

B. A mildly dilated LV with an EF of 60%, LV wall thickness of 15 mm, medial annular peak systolic tissue Doppler imaging of 12 cm per second, and e' velocity of 15 cm per second with a stroke volume index of 70 cc per m²

C. A normal LV size, left ventricular ejection fraction (LVEF) of 65%, left atrial volume index of 22 cm³ per m², a bicuspid aortic valve without stenosis or regurgitation, and a mid ascending aortic diameter of 52 mm

D. A normal LV size, LVEF 60%, cardiac output of 7.5 L per minute, normal aortic valve leaflet mobility, and transaortic time velocity integral of 110 cm

QUESTION 2. Based on review of his echocardiogram (**Videos 93-1 to 93-8** and Figs. 93-1 to 93-10), the likely finding on 12-lead ECG would be:

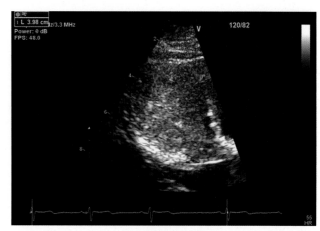

Figure 93-1

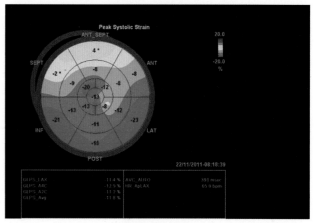

Figure 93-2

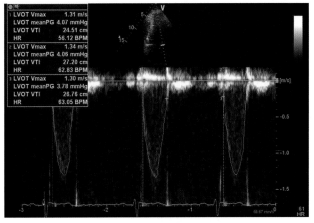

Figure 93-3

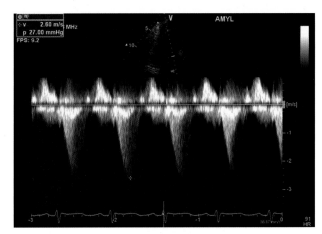

Figure 93-6

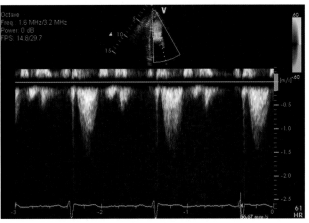

Figure 93-4

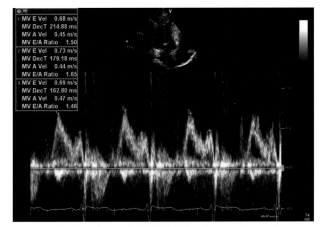

Figure 93-7

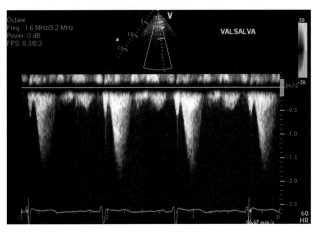

Figure 93-5

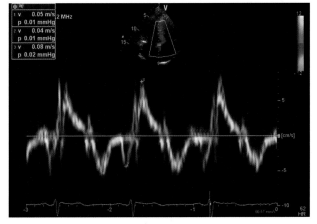

Figure 93-8

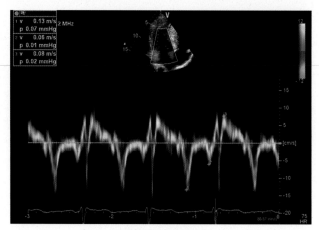

Figure 93-9

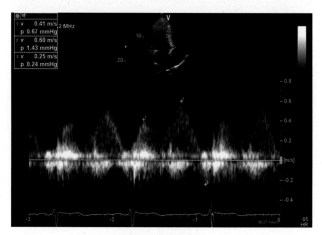

Figure 93-10

A. Low voltage
B. Deep symmetrical T wave inversions in the precordial leads
C. Diffuse ST segment elevation with PR segment depression
D. LV hypertrophy

QUESTION 3. Possible findings on genetic testing might include:

A. A defect in the gene encoding β-myosin heavy chain present in the patient and possibly a sibling
B. Genetic defect in cardiac troponin T in patient and in male but not in female relatives
C. Defect in the SCN5A cardiac sodium channel
D. Desmin gene mutation
E. Genetic testing would most likely be negative

QUESTION 4. Based on the two-dimensional (2D) images and Doppler findings at rest (Fig. 93-6), Valsalva (Fig. 93-7), and following amyl nitrate (Fig. 93-8), which of the following management strategies is preferred?

A. Alcohol septal ablation
B. Surgical myectomy
C. Diuretic therapy
D. β-Blocker therapy
E. Dihydropyridine calcium channel blocker, for example, amlodipine

QUESTION 5. The degree of septal hypertrophy (Fig. 93-1) correlates with the risk of sudden cardiac death.

A. True
B. False

QUESTION 6. Which of the following management steps is most appropriate?

A. Stop the metoprolol and arrange outpatient follow-up
B. Increase the metoprolol for presumed worsening outflow tract obstruction
C. Repeat transthoracic echocardiography
D. Obtain transesophageal echocardiography

QUESTION 7. He proceeds for elective placement of an implantable cardiac defibrillator, initiation of metoprolol, and is counseled to avoid competitive athletics. One week later, he returns with increased shortness of breath and an episode of syncope. Interrogation of his device demonstrates no dysrhythmia. On examination, his heart rate is 100 beats per minute, blood pressure (BP) 90/50 mm Hg, neck veins are elevated, and no murmurs are audible (at rest or with Valsalva). Based on the images obtained (**Videos 93-9 to 93-12** and Figs. 93-11 and 93-12), the likely hepatic vein profile would demonstrate:

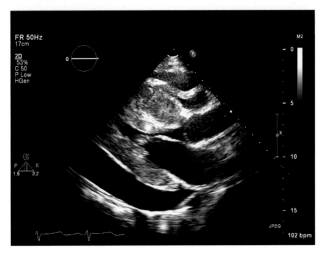

Figure 93-11

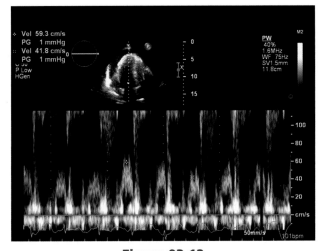

Figure 93-12

A. Systolic predominant forward flow with atrial flow reversals

B. Flow reversals in diastole that increase upon inspiration

C. Flow reversals in diastole that increase upon expiration

QUESTION 8. After ultrasound-guided pericardial access is obtained, the return is bloody. 10 cc of agitated saline is administered through the 16-gauge venous sheath (**Video 93-12**). Is it appropriate to proceed with placement of a sheath over a guidewire and a pericardial drain.

A. True

B. False

QUESTION 9. The laboratory findings (see table) on the pericardial fluid are most likely:

	Hemoglobin, g per dl	Total Nucleated Cells, per μl	Neutrophils, %	Lymphocytes, %	Glucose, mg per dl	Lactate Dehydrogenase, U per L
A.	0.8	11,000	90	1	69	
B.	0	180,000	98	0	<2	>10,000
C.	12	4,500	21	16		
D.	0.5	24,000	68	2	89	650
E.	0	160	15	75	100	700

ANSWER 1: B. After years of intense training, an athlete's heart may develop a global increase in LV wall thickness. This sometimes can be confused with hypertrophic cardiomyopathy (HCM). Unlike patients with HCM, an athlete's heart will tend to be upper normal in size or mildly enlarged with LV wall thicknesses no thicker than 17 mm with normal diastolic function, tissue Doppler, and strain imaging (e.g., option B, see example **Videos 93-13 to 93-15** and Fig. 93-13). This is in contrast to option A, where the LV is thick with global strain reduction describing a case of HCM. The presence of HCM is a contraindication to competitive athletics, and indeed HCM is the predominant abnormality that underlies sudden death in athletes. Other high risk factors include certain coronary anomalies and proarrhythmic conditions such as long QT syndrome or right ventricular (RV) dysplasia. Other conditions with which competitive athletes should be avoided include severe ascending aortic dilation (particularly in the setting of Marfan syndrome or bicuspid aortic valve, option C). Option D is concerning for severe sub- or supra-aortic stenosis.

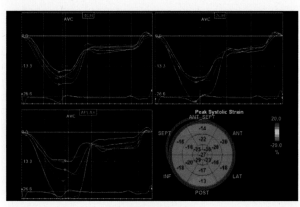

Figure 93-13

See *The Echo Manual, 3rd Edition,* discussion of athlete's heart versus HCM on page 267.

ANSWER 2: B. 2D echocardiography demonstrates global increase in LV mass with massive hypertrophy of the intraventricular septum. Evidence of LV hypertrophy would be expected on ECG. Low voltage would be expected in the setting of a large pericardial effusion or cardiac amyloidosis. ST segment elevation and PR depression is characteristic of acute pericarditis, and precordial T wave inversion is characteristic of apical variant of HCM.

ANSWER 3: A. Septal variant HCM is commonly associated with a gene defect and is typically autosomal dominant; hence, defects in male or female first-degree relatives are common. Hence, first-degree relatives require phenotypic and/or genetic screening. The most common defects are those encoding β-myosin heavy chain. Defects in cardiac troponin T are also well described. Defects in the SCN5A sodium channel gene are characteristic of Brugada syndrome, and desmin gene mutations are associated with RV dysplasia.

ANSWER 4: D. Despite the massive septal hypertrophy, there is little outflow tract obstruction at rest or inducible. Hence, there is no evidence to suggest a septal reduction procedure will provide any clinical benefit. Moreover, these procedures are reserved for symptomatic patients with significant outflow tract obstruction despite optimal medical therapy. Vasodilator agents such as diuretics or dihydropyridine calcium channel blocker should be avoided. The patient should be prescribed β-blocker therapy.

ANSWER 5: A. Echocardiography in this case demonstrates severe increase in LV wall thickness with massive thickening of the intraventricular septum (septal dimension of 43 mm). The degree of LV hypertrophy is associated with an increased risk of sudden cardiac death, particularly with a maximum thickness greater than 30 mm. Other frequently cited risk factors of sudden cardiac death in patients with HCM include an abnormal BP response to exercise, nonsustained ventricular tachycardia or frequent episodes of syncope, and a family history of sudden cardiac death.

The magnitude of hypertrophy is related directly to the risk of sudden death. The cumulative risk for sudden death is near 0% for a wall thickness of 19 mm or less and 40% for a thickness of 30 mm or more.

ANSWER 6: C. In a patient with a recent device placed who presents with shortness of breath, syncope, tachycardia, hypotension, and evidence of venous hypertension, one should consider transthoracic echocardiogram to evaluate for the presence of cardiac tamponade.

ANSWER 7: C. Echocardiography demonstrates a large circumferential pericardial effusion with features of tamponade. Best seen on **Video 93-9** and Figure 93-11, there is marked early diastolic RV collapse, consistent with elevated intrapericardial pressure. The inferior vena cava is plethoric with minimal respiratory change, also consistent with high right atrial pressure. The hallmark in the hepatic veins of cardiac tamponade is the presence of diastolic flow reversals that increase with expiration (Fig. 93-14).

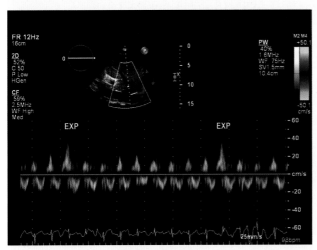

Figure 93-14

ANSWER 8: A. Whenever one gets a bloody return from pericardial access, it is critical to confirm that you are in the pericardial space rather than in an intracardiac chamber. Administration of agitated saline with echo imaging (**Video 93-12**) confirms a pericardial location. The agitated saline fails to rapidly pass throughout the pericardial space likely because of the bloody content.

See *The Echo Manual, 3rd Edition,* discussion of echocardiographically guided pericardiocentesis on page 293, and Figure 17-12 on page 296.

ANSWER 9: C. A large pericardial effusion occurring immediately after device placement is most likely related to lead perforation. In this insistence, a hemorrhagic effusion is expected. A hemoglobin in pericardial fluid >50% of the serum hemoglobin is consistent with a hemorrhagic effusion caused by perforation. This does not always require surgical management. If the site of perforation is small and patient is stable, following evacuation of the bloody effusion and maintenance of a dry pericardial space (through intermittent aspiration of the pericardial drain) will frequently allow the perforation site to heal. Blood in the pericardial space is very irritative. Patients frequently develop significant pericardial pain following aspiration and need aggressive treatment with intrapericardial lidocaine, oral and/or intravenous nonsteroidal anti-inflammatories and in are practice frequently also receive colchicine. As a precaution against the development of pericardial constriction, a course of maintenance scheduled anti-inflammatory therapy is used for 4 to 6 weeks following centesis. Options A and B are examples of the most common patterns with reasonably high levels of nucleated cells, mostly neutrophils, with low levels of hemoglobin, typically of effusions occurring in the setting of acute pericarditis. The pattern of a more chronic serous effusion is highlighted in option E with low cell counts, predominantly lymphocytes. Option B with a very high cell, lactate dehydrogenase count, and very low glucose occurs in the setting of highly inflammatory pericarditis because of a rheumatologic illness such as rheumatoid arthritis or systemic lupus erythematosus or an acute bacterial pericarditis.

References

Spirito P, Bellone P, Harris KM, et al. Magnitude of left ventricular hypertrophy and risk of sudden death in hypertrophic cardiomyopathy. *N Engl J Med.* 2000;342:1778–1785.

McKenna WJ, Behr ER. Hypertrophic cardiomyopathy: management, risk stratification, and prevention of sudden death. *Heart.* 2002;87:169.

Maron BJ, McKenna WJ, Danielson GK, et al. American College of Cardiology/European Society of Cardiology clinical expert consensus document on hypertrophic cardiomyopathy. A report of the American College of Cardiology Foundation Task Force on Clinical Expert Consensus Documents and the European Society of Cardiology Committee for Practice Guidelines. *J Am Coll Cardiol.* 2003;42:1687.

CASE 94

Murmur in a 38-Year-Old Patient

A 38-year-old patient presents for an echocardiogram to evaluate a murmur. Systemic blood pressure is 140/80 mm Hg. See **Videos 94-1 to 94-18** and Figures 94-1 to 94-9.

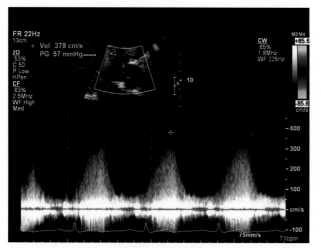

Figure 94-1

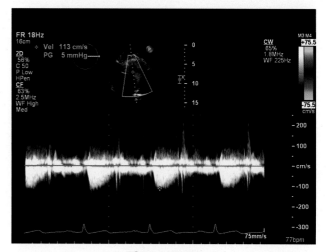

Figure 94-3

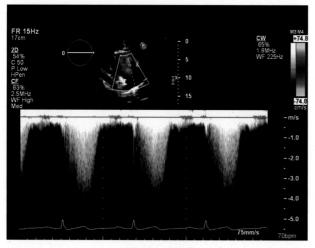

Figure 94-2

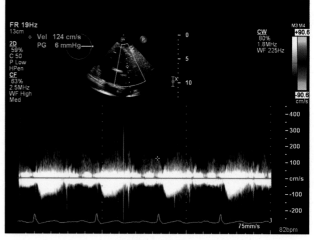

Figure 94-4

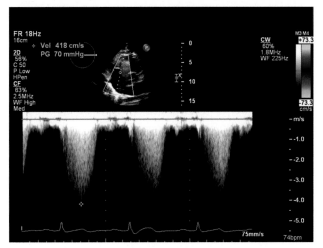

Figure 94-5

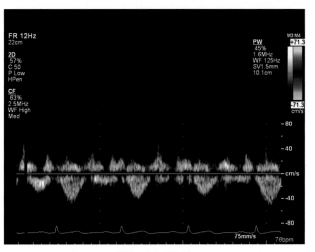

Figure 94-8

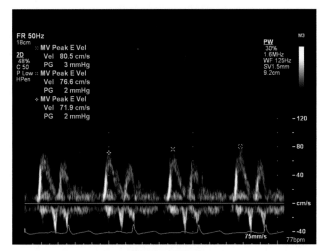

Figure 94-6

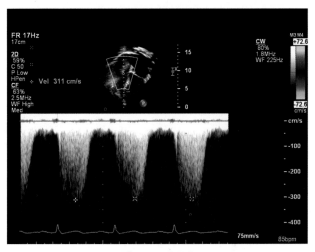

Figure 94-9

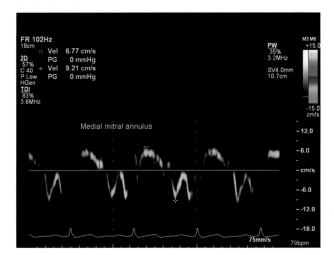

Figure 94-7

QUESTION 1. Which of the following defects is related to the abnormal flow?

- A. Atrial septal defect
- B. Gerbode defect
- C. Membranous ventricular septal defect (VSD)
- D. Ruptured sinus of Valsalva aneurysm

QUESTION 2. The expected physical examination finding is:

- A. A harsh pansystolic murmur
- B. A soft or potentially absent systolic murmur
- C. A midpeaking systolic ejection murmur
- D. A continuous murmur

QUESTION 3. The estimated right ventricular (RV) systolic pressure in this case is:

   A. 40 mm Hg
   B. 50 mm Hg
   C. 65 mm Hg
   D. 100 mm Hg

QUESTION 4. The likely grade of diastolic function/dysfunction based on the available data is:

   A. Normal
   B. Mild (grade 1) diastolic dysfunction
   C. Moderate (grade 2) diastolic dysfunction
   D. Severe (grade 3) diastolic dysfunction

QUESTION 5. Findings that would be attributable to this defect that warrants consideration of intervention include all of the following *except*:

   A. An elevated pulmonary vascular resistance
   B. Progressive RV dilation in the absence of pulmonary hypertension
   C. Severe tricuspid valve regurgitation (TR)
   D. Left ventricular (LV) dilation

ANSWER 1: C. There is evidence of left-right flow from LV to RV through a membranous VSD. This is the most common type of VSD seen in adult patients. A Gerbode defect is an unusual VSD communicating directly between the LV and the right atrium. This is often iatrogenic occurring at the time of valve replacement.

See *The Echo Manual, 3rd Edition,* discussion of types of VSDs and imaging notes on pages 337 to 344.

ANSWER 2: A. The murmur of a VSD is pansystolic with little if any diastolic component. It is mediated by the large pressure gradient in systole between the LV and RV. Unless the patient develops pulmonary hypertension and secondary RV hypertension, the murmur is typically loud as the gradient is high. An audible diastolic component suggests either there is an alternate communication rather than VSD, for example, aortic to atrial communication (e.g., sinus of Valsalva rupture), or there is an additional lesion.

ANSWER 3: A. In this patient, the TR Doppler profile is frequently contaminated by the Doppler signal from the VSD. Hence, one must be careful not to overestimate the TR velocity leading to an overestimate of pulmonary pressures. In a patient with a VSD, it is always prudent to assess pulmonary artery pressures by three methods:

(i) Based on the following equation:

RV systolic pressure = LV systolic pressure – peak VSD systolic gradient (in the absence of LV outflow tract obstruction peak LV systolic pressure = systolic blood pressure)

$$RV \text{ systolic pressure} = LV \text{ systolic pressure} - 4v^2$$
$$= LV \text{ systolic pressure} - 4(5)^2$$
$$= 140 - 100 = 40 \text{ mm Hg}$$

(ii) By the standard fashion ($4v^2$ + right atrial pressure (RAP), where v = peak TR velocity

(iii) Estimation of pulmonary artery diastolic pressure (PADP) by ($4v^2$ + RAP), where v = end PR velocity

The end PR velocity is quite normal (1 m per second) as is the estimated RA pressure with a normal sized inferior vena cava and a normal pulsed wave Doppler profile in the hepatic vein. Hence, the estimated PADP is normal at 9 to 10 mm Hg. This suggests against the presence of pulmonary hypertension.

On the basis of the estimated RV systolic pressure by the VSD gradient and the fact that pulmonary artery diastolic RA pressures are normal, we can work back and estimate that the transtricuspid (RA–RV) gradient is approximately 35 mm Hg, and hence the expected TR peak velocity is 3 m per second (Fig. 94-8).

Indeed, this corresponds with the one clear signal that appears uncontaminated.

See *The Echo Manual, 3rd Edition,* page 162 and Figure 10-11 on page 164.

ANSWER 4: A. The combination of a normal mitral inflow pattern (E/A ratio of 1.3), a normal deceleration time (200 milliseconds), and a normal E/e' ratio of 8.8 is compatible with normal diastolic function.

ANSWER 5: B. A small restrictive VSD like in this case rarely causes clinical complication, unless there is progressive valvular destruction, for example, TR in this case. A larger defect may lead to progressive pulmonary hypertension or LV dilation, either of which would be an indication of intervention. A VSD, however, should not cause isolated RV dilation, as the increased volume of blood enters the RV only during systole, where it passes directly through the open pulmonary valve into the pulmonary circulation. The presence of RV enlargement in the setting of a VSD should prompt the echocardiographer to seek an alternate explanation, for example, atrial septal defect, anomalous pulmonary vein, or pulmonary hypertension.

Systolic Murmur in a Female Phlebotomist

A 24-year-old female phlebotomist is referred for an echocardiogram (**Videos 95-1 to 95-12** and Figs. 95-1 to 95-11) after a systolic murmur was heard on a preemployment physical examination.

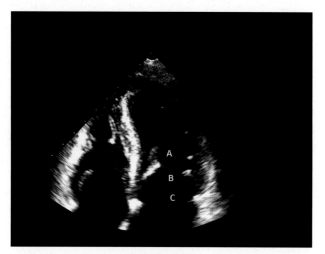

Figure 95-1

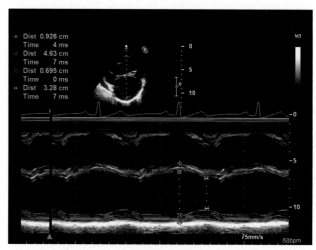

Figure 95-3

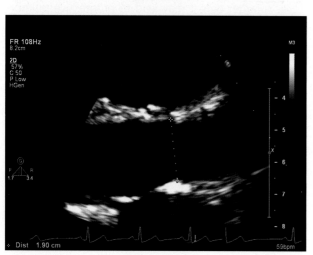

Figure 95-2

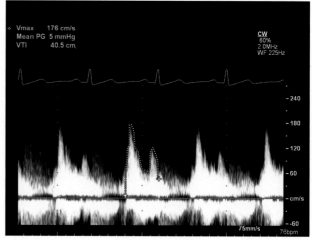

Figure 95-4

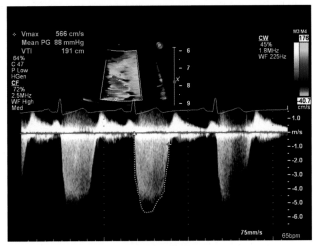

Figure 95-5

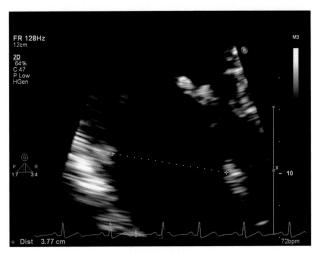

Figure 95-8

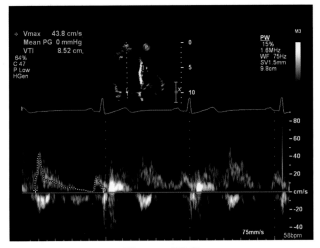

Figure 95-6

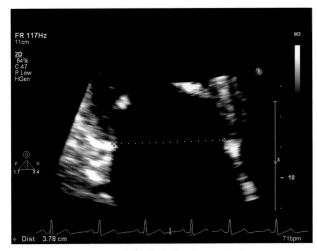

Figure 95-9

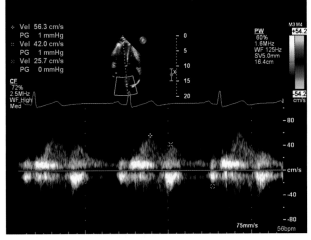

Figure 95-7

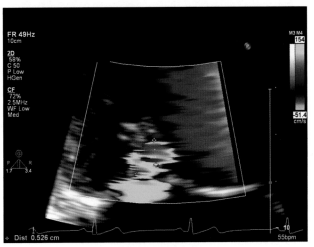

Figure 95-10

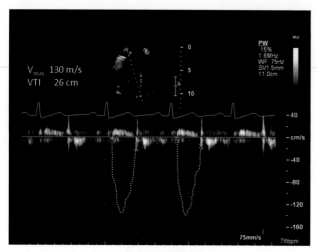

Figure 95-11

QUESTION 1. What condition is present?

A. Mitral valve (MV) prolapse

B. Rheumatic MV stenosis

C. Parachute MV

D. MV arcade (Hammock valve)

E. Cleft MV

QUESTION 2. This question relates to the quantification of mitral valve regurgitation (MR) by the volumetric or continuity method. What is the appropriate location of the sample volume to determine the time velocity integral (TVI) of transmitral flow (Fig. 95-1)?

A. Pulsed wave Doppler based on a sample volume in position A

B. Pulsed wave Doppler based on a sample volume in position B

C. Pulsed wave Doppler based on a sample volume in position C

D. Depth of sample volume not important as continuous wave Doppler should be used

QUESTION 3. This question also relates to the quantification of MR by the volumetric or continuity method. An inaccurately over measured mitral annulus diameter will lead to:

A. An overestimation of the MR

B. An underestimation of the MR

QUESTION 4. Quantify the severity of the MR.

A. Mild to moderate

B. Moderate to severe

C. Severe

QUESTION 5. The patient was referred for transesophageal echocardiography (**Videos 95-13 to 95-16**) that confirms the findings seen on the transthoracic echocardiogram. Based on the pulmonary vein pulsed wave Doppler interrogation (Fig. 95-12):

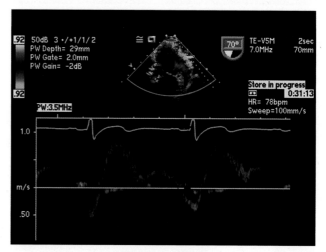

Figure 95-12

A. Findings are consistent with severe pulmonary hypertension

B. Findings are consistent with severe MR

C. Findings are consistent with elevated left atrial pressure

D. Doppler profile is normal

QUESTION 6. Based on Figure 95-13 (using a simplified version of the PISA method), what is the estimated MR volume?

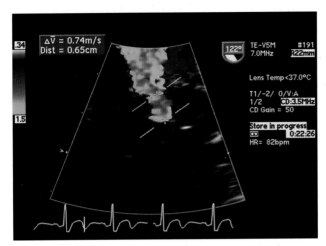

Figure 95-13

A. 20 cc

B. 30 cc

C. 40 cc

D. 50 cc

ANSWER 1: D. Two-dimensional images demonstrate thickened margins of the MV with restricted motion of the anterior MV leaflet. At first glance, one might suspect rheumatic MV stenosis with almost a "hockey stick" appearance to the anterior leaflet (**Video 95-1**). However, the leaflet itself is not thickened, and notably on short axis, there is no commissural fusion (**Videos 95-4 and 95-5**). It is apparent that the MV leaflets appear to directly insert into the papillary muscle with little, if any, chordae (**Video 95-2**). As we scan down to the mid left ventricle (**Video 95-6**), there are two normally positioned papillary muscles excluding a parachute MV. Apical views further underscore that the MV leaflets, particularly anterior leaflet, are inserting directly into the papillary muscles. The two-chamber views illustrate leaflets that directly insert into the papillary muscles, but also are attached with an echo bright, likely fibrous, band of tissue. This arc of tissue restricts leaflet, particularly anterior leaflet excursion. This may impede left ventricular filling or as in this case alter leaflet geometry and give rise to regurgitation.

MV arcade is a rare congenital anomaly of MV development, whereas in this case, the MV chordae are underdeveloped and either very short and thick or absent with the valve leaflet tips inserting directly into the papillary muscle. It is presumed that the lesion arises as an arrest in the normal MV development. Typically, the anterior leaflet is affected to a greater extent than the posterior leaflet. The valvular orifice, seen on short axis, is normal.

This should be recognized as being distinct from rheumatic mitral stenosis (**Videos 95-17 to 95-19**) or a parachute MV (**Videos 95-20 to 95-23**) for the reasons discussed.

ANSWER 2: C. Unlike the positioning of the sample volume for the assessment of diastolic function for the assessment of stroke volume through the MV, the sample must be placed at the mitral annulus (option C). Akin to the stroke volume calculation at the left ventricular outflow tract (LVOT) level, the stroke volume is calculated after the integration of the mitral annular area and the TVI.

ANSWER 3: A. The MR volume = the MV flow − left ventricular stroke volume

If the mitral annulus is overestimated, the MV flow is overestimated. As the radius of the mitral vale annulus is squared, error in measurement is multiplied in the calculation of flow.

See *The Echo Manual, 3rd Edition,* **discussion of volumetric method in the assessment of MR on page 213.**

ANSWER 4: A.

Quantifying MR by the PISA method

The regurgitant flow can be calculated as follows:

$$\text{Flow rate} = (r)^2 \times 6.28 \times \text{aliasing velocity}$$
$$= (0.53 \text{ cm})^2 \times 6.28 \times 51 \text{ cm per second}$$
$$= 90 \text{ cc per second}$$

Effective regurgitant orifice (ERO) = Flow rate/peak MR velocity

$$= 90 \text{ cc per second}/570 \text{ cm per second}$$
$$= 0.17 \text{ cm}^2$$

$$\text{MR volume} = \text{ERO} \times \text{MR}_{TVI}$$
$$= 0.17 \times 191 = 32 \text{ cc.}$$

See *The Echo Manual, 3rd Edition,* **discussion of PISA method on page 215.**

Quantifying MR by the volumetric method

$$\text{MR volume} = \text{MV flow} - \text{LVOT flow}$$
$$= (\text{Annulus D}^2 \times 0.785 \times \text{TVI})_{MV} - (\text{annulus D}^2 \times 0.785 \times \text{TVI})_{LVOT}$$
$$= (3.8^2 \times 0.785 \times 9)_{MV} - (1.9^2 \times 0.785 \times 26)_{LVOT}$$
$$= 102 - 74 = 28 \text{ cc}$$

Summary: The degree of MR by either the PISA or volumetric method is at the lower range of grade II/IV (mild to moderate) regurgitation.

ANSWER 5: D. In severe MR, there may be systolic flow reversal in the pulmonary vein; however, the absence of systolic flow reversal in the pulmonary vein does not exclude severe MR. The systolic forward flow into the left atrium is also blunted in other causes of elevated left atrial pressure.

See *The Echo Manual, 3rd Edition,* **Figure 12-34 on page 213, and discussion of pulmonary vein flow velocities on pages 126 and 127.**

ANSWER 6: B. The PISA method can be simplified, which is especially helpful when the peak velocity of the MR jet cannot be obtained.[1] In addition, simplification is helpful in determining the severity of MR intraoperatively when a surgical decision needs to be made without delay. The PISA method can be simplified in several different ways, and all the methods are based on the same formula.

See *The Echo Manual, 3rd Edition* on page 216.

The relation between the TVI and the peak velocity of MR has been shown to be relatively constant. Hence, usually

$$\frac{MR_{TVI}}{MR_{velocity}} = \frac{1}{3.25}$$

Therefore, one can simplify the equation as follows:

Mitral RegV = ERO × MRTVI

$$= \frac{6.28 \times r^2 \times \text{aliasing velocity} \times MR_{TVI}}{MR_{Velocity}}$$

$$= 6.28 \times r^2 \times \text{aliasing velocity} \times \frac{MR_{TVI}}{MR_{Velocity}}$$

Therefore,

$$MR\ RegV = \frac{6.28 \times r^2 \times \text{aliasing velocity}}{3.25}$$

$$= \frac{\text{PISA flow rate}}{3.25}$$

$$= 2r^2 \times \text{aliasing velocity}$$

$$= 2\ (0.65^2) \times 34$$

$$= 29\ \text{cc}$$

One can also estimate the ERO by assuming the MR velocity is 5 m per second as follows:

$$ERO = 6.28\ (r^2) \times \frac{\text{aliasing velocity}}{MR\ Velocity}$$

If one assumes the MR velocity is 500 cm per second, then

$$ERO = \frac{6.28 \times r^2 \times 36\ \text{cm per second}}{500\ \text{cm per second}} = 0.45\ (r^2)$$

$$= 0.2\ \text{cm}^2$$

Reference

1. Rossi A, Dujardin KS, Bailey KR, et al. Rapid estimation of regurgitant volume by the proximal isovelocity surface area method in mitral regurgitation: can continuous-wave Doppler echocardiography be omitted? *J Am Soc Echocardiogr.* 1998;11:138–148.

CASE 96

Exertional Shortness of Breath with Episode of Atrial Flutter

A 40-year-old man presents for the evaluation of symptoms of exertional shortness of breath. Over the past 9 months, he has had three episodes of symptomatic self-limited palpitations, one of which was documented as atrial flutter. He has no other cardiac history. On examination his blood pressure is 140/70 mm Hg. His jugular venous pulse is normal. He has a mild parasternal lift. Normal heart sounds and a 1–2/6 systolic ejection murmur along with the lower left sternal border.

QUESTION 1. Based on review of the transthoracic echo images (**Videos 96-1 to 96-11** and Figs. 96-1 to 96-6), which of the following statements is correct?

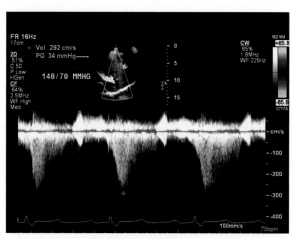

Figure 96-1

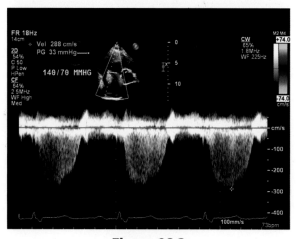

Figure 96-2

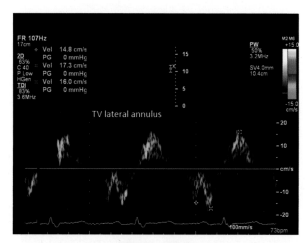

Figure 96-3

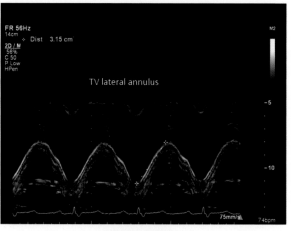

Figure 96-4

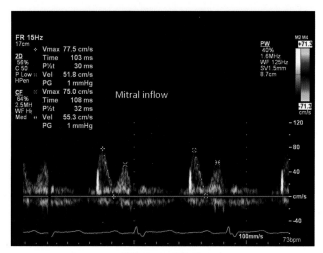

Figure 96-5

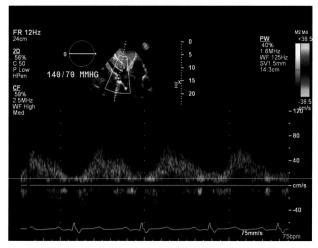

Figure 96-6

A. Normal right ventricular (RV) size
B. Mild to moderate RV enlargement
C. Moderate to severe RV enlargement

QUESTION 2. Based on Figures 96-3 and 96-4, which of the following statements is correct?

A. The tricuspid annular plane excursion (TAPSE) and RV tissue Doppler imaging TDI are both compatible with normal RV contractility
B. The TAPSE and RV TDI are both compatible with reduced RV contractility
C. The TAPSE but not the RV TDI is compatible with normal RV contractility
D. The RV TDI but not the TAPSE is compatible with normal RV contractility

QUESTION 3. The patient's symptoms are likely due to:

A. Pulmonary hypertension
B. Tricuspid valve prolapse
C. Sinus venosus atrial septal defect
D. Anomalous right-sided pulmonary venous drainage
E. RV cardiomyopathy

ANSWER 1: C. Echocardiographic images demonstrate moderate to severe enlargement in RV size. In the apical four-chamber view, the RV is similar or slightly larger the left ventricle.

ANSWER 2: A. The muscle fibers responsible for the majority of RV contractility are orientated in the longitudinal plane with the base of the RV moving down toward the apex during systole. Two simple measures of this longitudinal contractility are the TAPSE obtained by placing an M-mode cursor through the tricuspid annulus and measuring the distance of annular excursion during systole (normal excursion is greater than 20 mm). The other measure is achieved by placing a tissue Doppler sample volume at the tricuspid annulus and measuring the peak velocity of systolic annular excursion (normal being >14 to 15 cm per second). Both measures here are quite normal.

ANSWER 3: D. Echocardiography demonstrates moderate to severe RV enlargement with flattening of the interventricular septum during diastole compatible with RV volume overload. The tricuspid regurgitant velocity is upper normal and not the cause of the RV enlargement but rather a consequence of the lesion described below. Subcostal imaging demonstrates an abnormal vessel draining into the inferior vena cava opposite the hepatic vein. Color Doppler interrogation demonstrates flow into the IVC through both systole and diastole. Pulse wave interrogation confirms a pulmonary venous flow pattern. This lesion is referred to as the "Scimitar syndrome"[1] when the right lower pulmonary vein drains into the IVC inferior vena cava. The syndrome is so named, as the abnormal pulmonary vein(s) give a curvilinear pattern on chest X-ray resembling the middle Eastern sabre.

The lower right lung is commonly hypoplastic.

See *The Echo Manual, 3rd Edition*, discussion of anomalous pulmonary veins on pages 343 to 345.

Reference

Vida VL, Padalino MA, Boccuzzo G, et al. Scimitar syndrome. A European Congenital Heart Surgeons Association (ECHSA) multicentric study. *Circulation*. 2010;122(12):1159–1166.

CASE 97

Primary Biliary Cirrhosis

A 43-year-old woman with primary biliary cirrhosis is referred for echocardiography (Videos 97-1 to 97-9 and Figs. 97-1 to 97-8).

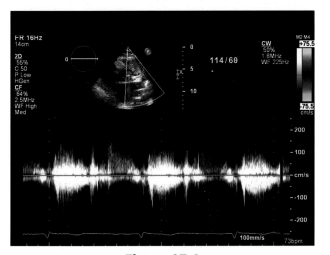

Figure 97-1

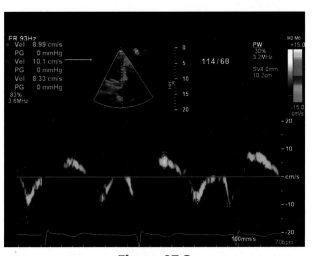

Figure 97-3

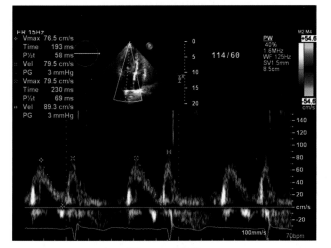

Figure 97-2

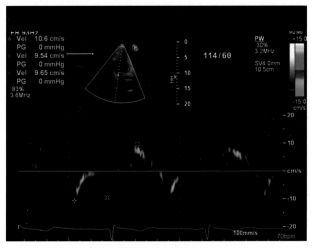

Figure 97-4

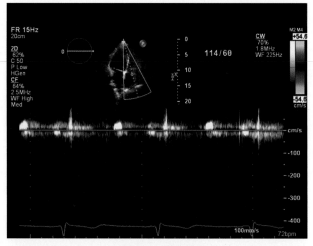

Figure 97-5

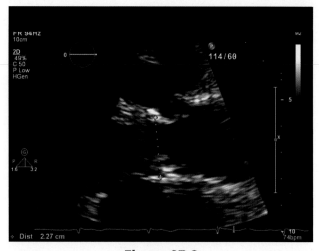

Figure 97-8

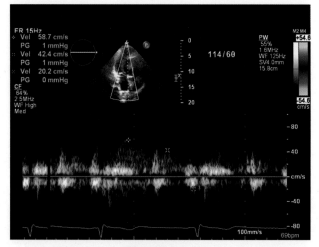

Figure 97-6

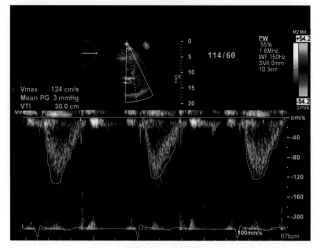

Figure 97-7

QUESTION 1. Appropriate indications for a transthoracic echocardiogram for patients with cirrhosis include:

A. Screen for the presence of pulmonary hypertension

B. Screen for the presence of intrapulmonary shunt

C. Evaluate an asymptomatic 2/6 systolic ejection murmur

D. Screen for the presence of pulmonary hypertension and intrapulmonary shunt

E. Screen for the presence of pulmonary hypertension and intrapulmonary shunt, and evaluate an asymptomatic 2/6 systolic ejection murmur

QUESTION 2. The cardiac index (body surface area = 1.5) in this case is:

A. In the expected range for patients with cirrhosis in patients with cirrhosis

B. Not in the range of what is expected in patients with cirrhosis

QUESTION 3. Agitated saline administration shows evidence of:

A. Intracardiac shunt

B. Persistent left superior vena cava

C. Intrapulmonary shunt

D. No right-left shunt

QUESTION 4. The significance of a large intrapulmonary shunt in patients with cirrhosis is:

A. A relative contraindication to liver transplantation
B. No impact on the timing of liver transplantation
C. A factor that may lead to an earlier transplant date

QUESTION 5. The presence of a right ventricular systolic pressure greater than 60 mm Hg in patients with cirrhosis is:

A. A relative contraindication to liver transplantation
B. No impact on the timing of liver transplantation
C. A factor that may lead to an earlier transplant date

QUESTION 6. A peak tricuspid regurgitant (TR) velocity/right ventricular outflow tract time velocity integral (RVOT TVI) greater than 0.12 in patients with cirrhosis:

A. Suggests portopulmonary hypertension
B. Suggests hepatopulmonary syndrome
C. Is typical
D. Is of little value

ANSWER 1: D. Patients with liver disease may commonly have evidence of pulmonary hypertension, intrapulmonary shunting, and systolic murmurs. Their significance is discussed in subsequent answers.

ANSWER 2: A. The hyperdynamic circulation associated with cirrhosis is typically characterized by high cardiac output and index as in this case.

Cardiac index = $[D^2 \times 0.785 \times TVI_{LVOT} \times HR]/BSA$

Cardiac index = $[2.3^2 \times 0.785 \times 30 \times 67]/1.5$
$= 5.2$ L/min/m^2

ANSWER 3: C. After administration of agitated saline, there is a delayed right-left shunt seen approximately 6 to 7 beats after saline first appears in the right-sided chambers, this is strongly suggestive of an intrapulmonary shunt.

Following agitated saline administration intravenously, if an atrial shunt is present, bubbles will appear immediately in the left atrium after being seen in the right atrium. In case of a left–right shunt, a negative contrast effect is seen. If the patient has an intrapulmonary shunt, more than three cardiac cycles may be needed for the bubbles to go through the pulmonary circulation before they appear in the left atrium.

Another indication for agitated saline is the evaluation of a persistent left superior vena cava that drains into the coronary sinus. In this case, agitated saline should be injected into a left arm vein. The enlarged coronary sinus in the left atrioventricular groove will be opacified first.

ANSWER 4: C. The evaluation for an intrapulmonary shunt is an important one as it is an indicator of possible hepatopulmonary syndrome, a pulmonary vasodilatory disorder that may complicate advanced liver disease.[1]

In patients who have evidence of delayed shunting on contrast echocardiography and have hypoxia (with normal chest X-ray and pulmonary function testing), a diagnosis of hepatopulmonary syndrome is made. Patients with hepatopulmonary syndrome do particularly poorly without liver transplantation, and hence patients may be given a higher priority for transplantation.

ANSWER 5: A. Another critical component of the echocardiographic assessment of patients with cirrhosis is an accurate assessment of pulmonary artery pressures. A significant minority of patients with cirrhosis have an elevated pulmonary artery systolic pressure. This is of major significance as patients with cirrhosis and uncontrolled pulmonary hypertension have an excessive perioperative transplant mortality. An estimated right ventricular systolic pressure greater than 50 mm Hg in a patient with cirrhosis (or unexplained right-sided chamber enlargement) should undergo confirmatory right heart catheterization to evaluate for the presence and severity of pulmonary hypertension. Catheterization will help distinguish a flow-mediated pulmonary hypertension (in the setting of high output) from a pulmonary arteriopathy with a high pulmonary vascular resistance (portopulmonary hypertension). The presence of portopulmonary hypertension is a contraindication for liver transplant, although selected patients may successfully receive a transplant if their pulmonary hypertension is controlled with therapy.

ANSWER 6: A. Although the majority of patients with cirrhosis have a high cardiac output and normal/low pulmonary vascular resistance, approximately 5% of patients with cirrhosis develop portopulmonary hypertension. An elevation in the ratio the of peak TR velocity to the RVOT TVI (>0.12) is associated with an elevated pulmonary vascular resistance on cardiac catheterization.[2]

References

1. Rodriguez-Roisin R, Krowka MJ. Hepatopulmonary syndrome. *N Engl J Med.* 2008;358:2378–2387.

2. Farzaneh-Far R, McKeown BH, Dang D, et al. Accuracy of Doppler-estimated pulmonary vascular resistance in patients before liver transplantation. *Am J Cardiol.* 2008;101(2):259–262.

CASE 98

Exertional Dyspnea following Mitral and Aortic Valve Replacements

A 55-year-old woman presents 3 years post mitral and aortic valve replacements with tissue prostheses with exertional dyspnea. She undergoes transthoracic echocardiography (**Videos 98-1 to 98-8** and Figs. 98-1 to 98-6).

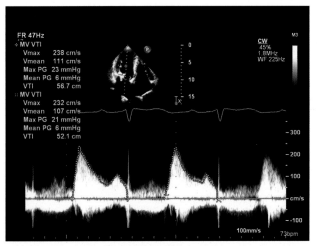

Figure 98-1

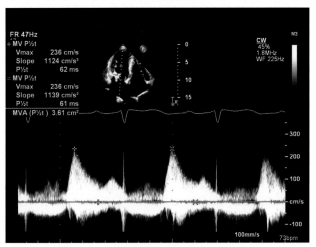

Figure 98-2

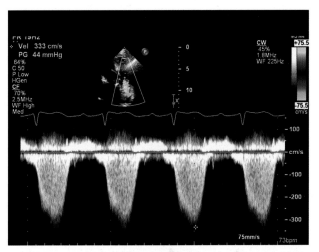

Figure 98-3

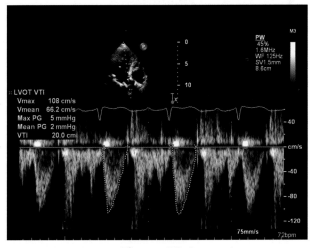

Figure 98-4

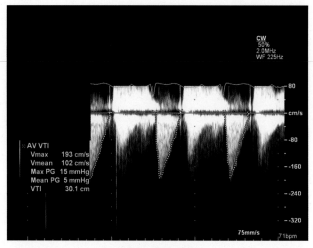

Figure 98-5

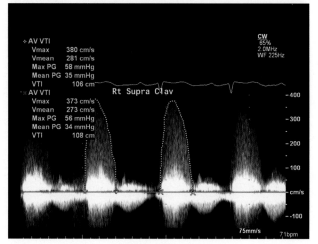

Figure 98-6

QUESTION 1. Calculate the aortic valve prosthesis orifice area, assuming a sewing ring inner diameter of 25 mm and an outer diameter of 28 mm.

    A. 1.0 cm^2

    B. 1.25 cm^2

    C. 2.2 cm^2

    D. 3.0 cm^2

    E. 3.7 cm^2

QUESTION 2. The best equation for calculating the mitral prosthesis effect orifice area is:

    A. 220/pressure halftime (PHT)

    B. 758/deceleration time (DT)

    C. 150/PHT

    D. PHT and/or DT are not helpful in the assessment of mitral valve prosthetic area

QUESTION 3. Based on the transthoracic echocardiogram, the mitral valve prosthesis likely has:

    A. Normal function

    B. Stenosis/obstruction

    C. Regurgitation

QUESTION 4. The patient is referred for transesophageal echocardiography (**Videos 98-9 to 98-16** and Figs. 98-7 to 98-9). Doppler imaging of left and right pulmonary veins are compatible with severe mitral valve regurgitation.

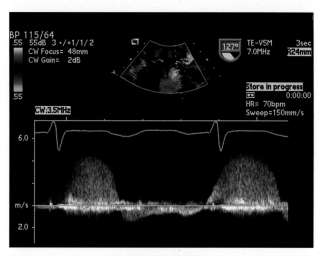

Figure 98-7

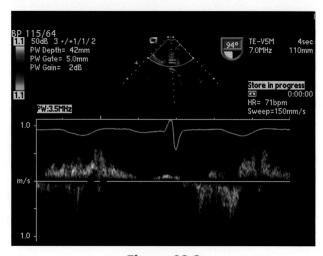

Figure 98-8

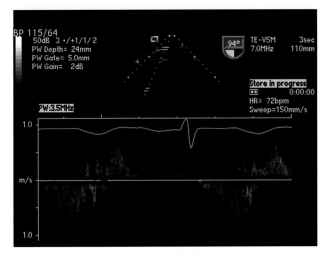

Figure 98-9

A. True
B. False

QUESTION 5. The mechanism of the tricuspid valve regurgitation is:

A. Tricuspid valve leaflet prolapse
B. Tricuspid annular dilatation
C. Tricuspid leaflet perforation

QUESTION 6. Before consideration of periprosthetic leak closure, the patient developed fever and chills. Blood cultures grew out *Streptococcus bovis.* With which of the following medical conditions is *S. bovis* associated?

A. Rheumatoid arthritis
B. Lung cancer
C. Colon cancer
D. Recent dental extraction

QUESTION 7. Repeat transesophageal echocardiography was performed (**Videos 98-17 to 98-24**). Based on the echocardiographic evidence, infective endocarditis is:

A. Unlikely
B. Possible
C. Likely

QUESTION 8. The mitral prosthetic surface seen in **Video 98-25** is:

A. Atrial
B. Ventricular

ANSWER 1: B. The area of an aortic prosthesis may be calculated by the continuity method similar to the way aortic valve area is calculated in an aortic stenosis case.

$$
\begin{aligned}
\text{Aortic prosthesis area} &= \text{LVOT area} \times \text{LVOT TVI/AP TVI} \\
&= \text{SROD}^2 \times 0.785 \times \text{LVOT TVI/} \\
&\quad \text{AP TVI} \\
&= 2.8^2 \times 0.785 \times 20/100 \\
&= 1.25 \text{ cm}^2
\end{aligned}
$$

where SROD, sewing ring outer diameter.

In this case, two different signals are obtained of the aortic valve gradients. The first from the apical long axis is clearly suboptimal with the peak signals obtained from the right supraclavicular location. As with aortic stenosis cases, it is critical to perform a complete Doppler interrogation, with Doppler samples taken from all locations not just from the apex, including with the nonimaging probe.

ANSWER 2: D. A native mitral valve area may be estimated by using either the equation 220/pressure halftime or 758/deceleration time. However, the PHT (or DT) should not be used to calculate prosthetic areas as these equations are inaccurate.

ANSWER 3: C. The early mitral inflow (E) velocity is very high. Although this may simply represent very high left ventricular filling pressures (in the absence of valve dysfunction), a velocity of >2 m per second typically indicates valve dysfunction. However, this may reflect stenosis, regurgitation, or both. Little, if any, regurgitation is seen on 2D color Doppler imaging; however, there is significant acoustic shadowing of the left atrium. A helpful indicator is the pressure halftime. Here the pressure halftime is short (60 milliseconds), and this suggests that the elevated E velocity is likely related to regurgitation rather than obstruction (associated with a prolonged pressure halftime) if the valve is dysfunctional. Finally, a high output state may give rise to a high E velocity even in the absence of prosthesis dysfunction. However, the normal LVOT TVI (20 cm) in the setting of a normal heart rate (77 beats per minute) excludes a high output state.

ANSWER 4: A. Both pulmonary veins imaged demonstrate the presence of systolic flow reversals, which are a specific (although not sensitive) sign of severe mitral valve regurgitation.

See *The Echo Manual, 3rd Edition,* **discussion of signs that suggest severe MR on page 218.**

ANSWER 5: B. As is indicated on both the transthoracic (**Videos 98-8 and 98-25**) and transesophageal (**Videos 98-15 and 98-16**) echocardiograms, there is severe central tricuspid valve regurgitation secondary to lack of leaflet coaptation with underlying annular dilatation.

ANSWER 6: C. S. bovis is a gram positive bacillus bacteria that is found typically in the lower gastrointestinal tract. There is a correlation between colonic abnormalities, particularly colon carcinoma and *S. bovis* infection. The identification of *S. bovis* infection should prompt a colonoscopy to evaluate for possible colon cancer.[1]

ANSWER 7: C. In the setting of prosthetic valvular dysfunction, fever chills, and positive bacteremia (with an organism commonly associated with infective endocarditis), the pretest probability for infective endocarditis is very high. Moreover, on TEE imaging, there is a new mobile mass (presumed vegetation) attached to the anterolateral mitral annulus in the location of the periprosthetic regurgitation.

ANSWER 8: B. Three-dimensional imaging (**Video 98-25**) illustrates the ventricular aspect of the mitral prosthesis. The patient went on to redo surgery with mitral valve re-replacement.

Reference

1. Alazmi W, Bustamante M, O'Loughlin C, et al. The association of *Streptococcus bovis* bacteremia and gastrointestinal diseases: a retrospective analysis. *Dig Dis Sci.* 2006;51(4):732–736.

Exertional Shortness of Breath and Chest Pain in a 30-Year-Old Woman

*A*30-year-old woman presents for a transthoracic echocardiogram (Videos 99-1 to 99-12 and Figs. 99-1 to 99-9) with exertional shortness of breath and chest pain.

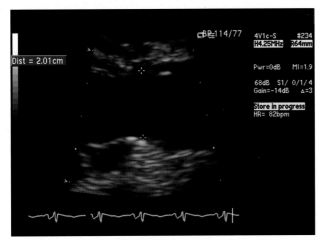

Figure 99-1

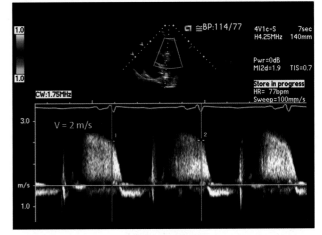

Figure 99-3

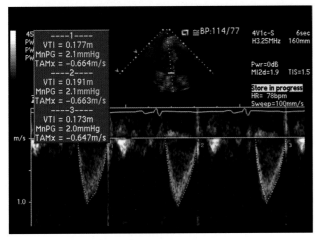

Figure 99-2

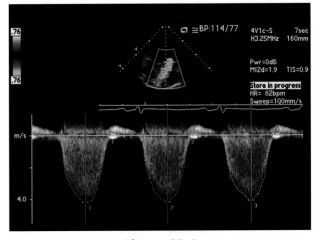

Figure 99-4

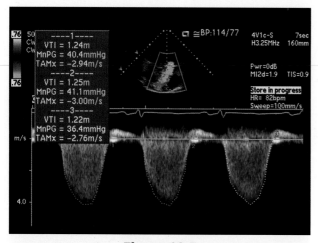

Figure 99-5

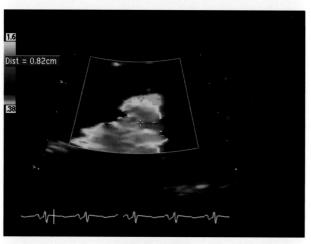

Figure 99-6

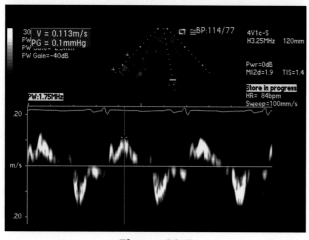

Figure 99-7

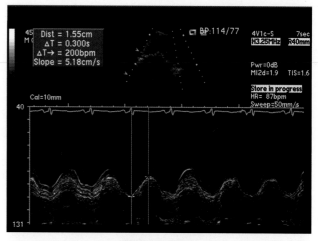

Figure 99-8

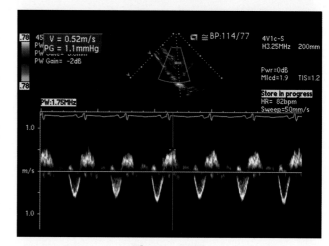

Figure 99-9

QUESTION 1. Which of the following dimensions indicates right ventricular (RV) enlargement?

   A. Mid RV diameter >35 mm from the apical four-chamber view

   B. Basal RV diameter >35 mm from the apical four-chamber view

   C. RV long-axis length >75 mm from the apical four-chamber view

   D. RV outflow tract diameter from the parasternal short axis (at the aortic valve level) >23 mm

QUESTION 2. Which of the following clinical scenarios best explains the echocardiographic findings?

A. Acute saddle pulmonary embolism
B. Pulmonary venous hypertension secondary to left-sided valvular disease
C. Chronic thromboembolic disease leading to pulmonary hypertension and right heart failure
D. Extrinsic pulmonary arterial compression leading to secondary RV dysfunction
E. Primary severe tricuspid valve regurgitation (TR) leading to secondary RV dysfunction

QUESTION 3. The hepatic vein Doppler pattern is consistent with all of the following *except*:

A. Marked V waves on examination of the jugular venous pressure
B. Severe TR
C. Kussmaul sign
D. Marked RV dysfunction

QUESTION 4. The severity and mechanism of the TR is:

A. Moderate regurgitation secondary to bileaflet prolapse
B. Severe regurgitation secondary to bileaflet prolapse
C. Tricuspid annulus dilation with secondary (functional) moderate regurgitation
D. Tricuspid annulus dilation with secondary (functional) severe regurgitation

QUESTION 5. The calculated cardiac output equals:

A. 3.8 L per minute
B. 4.4 L per minute
C. 5.6 L per minute
D. 6.4 L per minute

QUESTION 6. The estimated pulmonary arterial pressures in this case are:

A. 36/24 mm Hg
B. 64/16 mm Hg
C. 74/26 mm Hg
D. 84/36 mm Hg

QUESTION 7. Calculate the pulmonary artery (PA) capacitance.

A. 0.6
B. 0.8
C. 1.0
D. 1.2

QUESTION 8. Which of the following measures is normal in this patient?

A. Tricuspid annular systolic plane excursion (TAPSE) of 16 mm
B. Peak systolic tricuspid annular tissue velocity of 11 cm per second
C. A right index of myocardial performance by pulsed wave Doppler of 0.7
D. A RV fractional area change of 42%

QUESTION 9. Based on the findings, the appropriate management step should include all of the following *except*:

A. Lifelong warfarin anticoagulation
B. Consideration of surgical thromboendarterectomy
C. Thrombolytic therapy
D. Placement of a vena caval filter

ANSWER 1: A. Recently published guidelines on the echocardiographic assessment of the RV indicate that the "RV dimension is best estimated at end-diastole from a right ventricle–focused apical four-chamber view. Either the diameter >42 mm at the base and [or] > 35 mm at the mid level indicates RV dilatation. Similarly, longitudinal dimension >86 mm or the diameter of the RV outflow tract from the para-sternal short-axis view >27 mm indicates RV enlargement."[1]

ANSWER 2: C. The echocardiographic findings are of marked RV enlargement and dysfunction in the setting of severe pulmonary hypertension. Imaging of the pulmonary arterial bifurcation indeed demonstrates evidence of thrombus, the likely mechanism of the pulmonary hypertension. However, the degree of pulmonary hypertension suggests significant chronicity to the process. The RV is exquisitely sensitive to acute changes in RV afterload and in the acute setting is unable to support a right ventricular systolic pressure (RVSP) higher than 50 to 60 mm Hg. A RVSP higher than this range suggests a chronic process.

See *The Echo Manual, 3rd Edition*, discussion of chronic thromboembolic pulmonary hypertension on page 151.

ANSWER 3: C. The presence of marked systolic flow reversals may occur in the setting of severe TR and/ or RV dysfunction (the earlier peaking of the reversal in this case suggests the mechanism is more the latter, as reversals due to severe TR tend to be more late peaking). The venous reversal of flow in systole can be appreciated on examination as prominent V waves on clinical examination. Kussmaul sign (an increase in venous pressure on inspiration) is sign with constrictive pericarditis, which is associated with prominent *diastolic* flow reversals with expiration.

ANSWER 4: D. The tricuspid valve leaflets are normal, but are pulled apart by dilation of the tricuspid valve annulus secondary to RV enlargement. This leads to poor leaflet coaptation and functional regurgitation. A number of factors present here suggest the presence of severe TR. These include (1) color flow regurgitant jet area ≥30% of the right atrial (RA) area, (2) dense continuous wave Doppler signal, (3) annulus dilatation (≥40 mm) and inadequate cusp coaptation, (4) an effective regurgitant orifice (ERO) ≥0.4 cm², and (5) a regurgitant volume ≥45 ml.

The regurgitant flow can be calculated as follows:

Flow rate = $(r)^2$ × 6.28 × aliasing velocity × angle correction factor*

= $(0.8cm)^2$ × 6.28 × 38 cm per second × 220/180

= 187 cc per second

*Unlike the flat leaflets of mitral valve, the tricuspid valve leaflets are funnel shaped. This needs to be accounted for when calculating PISA. The assumption of a hemispheric shape of the flow convergence needs to be corrected for by measuring the angle of the leaflets. Typically, the angle of the tricuspid leaflets is 220° rather than the 180° of the mitral valve. Without this adjustment, the additional area of flow convergence would not be accounted for if the angle of the leaflets were not measured, which would lead to underestimation of the regurgitation severity.

ERO = Flow rate/peak TR velocity

= 187 cc per second/400 cm per second

= 0.47 cm²

Regurgitant volume = ERO × regurgitant time velocity integral (TVI)

= 0.47 cm² × 120 cm

= 56 cc

See *The Echo Manual, 3rd Edition*, discussion of PISA method on page 215, and discussion of tricuspid valve regurgitation on pages 219 and 220.

ANSWER 5: B. Stroke volume (SV) is calculated from the left ventricular outflow tract (LVOT) as a product of the LVOT area (LVOT diameter × 0.785) and the LVOT TVI.

Here SV = $(2.0 cm)^2$ × 0.785 × 18 cm = 57 ml at a heart rate of 78 beats per minute = 4.4 L per minute.

See *The Echo Manual, 3rd Edition*, Figure 4-16 on page 71.

ANSWER 6: D. There are three key parameters in the assessment of PA pressures. In the absence of RV outflow tract obstruction, RVSP is equivalent to the pulmonary artery systolic pressure (PASP). This can be estimated based on the modified Bernoulli equation: $4v^2$ + an estimate of RA pressure (where the v = peak TR systolic velocity). Similarly, the gradient at end diastole across the pulmonary valve (end-diastolic pulmonary regurgitant velocity) can be used to estimate the pulmonary artery diastolic pressure (PADP). In this case, the dilated inferior vena cava with little, if any, collapsibility with respiration suggests a marked elevation in RA pressure (conventionally estimated at 20 mm Hg). The hepatic vein Doppler demonstrates systolic flow reversals with only diastolic forward flow (also findings that suggest a high RA pressure).

$$PASP = RVSP = 4 (4)^2 + 20 = 84 \text{ mm Hg}$$

$$= 4 (2)^2 + 20 = 36 \text{ mm Hg}$$

See *The Echo Manual, 3rd Edition*, **discussion of tricuspid regurgitant and pulmonary regurgitant velocities on pages 144 to 147.**

ANSWER 7: D. Estimated by either echocardiography or catheterization, PA capacitance (PA CAP) is likely a better measure of the severity of disease in pulmonary hypertension than pulmonary vascular resistance, as it incorporates the pulsatile component of changes in pulmonary arterial pressure and flow, which is up to one half of the power transferred from the RV to the pulmonary vascular bed. PA CAP is defined as the ratio of cardiac stroke volume (SV) to PA pulse pressure which can be derived from the peak tricuspid regurgitant (TR) and the end diastolic pulmonary regurgitant (PR_{end}) velocities (V_{max}). SV was calculated in the answer to Question 2.

$$\begin{aligned}
\text{PV capacitance} &= \text{SV/PA pulse pressure} \\
&= (\text{LVOT area} \times \text{TVI})/4 \, (\text{TR } V_{max}^2 - PR_{end} \, V_{max}^2) \\
&= 57/4(4^2 - 2^2) \\
&= 57/48 \\
&= 1.2
\end{aligned}$$

ANSWER 8: D. Measures of RV longitudinal systolic function are important parameters to obtain in the assessment of RV systolic function in patients with pulmonary hypertension. Measures of 16 mm for TAPSE and 11 cm per second for peak systolic tricuspid valve annular velocities are both reduced particularly for a young patient where they are typically much higher (TAPSE >18 to 20 and systolic tissue Doppler imaging (TDI) >15). Not measured here, the right index of myocardial performance (an integrative marker of systolic and diastolic function but prone to error in the setting of marked RA hypertension) greater than 0.4 is abnormal. The RV fractional area change is normally greater than that of 35%.

ANSWER 9: C. On the basis of the chronicity of the event, there will be little gained by thrombolytic therapy as the venous clot will have become scarred and fibrotic. Anticoagulation and filter placement are indicated, although their role is prevention of further embolic events. Consideration of thromboendarterectomy by an experienced surgeon in an experienced center is critical as outcomes for the patients may be dramatically improved. Here this patient did proceed with successful thromboendarterectomy (Fig. 99-10) with resolution of symptoms and pulmonary hypertension on follow-up.

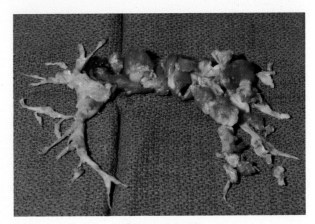

Figure 99-10

References

Rudski LG, Lai WW, Afilalo J, et al. Guidelines for the echocardiographic assessment of the right heart in adults: a report from the American Society of Echocardiography. *J Am Soc Echocardiogr.* 2010;23:685–713.

Mahapatra S, Nishimura RA, Oh JK, et al. The prognostic value of pulmonary vascular capacitance determined by Doppler echocardiography in patients with pulmonary arterial hypertension. *J Am Soc Echocardiogr.* 2006;19:1045–1050.

Exertional Dyspnea with Systemic Hypertension

*A*n 80-year-old man is referred for an evaluation of exertional dyspnea. He has a medical history of systemic hypertension treated with lisinopril and hydrochlorothiazide. Over the past 2 years, he describes progressive limiting exertional shortness of breath. Work-up to date includes a normal chest X-ray, pulmonary function tests, coronary angiogram, and right heart catheterization.

QUESTION 1. There is echocardiographic evidence of (**Videos 100-1 to 100-8** and Figs. 100-1 to 100-10):

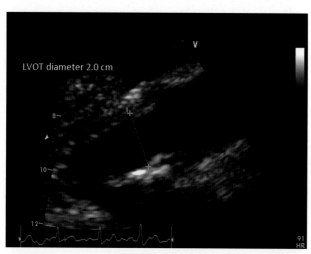

Figure 100-1

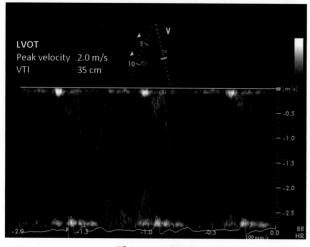

Figure 100-2

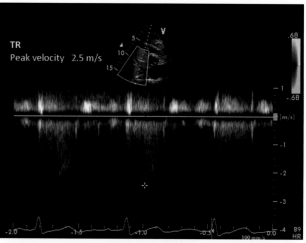

Figure 100-3

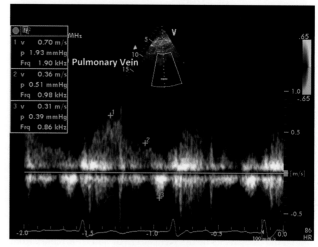

Figure 100-4

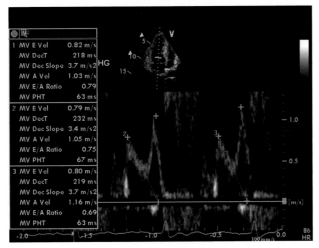

Figure 100-5

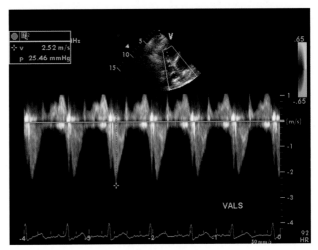

Figure 100-8

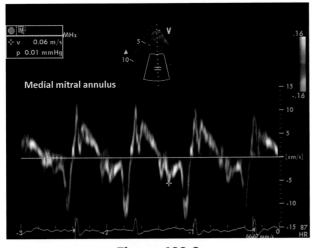

Figure 100-6

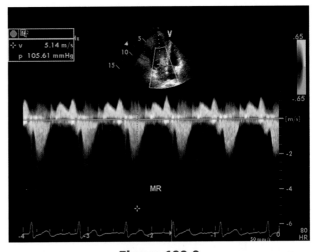

Figure 100-9

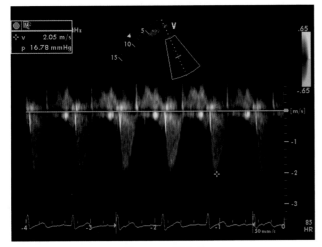

Figure 100-7

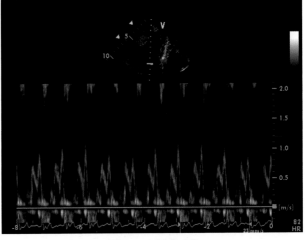

Figure 100-10

A. Pulmonary hypertension
B. Normal ejection fraction low output cardiomyopathy
C. Constrictive pericarditis
D. Aortic stenosis
E. Hypertensive heart disease

QUESTION 2. The pulmonary vein profile (Fig. 100-4) suggests:

A. The absence of left atrial (LA) mechanical function
B. The presence of normal LA pressure
C. The presence of pulmonary arterial hypertension
D. The presence of pulmonary vein stenosis

QUESTION 3. If the systemic blood pressure is 100/60 mm Hg, then the LA pressure is approximately:

A. 9 to 11 mm Hg
B. 14 to 16 mm Hg
C. 19 to 21 mm Hg
D. 25 to 28 mm Hg

QUESTION 4. Which of the following investigations is most likely to give the diagnosis?

A. Cardiac MRI
B. Transesophageal echocardiography
C. Dobutamine stress echocardiography
D. Exercise echocardiography
E. Repeat coronary angiography
F. Pulmonary consultation

QUESTION 5. Based on your review of the images (**Videos 100-9 to 100-12** and Figs. 100-11 and 100-12), what would be the expected clinical findings?

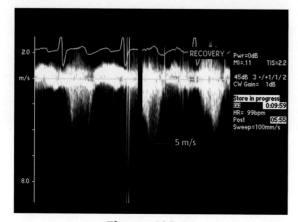

Figure 100-11

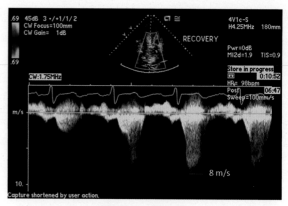

Figure 100-12

A. Harsh systolic murmur
B. Systemic hypertension (systolic blood pressure [SBP] >160 mm Hg)
C. No audible murmurs
D. Irregularly irregular pulse

QUESTION 6. What is the recommended management strategy?

A. Refer to cardiac surgeon
B. Refer to interventional cardiologist
C. Change in medical therapy
D. No change, routine follow-up

ANSWER 1: E. The inferior vena cava (IVC) is of normal size and collapses normally with inspiration suggesting normal right atrial pressure (e.g., 5 mm Hg) and making constriction quite unlikely. Coupled with a peak tricuspid regurgitant velocity of 2.5 m per second, the estimated right ventricular (RV) systolic pressure is equal to $4(2.5)^2 + 5 = 30$ mm Hg (i.e., normal pulmonary pressures). The calculated cardiac output is equal to $0.785 \times (2)^2 \times 35 \times 88 = 9.7$ L per minute (i.e., if anything, high output not low output). Constriction is unlikely with a normal IVC and a "nonrestrictive" mitral inflow pattern that does not change with respiration. The aortic valve seen in short axis (**Video 100-2**) opens normally without restriction, and the mildly elevated gradient obtained by continuous wave Doppler through the left ventricular outflow tract (LVOT) is late peaking, consistent with dynamic outflow tract obstruction rather than fixed valvular obstruction. The upper normal wall thicknesses and basal septal hypertrophy are findings consistent with an elderly patient with a history of systemic hypertension.

ANSWER 2: B. Pulmonary vein Doppler recordings show four distinct velocity components (Fig. 100-11): two systolic velocities (PVS1 and PVS2), diastolic velocity (PVd), and atrial flow reversal velocity (PVa). The first systolic forward flow, PVS1, occurs early in systole and is related to atrial relaxation, which decreases LA pressure and fosters pulmonary venous flow into the LA. The second systolic forward flow, PVS2, occurs in mid to late systole and is produced by the increase in pulmonary venous pressure. At normal LA pressure, the late systolic increase in pulmonary venous pressure is larger and more rapid than LA pressure. However, at elevated filling pressures, the late systolic pressure increase in the LA is equal to or more rapid than that in the pulmonary vein, resulting in earlier peak velocity of PVS2. The remaining pulmonary vein flow velocity components (PVd, PVa, and PVS1) follow phasic changes in LA pressure.

With normal atrioventricular conduction, the systolic components are closely connected, and a distinct PVS1 peak velocity may not be identified in 70% of patients (as in this case). During diastole, forward flow velocity (PVd) occurs after opening of the mitral valve and in conjunction with the decrease in LA pressure. With atrial contraction, the increase in LA pressure may result in flow reversal into the pulmonary vein. The extent and duration of the flow reversal are related to left ventricular (LV) diastolic pressure, LA compliance, and heart rate. The diastolic phase of

pulmonary venous flow resembles early mitral flow. The peak velocity and deceleration time correlate well with those of mitral E velocity because the LA functions mainly as a passive conduit for flow during early diastole. The analysis of pulmonary vein flow velocities complements the assessment of the mitral flow velocity pattern. This is especially true if the mitral E and A waves fuse. In this situation, the ratio between pulmonary vein systolic and diastolic flow velocities can be helpful in characterizing diastolic filling in patients with sinus rhythm (PVS2 >> PVd in impaired relaxation and PVS2 << PVd in restrictive filling).

ANSWER 3: A. The LA pressure may be estimated based on a calculation of LV pressure (LAP) using the peak mitral regurgitant (MR) velocity to estimate LV systolic pressure (LVSP) just as one uses the peak tricuspid regurgitant velocity to calculate RV systolic pressure.

LVSP = $4(\text{Peak MR vel})^2 + \text{LAP}$

LVSP also = Systemic SBP + LVOT peak gradient
= $100 + 4(2.05)^2$
= $100 + 16.78 = 117$ mm Hg
$117 = 4 (\text{Peak MR vel.})^2 + \text{LA pressure}$
$117 = 4(5.14)^2 + \text{LA pressure}$
$117 = 106 + \text{LA pressure}$

LA pressure = 11 mm Hg

ANSWER 4: D. Echocardiography demonstrates a small LV cavity with hyperdynamic LV systolic function (high LV ejection fraction and high cardiac output). The LV global thickness is normal, but there is hypertrophy of the basal septum. There is associated LVOT obstruction with systolic anterior motion of the mitral apparatus with mild to moderate MR. At rest there is a peak gradient of 18mm Hg, which increases to 25 mm Hg with Valsalva. It is important to assess whether there is evidence of increasing outflow tract obstruction with exercise.

ANSWER 5: A. Post stress, there was significant dynamic LVOT obstruction with severe MR. In recovery (with patient standing), the amount of mitral apparatus systolic anterior motion increased even further and the amount of MR becomes very severe; this was associated with a symptomatic drop in SBP from 127 mm Hg to 94 mm Hg.

On the basis of the available Doppler data, the peak LVOT velocity of 5 m per second at a time when the corresponding peak MR velocity was 8 m per second suggests the systemic blood pressure is not high.

Similar to the method in the answer to 3,

$$LVSP = 4 \text{ (Peak MR vel)}^2 + LA \text{ pressure}$$

$$LVSP \text{ also} = \text{Systemic SBP} + LVOT \text{ peak gradient}$$

$$4 \text{ (Peak MR vel)}^2 + LA \text{ pressure} = SBP + LVOT \text{ peak gradient}$$

$$4 \text{ (Peak MR vel)}^2 - LVOT \text{ peak gradient} = SBP - LA \text{ pressure}$$

$$4 (8)^2 - 4(5)^2 = SBP - LA \text{ pressure}$$

$$256 - 100 = 156 = SBP - LA \text{ pressure}$$

In the setting of severe LVOT obstruction and severe acute MR, the LA pressure would be expected to be very high. Indeed, the measured SBP was 127 mm Hg. i.e. a calculated LA pressure of 156-127 = 29 mm Hg.

ANSWER 6: C. Although a septal reduction procedure either myectomy or septal ablation is a consideration, this should be reserved for patients who fail medical therapy. Currently the patient is on two vasodilators. These were stopped and in their place a negative inotropic antihypertensive (β-blocker) started. Within weeks, the patient's symptoms had entirely resolved.

Index

Note: Page number followed by '*f*' indicate figures.